5TH EDITION

Winningham's CRITICAL THINKING CASES IN NURSING

Medical-Surgical, Pediatric, Maternity, and Psychiatric

MARIANN HARDING, MSN, RN
Associate Professor
Department of Nursing
Kent State University at Tuscarawas
New Philadelphia, Ohio

JULIE S. SNYDER, MSN, RN-BC
Adjunct Faculty
School of Nursing
Old Dominion University
Norfolk, Virginia

BARBARA A. PREUSSER[†], PHD, FNPC
Family Nurse Practitioner
Veterans Administration Medical Center
Salt Lake City, Utah

[†]*Deceased*

3251 Riverport Lane
St. Louis, Missouri 63043

WINNINGHAM'S CRITICAL THINKING CASES IN NURSING:
MEDICAL-SURGICAL, PEDIATRIC, MATERNITY, AND PSYCHIATRIC   ISBN: 978-0-323-08325-6

Previous editions copyrighted 2009, 2005, 2001, 1996

Library of Congress Cataloging-in-Publication Data
Harding, Mariann.
   Winningham's critical thinking cases in nursing : medical-surgical, pediatric, maternity, and psychiatric / Mariann Harding, Julie S. Snyder, Barbara A. Preusser. – 5th ed.
      p. ; cm.
   Critical thinking cases in nursing
   Rev. ed. of: Critical thinking in medical-surgical settings / Maryl L. Winningham and Barbara A. Preusser. 2nd ed. c2011.
   Includes bibliographical references.
   ISBN 978-0-323-08325-6 (pbk. : alk. paper)
   I. Snyder, Julie S. II. Preusser, Barbara A. III. Winningham, Maryl Lynne, 1947–2001. Critical thinking in medical-surgical settings. IV. Title. V. Title: Critical thinking cases in nursing.
   [DNLM: 1. Nursing Process–Case Reports. 2. Nursing Process–Problems and Exercises. 3. Nursing Care–Case Reports. 4. Nursing Care–Problems and Exercises. WY 18.2]
   610.73–dc23   2012003221

Executive Content Strategist: Lee Henderson
Content Development Specialist: Jacqueline Twomey
Publishing Services Managers: Hemamalini Rajendrababu & Deborah L. Vogel
Project Managers: Anitha Sivaraj & John W. Gabbert
Design Direction: Karen Pauls

Printed in the United States of America

Last digit is the print number: 9 8 7 6 5 4 3 2 1

To Drs. Maryl L. Winningham and Barbara A. Preusser

Drs. Winningham and Preusser, authors of this text for the previous four editions, dedicated their lives to the care of others and the pursuit of excellence in nursing practice. They have bequeathed a nursing heritage of integrity, excellence, courage, and service to their students, colleagues, and readers.

Contributors

Ann Campbell, RN, MSN, CPNP
Faculty
School of Nursing
Old Dominion University
Norfolk, Virginia

Sara B. Forbus, MSN, RN
Faculty
School of Nursing
Old Dominion University
Norfolk, Virginia

Contributors to Previous Editions

Elizabeth Jane Bell, MSN, ANPc

Lesley A. Black, BSN, MS, ANPc, CWOCN

Kent Blad, MS, FNPc, ACNP-C, FCCM

Jamie Clinton-Lont, BSN, FNPc

Susan L. Croft, BSN, MS

Joyce Foster, PhD, CNM, FACNM, FAAN

Shellagh Gutke, BSN, CWOCN

Nancy Hayden, MSN, FNPc

Sondra Heaston, MS, FNPc, CEN

Janice Hulbert, RN, MS

Lisa Jensen, BSN, MS, APRN, CS

Stephanie C. Kettendorf, MS, RN, CNS, NCBF

Julie Killebrew, BSN, MS

Karen Kone, BSN, ACRN

Kathleen Kuntz, MSN, APRN, SANE

Janet G. Madsen, PhD

Debra Ann Mills, RN, MS

Jeanie O'Donnell, MSN

Deb Plasman-Coles, PAc

Laura Lee Scott, MSN, FNPc

Mary Seegmiller, MSN

Sandra Smeeding, MS, FNPc

Deborah D. Smith, BSN

Ann Speirs, BSN

Ronald Ulberg, BSN, MSN

Kristy Vankatwyk, MSN, FNPc

Annette S. Wendel, BSN

Wendy Whitney, MSN, FNPc, CANP

Mary Youtsey, BSN, CDE

Reviewers

Diane K. Daddario, MSN, ACNS-BC, RN, BC, CMSRN
Nurse Specialist
Geisinger Medical Center
Danville, Pennsylvania;
Staff Nurse
Evangelical Community Hospital
Lewisburg, Pennsylvania;
Nursing Instructor
Pennsylvania College of Technology
Williamsport, Pennsylvania

Jennifer Duhon, RN, MS
Director of Health Services
Lutheran Senior Services
Peoria, Illinois

Sara B. Forbus, MSN, RN
Faculty
School of Nursing
Old Dominion University
Norfolk, Virginia

Mimi Haskins, MS, RN, CMSRN
Nursing Staff Development Instructor
Roswell Park Cancer Institute
Buffalo, New York

Suzanne Jed, MSN, APRN-BC
Clinical Instructor, Family Medicine
Keck School of Medicine
University of Southern California
Los Angeles, California

Jamie Lynn Jones, MSN, RN
Assistant Professor, Nursing
University of Arkansas at Little Rock
Little Rock, Arkansas

Tamara M. Kear, PhD, MSN, RN
Assistant Professor of Nursing
Villanova University
Villanova, Pennsylvania

Cheryl A. Lehman, PhD, RN, CNS-BC, RN-BC, CRRN
CNS Program Coordinator
Department of Health Restoration &
    Care Systems Management (HRCSM)
Clinical Associate Professor
The University of Texas Health Science
    Center at San Antonio
San Antonio, Texas

Casey Norris, MSN, BSN
Adjunct Instructor, Nursing
South College
Pulmonary Clinical Nurse Specialist
East Tennessee Children's Hospital
Knoxville, Tennessee

Brenda K. Shelton, MS, RN, CCRN, AOCN
The Sidney Kimmel Cancer Center at Johns
    Hopkins
Baltimore, Maryland

Introduction

There is an urgent need for nurses with well-practiced critical thinking skills. As new graduates, you will make decisions and take actions of an increasingly sophisticated nature. You will encounter problems you have never seen or heard about during your classroom and clinical experiences. You are going to have to make complex decisions with little or no guidance and limited resources.

We want you to be exposed to as much as possible during your student days, but more importantly, we want you to learn to *think*. You cannot memorize your way out of any situation, but you can *think* your way out of any situation. We know that students often learn more and faster when they have the freedom to make mistakes. This book is designed to allow you to experiment with finding answers without the pressure of someone's life hanging in the balance. We want you to do well. We want you to be the best. It is our wish for you to grow into confident, competent professionals. After all, someday we will be one of those people you care for, and when that day comes, we want you to be very, very good at what you do!

What Is Critical Thinking?

Critical thinking is *not* memorizing lists of facts or the steps of procedures. Instead, critical thinking is an analytical process that can help you think through a problem in an organized and efficient manner. Five steps are involved in critical thinking. Thinking about these steps may help you when you work through the questions in your cases. Here are the five steps with an explanation of what they mean.

1. Recognize and define the problem by asking the right questions: Exactly what is it you need to know? What is the question asking?
2. Select the information or data necessary to solve the problem or answer the question: First you have to ask whether all the necessary information is there. If not, how and where can you get the additional information? What other resources are available? This is one of the most difficult steps. In real clinical experiences, you rarely have all of the information, so you have to learn where you can get necessary data. For instance, patient and family interviews, nursing charting, the patient medical chart, laboratory data on your computer, your observations, and your own physical assessment can help you identify important clues. Of course, information can rapidly become outdated. To make sure you are accessing the most current and accurate information, you will occasionally need to use the Internet to answer a question.
3. Recognize stated and unstated assumptions; that is, what do you think is or is not true? Sometimes answers or solutions seem obvious; just because something seems obvious doesn't mean it is correct. You may need to consider several possible answers or solutions. Consider all clues carefully and *do not dismiss a possibility too quickly*. Remember, "*You never find an answer you don't think of.*"

4. Formulate and select relevant and/or potential decisions. Try to think of as many possibilities as you can. Consider the pros and cons of the consequences of making each decision. What is the best answer/solution? What could go wrong? This requires considering many different angles. In today's health care settings, decision-making often requires balancing the well-being needs of the patient, the preferences and concerns of the patient and caregiver, and financial limitations imposed by the reimbursement system. In making decisions, you need to take into account all relevant factors. Remember, you may need to explain why you rejected other options.

5. Draw a valid, informed conclusion: Consider all data; then determine what is relevant and what makes the most sense. Only then should you draw your conclusion.

It may look as if this kind of thinking comes naturally to instructors and experienced nurses. You can be certain that even experienced professionals were once where you are now. The rapid and sound decision-making that is essential to good nursing requires years of practice. The practice of good clinical thinking leads to good thinking in clinical practice. This book will help you practice the important steps in making sound clinical judgments until the process starts to come naturally.

The practice of good clinical thinking leads to good thinking in clinical practice.

The "How to" of Case Studies

When you begin each case, read through the whole story once, from start to finish, getting a general idea of what it is about. Write down things you have to look up. This will help you move through the case smoothly and get more out of it. How much you have to look up will depend on where you are in your program, what you know, and how much experience you already have. Preparing cases will become easier as you advance in your program.

Acknowledgments

We would like to express our appreciation to the editorial Elsevier staff—Kristen Geen, Lee Henderson, Jamie Horn, and Jacqueline Twomey—for their professional support and contributions in guiding this text to publication. We extend a special thanks to our reviewers who gave us helpful suggestions and insights as we developed this edition.

Mariann's gratitude goes to the most important people in her life—her husband, Jeff, and her daughters, Kate and Sarah—for their giving of love, support, and time during the months of writing. She gives a special thanks to her students, colleagues, and patients; each has taught her much and fueled her passion for nursing and education. Finally, Mariann gives her thanks to God, who made all things possible.

Julie thanks her husband, Jonathan, for his love, support, and patience during this project. She is grateful for the encouragement from daughter Emily, son-in-law Randy, and parents Willis and Jean Simmons. Julie appreciates the hard work of colleagues Ann Campbell and Sara Forbus as contributors to this edition. She is especially thankful to the students, whose eagerness to learn is an inspiration. Most importantly, Julie gives thanks to God, our source of hope and strength.

Contents

CONTENTS

PART ONE *Medical-Surgical Cases*
Cardiovascular Disorders

Case Study 1

Name _____ Class/Group _____ Date _____

Group Members _____

INSTRUCTIONS All questions apply to this case study. Your responses should be brief and to the point. When asked to provide several answers, list them in order of priority or significance. Do not assume information that is not provided. Please print or write clearly. If your response is not legible, it will be marked as ? and you will need to rewrite it.

▶ Scenario

M.G., a "frequent flier," is admitted to the emergency department (ED) with a diagnosis of heart failure (HF). She was discharged from the hospital 10 days ago and comes in today stating, "I just had to come to the hospital today because I can't catch my breath and my legs are as big as tree trunks." After further questioning, you learn she is strictly following the fluid and salt restriction ordered during her last hospital admission. She reports gaining 1 to 2 pounds every day since her discharge.

1. What error in teaching most likely occurred when M.G. was discharged 10 days ago?

CASE STUDY PROGRESS

During the admission interview, the nurse makes a list of the medications M.G. took at home.

■ Chart View

Nursing Assessment: Medications Taken at Home

Enalapril (Vasotec) 5 mg PO bid
Pioglitazone (Actos) 45 mg PO every morning
Furosemide (Lasix) 40 mg/day PO
Potassium chloride 20 mEq/day PO

---

2. Which of these medications may have contributed to M.G.'s heart failure? Explain.

3. How do angiotensin-converting enzyme (ACE) inhibitors, such as enalapril (Vasotec), work to reduce heart failure? (Select all that apply.) ACE inhibitors:
   a. prevent the conversion of angiotensin I to angiotensin II.
   b. cause systemic vasodilation.
   c. promote the excretion of sodium and water in the renal tubules.
   d. reduce preload and afterload.
   e. increase cardiac contractility.
   f. block sympathetic nervous system stimulation to the heart.

CASE STUDY PROGRESS

After reviewing M.G.'s medications, the physician writes these medication orders:

▉ Chart View

Medication Orders

Enalapril (Vasotec) 5 mg PO bid
Carvedilol (Coreg) 100 mg PO every morning
Glipizide (Glucotrol) 10 mg PO every morning
Furosemide (Lasix) 80 mg IV push (IVP) now, then 40 mg/day IVP
Potassium chloride (K-Dur) 20 mEq/day PO

4. What is the rationale for changing the route of the furosemide (Lasix)?

5. You administer furosemide (Lasix) 80 mg IVP. Identify three parameters you would use to monitor the effectiveness of this medication.

6. What laboratory tests should be ordered for M.G. related to the order for furosemide (Lasix)? (Select all that apply.)
   a. Magnesium level
   b. Sodium level

c. Complete blood count (CBC)
d. Serum glucose levels
e. Potassium level
f. Coagulation studies

7. What is the purpose of the beta blocker carvedilol? It is given to:
   a. increase the contractility of the heart
   b. cause peripheral vasodilation
   c. increase urine output
   d. reduce cardiac stimulation by catecholamines

CASE STUDY PROGRESS

The next day, M.G. has shown only slight improvement, and digoxin (Lanoxin) 125 mcg PO daily is added to her orders.

8. What is the action of the digoxin? Digoxin:
   a. causes systemic vasodilation.
   b. promotes the excretion of sodium and water in the renal tubules.
   c. increases cardiac contractility and cardiac output.
   d. blocks sympathetic nervous system stimulation to the heart.

9. Which findings from M.G.'s assessment would indicate an increased possibility of digoxin toxicity? Explain your answer.
   a. Serum potassium level of 2.2 mEq/L
   b. Serum sodium level of 139 mEq/L
   c. Apical heart rate of 64 beats/minute
   d. Digoxin level 1.6 ng/mL

10. When you go to give the digoxin, you notice that it is available in milligrams (mg) not micrograms (mcg). Convert 125 mcg to mg.

1 Cardiovascular

11. M.G.'s symptoms improve with IV diuretics and the digoxin. She is placed back on oral furosemide (Lasix) once her weight loss is deemed adequate to achieve a euvolemic state. What will determine whether the oral dose will be adequate to consider her for discharge?

12. M.G. is ready for discharge. Using the mnemonic MAWDS, what key management concepts should be taught to prevent relapse and another admission?

Case Study 2

Name _____ Class/Group _____ Date _____

Group Members _____

INSTRUCTIONS All questions apply to this case study. Your responses should be brief and to the point. When asked to provide several answers, list them in order of priority or significance. Do not assume information that is not provided. Please print or write clearly. If your response is not legible, it will be marked as ? and you will need to rewrite it.

▶ Scenario

M.P. is a 65-year-old African-American woman who comes to your clinic for a follow-up visit. She was diagnosed with hypertension (HTN) 2 months ago and was given a prescription for a thiazide diuretic but stopped taking it 2 weeks ago because "it made me dizzy and I kept getting up during the night to empty my bladder." During today's clinic visit, she expresses fear because her mother died of a cerebrovascular accident (CVA, stroke) at her age, and M.P. is afraid she will suffer the same fate. She states, "I've never smoked and I don't drink, but I am so afraid of this high blood pressure." You review the data on her past clinic visits.

■ Chart View

Family History

Mother, died at age 65 years of CVA
Father, died at age 67 years of myocardial infarction (MI)
Sister, alive and well, age 62 years
Brother, alive, age 70 years, has coronary artery disease, HTN, type II diabetes mellitus (DM)

Patient Past History

Married for 45 years, two children, alive and well, six grandchildren
Cholecystectomy, age 42 years
Hysterectomy, age 48 years

Blood Pressure Assessments

January 2: 150/92
January 31: 156/94 (Given prescription for hydrochlorothiazide [HCTZ] 25 mg PO every morning)
February 28: 140/90

1. According to the most recent Joint National Committee on Prevention, Detection, Evaluation, and Treatment of High Blood Pressure, M.P.'s blood pressure falls under which classification?

2. What could M.P. be doing that is causing her nocturia?

CASE STUDY PROGRESS

During today's visit, M.P.'s vital signs were BP: 162/102, P: 78, R: 16, T: 98.2° F (36.8° C). Her most recent basic metabolic panel (BMP) and fasting lipids were within normal limits. Her height is 5 ft, 4 in., and she weighs 110 lb. She tells you that she tries to go on walks but does not like to walk alone so has done so only occasionally.

3. What risk factors does M.P. have that increase her risk for cardiovascular disease?

CASE STUDY PROGRESS

Because M.P.'s BP continues to be high, the internist decides to put her on another drug and recommends that she try again with the HCTZ.

4. According to national guidelines, what drug category or categories are recommended for M.P. at this time?

5. M.P. goes on to ask whether there is anything else she should do to help with her HTN. She asks, "Do I need to lose weight?" Look up her height and weight for her age on a body mass index chart. Is she considered overweight?

6. What nonpharmacologic lifestyle alteration measures might help someone like M.P. control her BP? (List two examples and explain.)

CASE STUDY PROGRESS

The internist decreases M.P.'s HCTZ dosage to 12.5 mg PO daily and adds a prescription for benazepril (Lotensin) 5 mg daily. M.P. is instructed to return to the clinic in 1 week to have her blood work checked. She is also instructed to monitor her BP at least twice a week and return for a medication management appointment in 1 month with her list of BP readings.

7. Why did the internist decrease the dose of the HCTZ?

8. You provide M.P. with education about the common side effects of benazepril, which can include which conditions? (Select all that apply.)
   a. Headache
   b. Cough
   c. Shortness of breath
   d. Constipation
   e. Dizziness

9. It is sometimes difficult to remember whether you've taken your medication. What techniques might you teach M.P. to help her remember to take her medication each day? (Name at least two.)

10. After the teaching session, which statement by M.P. indicates a need for further instructions?
   a. "I need to rise up slowly when I get out of bed or out of a chair before standing up."
   b. "I will leave the salt shaker off the table and not salt my food when I cook."
   c. "It's okay to skip a few doses if I am feeling bad as long as it's just for a few days."
   d. "I will call if I feel very dizzy, weak, or short of breath while on this medicine."

CASE STUDY PROGRESS

M.P. returns in 1 month for her medication management appointment. She tells you she is feeling fine and does not have any side effects from her new medication. Her BP, checked twice a week at the senior center, ranges from 132 to 136/78 to 82 mm Hg.

11. When someone is taking HCTZ and an ACE inhibitor, such as benazepril, what laboratory tests would you expect to be monitored?

■ Chart View

Laboratory Test Results (Fasting)

Potassium	3.6 mEq/L
Sodium	138 mEq/L
Chloride	100 mEq/L
CO_2	28 mEq/L
Glucose	112 mEq/L
Creatinine	0.7 mg/dL
BUN	18 mg/dL
Magnesium	1.9 mEq/L

12. What lab results, if any, are of concern at this time?

13. You take M.P.'s BP and get 134/82 mm Hg. She asks whether these BP readings are okay. On what do you base your response?

14. List at least three important ways you might help her maintain her success.

CASE STUDY OUTCOME

M.P. comes in for a routine follow-up visit 3 months later. She continues to do well on her daily BP drug regimen, with average BP readings of 130/78 mm Hg. She participates in a senior citizens group-walking program at the local mall. She admits she has not done as well with decreasing her salt intake but that she is trying. She tells you she was recently at a luncheon with her garden club and that most of those women take different BP pills than she does. She asks why their pills are different shapes and colors.

15. How can you explain the difference to M.P.?

Case Study **3**

Name _____ Class/Group _____ Date _____

Group Members _____

INSTRUCTIONS All questions apply to this case study. Your responses should be brief and to the point. When asked to provide several answers, list them in order of priority or significance. Do not assume information that is not provided. Please print or write clearly. If your response is not legible, it will be marked as ? and you will need to rewrite it.

▶ Scenario

You are a nurse at a freestanding cardiac prevention and rehabilitation center. Your new patient in risk-factor modification is B.T., a 41-year-old traveling salesman, who is married and has three children. He tells you that his work does not let him slow down. During a recent evaluation for chest pain, he underwent a cardiac catheterization procedure that showed moderate single-vessel disease with a 50% stenosis in the mid right coronary artery (RCA). He was given a prescription for sublingual (SL) nitroglycerin (NTG), told how to use it, and referred to your cardiac rehabilitation program for sessions of 3 days a week. B.T.'s wife comes along to help him with healthy lifestyle changes. You take a nursing history, as indicated in the following.

■ Chart View

Family History

Father died suddenly at age 42 of a myocardial infarction (MI)
Mother (still living) had a quadruple coronary artery bypass graft (CABG × 4) at age 52

Past History and Current Medications

Metoprolol (Lopressor) 25 mg PO every 12 hours
Aspirin (ASA) 325 mg per day PO
Simvastatin (Zocor) 20 mg PO every evening

Lifestyle Habits

Smokes an average of 1½ packs of cigarettes per day (PPD) for the past 20 years
Drinks an "occasional" beer, and "a 6-pack every weekend when watching football"
Dietary history: High in fried and fast foods because of his traveling
Exercise: "I don't have time to take walks."

General Assessment

White Male

Weight	235 lb
Height	5 ft, 8 in.
Waist circumference	48 in.
Blood pressure	148/88 mm Hg
Pulse	82 beats/min
Respiratory rate	18 breaths/min
Temperature	98.4° F (36.9° C)

1. Calculate B.T.'s smoking history in terms of pack-years.

2. There are several risk factors for coronary artery disease (CAD). For each risk factor listed, mark whether it is nonmodifiable or modifiable.
   a. Age
   b. Smoking
   c. Family history of CAD
   d. Obesity
   e. Physical inactivity
   f. Gender
   g. Hypertension
   h. Diabetes mellitus
   i. Hyperlipidemia
   j. Ethnic background
   k. Stress
   l. Excessive alcohol use

3. Circle the nonmodifiable and modifiable risk factors that apply to B.T.

CASE STUDY PROGRESS

You review B.T.'s most recent lab results.

▪ Chart View

Laboratory Testing (Fasting)

Total cholesterol	240 mg/dL
HDL	35 mg/dL
LDL	112 mg/dL
Triglycerides	178 mg/dL

4. Which lab values are of concern at this time? Explain your answers.

1 Cardiovascular

5. B.T. asks you, "So, how is my 'good cholesterol' doing today?" Which is considered the "good cholesterol," and why? What do his HDL and LDL levels indicate to you?

CASE STUDY PROGRESS

B.T. laughingly tells you he believes in the five all-American food groups: salt, sugar, fat, chocolate, and caffeine.

6. Identify health-related problems in this case description; the problem that is potentially life threatening should be listed first.

7. Of all of his behaviors, which one is the most significant in promoting cardiac disease?

8. What is the highest priority problem that you need to address with B.T.? How will you determine this? Identify the teaching strategy you would use with him.

9. What is the second problem you would work with B.T. to change? Identify an appropriate strategy to resolve the problem.

1 Cardiovascular

1 Cardiovascular

10. B.T.'s wife takes you aside and tells you, "I'm so worried for B. I grew up in a really dysfunctional family where there was a lot of violence. B. has been so good to the kids and me. I'm so worried I'll lose him that I have nightmares about his heart stopping. I find myself suddenly awakening at night just to see if he's breathing." How are you going to respond?

CASE STUDY PROGRESS

Six weeks after you start working with B.T., he admits that he has been under a lot of stress. He is walking on the treadmill and rubs his chest and says, "It feels really heavy on my chest right now." You feel his pulse and note that his skin is slightly diaphoretic and that he is agitated and appears to be anxious.

11. What is the first action you are going to do? What other information will you obtain? Explain.

12. B.T. is still uncomfortable, and he has an unopened bottle of sublingual nitroglycerin (SL NTG) tablets. You decide to give him one tablet. After 5 minutes, which is the appropriate action to take?
a. If the chest discomfort is relieved, call 911.
b. If the chest discomfort is not relieved, give another SL NTG tablet, and wait 5 minutes more.
c. If the chest discomfort is not relieved, have someone else call 911, while you give B.T. another SL NTG tablet.
d. If the chest discomfort is not relieved, do a 12-lead electrocardiogram (ECG) to look for ischemic changes, and call 911.

13. What other actions will you take at this time?

14. Five minutes after the first NTG tablet, B.T. states that the discomfort is still there and only slightly relieved. Explain what you can expect to be doing while waiting for emergency medical system (EMS) to arrive.

CASE STUDY OUTCOME

B.T. is transported to the ED of a local hospital and undergoes another cardiac catheterization with coronary stent placement.

Case Study **4**

Name_____ Class/Group_____ Date_____

Group Members _____

INSTRUCTIONS All questions apply to this case study. Your responses should be brief and to the point. When asked to provide several answers, list them in order of priority or significance. Do not assume information that is not provided. Please print or write clearly. If your response is not legible, it will be marked as ? and you will need to rewrite it.

▶ Scenario

S.P. is a 68-year-old retired painter who is experiencing right leg calf pain. The pain began approximately 2 years ago but has become significantly worse in the past 4 months. The pain is precipitated by exercise and is relieved with rest. Two years ago, S.P. could walk two city blocks before having to stop because of leg pain. Today, he can barely walk across the yard. S.P. has smoked two to three packs of cigarettes per day (PPD) for the past 45 years. He has a history of coronary artery disease (CAD), hypertension (HTN), peripheral vascular disease (PVD), and osteoarthritis. Surgical history includes quadruple coronary artery bypass graft (CABG × 4) 3 years ago. He has had no further symptoms of cardiopulmonary disease since that time, even though he has not been compliant with the exercise regimen his cardiologist prescribed, he continues to eat anything he wants, and continues to smoke two to three PPD. Other surgical history includes open reduction internal fixation of the right femoral fracture 20 years ago.

S.P. is in the clinic today for a routine semiannual follow-up appointment with his primary care provider. As you take his vital signs, he tells you that, besides the calf pain, he is experiencing right hip pain that gets worse with exercise, the pain doesn't go away promptly with rest, some days are worse than others, and his condition is not affected by a resting position.

■ Chart View

General Assessment

Weight	261 lb
Height	5 ft, 10 in.
Blood pressure	163/91 mm Hg
Pulse	82 beats/min
Respiratory rate	16 breaths/min
Temperature	98.4° F (36.9° C)

Laboratory Testing (Fasting)

Cholesterol	239 mg/dL
Triglycerides	150 mg/dL
HDL	28 mg/dL
LDL	181 mg/dL

Current Medications

Lisinopril (Zestril)	20 mg/day
Metoprolol (Lopressor)	25 mg twice a day
Aspirin	325 mg/day
Simvastatin (Zocor)	20 mg/day

1. What are the likely sources of his calf pain and his hip pain?

2. S.P. has several risk factors for claudication. From his history, list two risk factors, and explain the reason they are risk factors.

3. You decide to look at S.P.'s lower extremities. What signs do you expect to find with intermittent claudication? (Select all that apply.)
   a. Cool or cold extremity
   b. Thin, dry, and scaly skin
   c. Brown discoloration of the skin
   d. Decreased or absent pedal pulses
   e. Ankle edema
   f. Thick, brittle nails

4. Where would you expect S.P. to complain of pain if he had superficial femoral artery stenosis? Popliteal stenosis?

5. What is the purpose of the daily aspirin listed in his current medication?

CASE STUDY PROGRESS

S.P.'s primary care provider has seen him and wants you to schedule the patient for an ankle-brachial index (ABI) test to determine the presence of arterial blood flow obstruction. You confirm the time and date of the procedure and then call S.P. at home.

6. What will you tell S.P. to do to prepare for the tests?

CASE STUDY PROGRESS

S.P.'s ABI results showed 0.43 right (R) leg and 0.59 left (L) leg. His primary care provider discusses these results with him and decides to wait 2 months to see whether his symptoms improve with medication changes and risk factor modification before deciding about surgical intervention. S.P. receives a prescription for clopidogrel (Plavix) 75 mg daily and is told to discontinue the daily aspirin. In addition, S.P. received a consult for physical therapy.

7. What do these ABI results indicate?

8. You counsel S.P. on risk factor modification. What would you address, and why?

9. How will the physical therapy help?

10. In addition to risk factor modification, what other measures to improve tissue perfusion or to prevent skin damage should you recommend to S.P.?

11. S.P. tells you his neighbor told him to keep his legs elevated higher than his heart and ask for compression stockings to keep swelling down in his legs. How should you respond?

12. S.P. has been on aspirin therapy and now will be taking clopidogrel. What is the most important aspect of patient teaching that you will emphasize with this drug?

CASE STUDY OUTCOME

S.P. asks for nicotine patches to assist with smoking cessation and makes an appointment for a physical therapy evaluation and a nutritional assessment. He assures you he doesn't want to lose his leg and will be more careful in the future.

Case Study **5**

Name _____ Class/Group _____ Date _____

Group Members _____

INSTRUCTIONS All questions apply to this case study. Your responses should be brief and to the point. When asked to provide several answers, list them in order of priority or significance. Do not assume information that is not provided. Please print or write clearly. If your response is not legible, it will be marked as ? and you will need to rewrite it.

▶ Scenario

You are the nurse working in an anticoagulation clinic. One of your patients is K.N., who has a long-standing history of an irregularly irregular heartbeat (atrial fibrillation, or A-fib) for which he takes the oral anticoagulant warfarin (Coumadin). Recently, K.N. had his mitral heart valve replaced with a mechanical valve.

1. How does atrial fibrillation differ from a normal heart rhythm?

2. What is the purpose of the warfarin (Coumadin) in K.N.'s case?

CASE STUDY PROGRESS

K.N. calls your anticoagulation clinic to report a nosebleed that is hard to stop. You ask him to come into the office to check his coagulation levels. The laboratory technician draws a PT/INR test.

3. What is a PT/INR test, and what are the expected levels for K.N.? What is the purpose of the INR?

4. When you get the results, his INR is critical at 7.2. What is the danger of this INR level?

1 Cardiovascular

CASE STUDY PROGRESS

The health care provider does a brief focused history and physical examination, orders additional lab tests, and determines that there are no signs of bleeding other than the nosebleed, which has stopped. The provider discovers that K.N. recently went to the local urgent care center for a sinus infection and had received a prescription for the antibiotic co-trimoxazole (sulfamethoxazole-trimethoprim) (Septra).

5. What happened when K.N. began taking the antibiotic?

6. What should K.N. have done to prevent this problem?

7. The provider gives K.N. a low dose of vitamin K orally, asks him to hold his warfarin dose that evening, and asks him to come back tomorrow for another PT/INR blood draw. Why do you tell K.N. to take the vitamin K?

8. You want to make certain K.N. knows what "hold the next dose" means. What should you tell him?

9. K.N. asks you why his PT/INR has to be checked so soon. How will you respond?

CASE STUDY PROGRESS

K.N.'s INR the next day is 3.7, and the health care provider made no further medication changes. K.N. is instructed to finish the remaining 2 days of antibiotics and return again in 7 days to have another PT/INR drawn.

10. Why should the INR be checked again so soon instead of the usual monthly follow-up?

11. K.N. grumbles about all of the lab tests but agrees to follow through. You provide patient education to K.N. and start with reviewing the signs and symptoms (S/S) of bleeding. What are potential S/S of bleeding that should be taught to K.N.? (Select all that apply.)
   a. Black, tarry stool
   b. Stool that is pale in color
   c. New onset of dizziness
   d. Insomnia

    e. New joint pain or swelling

    f. Unexplained abdominal pain

12. What other patient education needs to be stressed at this time? (Identify two.)

13. Four months later, K.N. informs you that he is going to have a knee replacement next month. What will you do with this information?

CASE STUDY PROGRESS

You know that sometimes the only needed action is to stop the warfarin (Coumadin) several days before the surgery. Other times, the provider initiates "bridging therapy," or stops the warfarin and provides anti-coagulation protection by initiating low-molecular-weight heparin. After reviewing all of his anticoagulation information, the provider decides that K.N. will need to stop the warfarin (Coumadin) 1 week before the surgery and, in its place, be started on enoxaparin (Lovenox) therapy.

14. Compare the duration of action of warfarin (Coumadin) and enoxaparin (Lovenox), and explain the reason the provider switched to enoxaparin at this time.

CASE STUDY PROGRESS

K.N. is in the office and ready for his first enoxaparin (Lovenox) injection.

15. Which nursing interventions are appropriate when administering enoxaparin? (Select all that apply.)
   a. Monitor activated partial thromboplastin (aPTT) levels.
   b. Administer via intramuscular (IM) injection into the deltoid muscle.
   c. The preferred site of injection is the lateral abdominal fatty tissue.
   d. Massage the area after the injection is given.
   e. Hold extra pressure over the site after the injection.

CASE STUDY OUTCOME

K.N. undergoes knee surgery without complications and does not experience any thrombotic events or bleeding episodes during his recovery.

Case Study 6

Name _____   Class/Group _____   Date _____

Group Members _____

INSTRUCTIONS All questions apply to this case study. Your responses should be brief and to the point. When asked to provide several answers, list them in order of priority or significance. Do not assume information that is not provided. Please print or write clearly. If your response is not legible, it will be marked as ? and you will need to rewrite it.

▶ Scenario

You are working in the internal medicine clinic of a large teaching hospital. Today your first patient is 70-year-old J.M., a man who has been coming to the clinic for several years for management of coronary artery disease (CAD) and hypertension (HTN). A cardiac catheterization done a year ago showed 50% stenosis of the circumflex coronary artery. He has had episodes of dizziness for the past 6 months and orthostatic hypotension, shoulder discomfort, and decreased exercise tolerance for the past 2 months. On his last clinic visit 3 weeks ago, a chest x-ray (CXR) showed cardiomegaly, and a 12-lead electrocardiogram (ECG) showed sinus tachycardia with left bundle branch block (LBBB). You review his morning blood work and initial assessment.

■ Chart View

Laboratory Testing

Chemistry

Sodium	142 mEq/L
Chloride	95 mEq/L
Potassium	3.9 mEq/L
Creatinine	0.8 mg/dL
Glucose	82 mg/dL
BUN	19 mg/dL

CBC

WBC	5400/mm³
Hgb	13 g/dL
Hct	41%
Platelets	229,000/mm³

Initial Assessment

Complains of increased fatigue and shortness of breath, especially with activity, and "waking up gasping for breath" at night, for the past 2 days.

Vital Signs

Temperature	97.9° F (36.6° C)
Blood pressure	142/83 mm Hg
Heart rate	105 beats/min
Respiratory rate	18 breaths/min

1. As you review these results, which ones are of possible concern, and why?

2. Knowing his history and seeing his condition this morning, what further questions are you going to ask J.M. and his daughter?

CASE STUDY PROGRESS

J.M. tells you he becomes exhausted and has shortness of breath climbing the stairs to his bedroom and has to lie down and rest ("put my feet up") at least an hour twice a day. He has been sleeping on two pillows for the past 2 weeks. He has not salted his food since the physician told him not to because of his high blood pressure, but he admits having had ham and a whole bag of salted peanuts 3 days ago. He denies having palpitations but has had a constant, irritating, nonproductive cough lately.

3. You think it's likely that J.M. has heart failure (HF). From his history, what do you identify as probable causes for his HF?

4. You are now ready to do your physical assessment. For each potential assessment finding for HF, indicate whether the finding indicates left-sided heart failure (L) or right-sided heart failure (R).

_____ 1. Fatigue, weakness, especially with activity
_____ 2. Jugular (neck) vein distention
_____ 3. Dependent edema (legs and sacrum)

_____ 4. Hacking cough, worse at night
_____ 5. Enlarged liver and spleen
_____ 6. Exertional dyspnea
_____ 7. Distended abdomen
_____ 8. Weight gain
_____ 9. S3/S4 gallop
_____10. Crackles/wheezes in lungs

■ Chart View

Medication Orders

Enalapril (Vasotec) 10 mg PO twice a day
Furosemide (Lasix) 20 mg PO every morning
Carvedilol (Coreg) 6.25 mg PO twice a day
Digoxin (Lanoxin) 0.5 mg PO now, then 0.125 mg PO daily
Potassium chloride 10 mEq tablet PO once a day

CASE STUDY PROGRESS

The physician confirms your suspicions and indicates that J.M. is experiencing symptoms of early left-sided heart failure. Medication orders are written.

5. For each medication listed, identify its class, and describe its purpose for the treatment of HF.

6. When you go to remove the medications from the automated dispensing machine, you see that carvedilol (Coreg CR) is stocked. Will you give it to J.M.? Explain.

7. As you remove the digoxin tablet from the automated medication dispensing machine, you note that the dosage on the tablet label is 250 mcg. How many tablets would you give?

8. Based on the new medication orders, which blood test or tests should be monitored carefully? Explain your answer.

9. When you give J.M. his medications, he looks at the potassium tablet, wrinkles his nose, and tells you he "hates those horse pills." He tells you a friend of his said he could eat bananas instead. He says he would rather eat a banana every day than take one of those pills. How will you respond?

CASE STUDY PROGRESS

This is J.M.'s first episode of significant HF. Before he leaves the clinic, you want to teach him about life-style modifications he can make and monitoring techniques he can use to prevent or minimize future problems.

10. List five suggestions you might make and the rationale for each.

11. You tell J.M. the combination of high-sodium foods he had during the past several days might have contributed to his present episode of HF. He looks surprised. J.M. says, "But I didn't add any salt to them!" To what health care professional could J.M. be referred to help him understand how to prevent future crises? State your rationale.

12. You also include teaching about digoxin toxicity. When teaching J.M. about the signs and symptoms of digoxin toxicity, which should be included? (Select all that apply.)
a. Dizziness when standing up
b. Visual changes
c. Loss of appetite or nausea
d. Increased urine output
e. Diarrhea

CASE STUDY OUTCOME

J.M.'s condition improves after 5 days of treatment, and he is discharged to home. He has a follow-up appointment with a cardiologist in 2 weeks.

Case Study 7

Name _____ Class/Group _____ Date _____

Group Members _____

INSTRUCTIONS All questions apply to this case study. Your responses should be brief and to the point. When asked to provide several answers, list them in order of priority or significance. Do not assume information that is not provided. Please print or write clearly. If your response is not legible, it will be marked as ? and you will need to rewrite it.

▶ **Scenario**

It is midmorning on the cardiac unit where you work, and you are getting a new patient. G.P. is a 60-year-old retired businessman, who is married and has three grown children. As you take his health history, he tells you that he began feeling changes in his chest about 10 days ago. He has hypertension (HTN) and a 5-year history of angina pectoris. During the past week, he has had frequent episodes of mid-chest discomfort. The chest pain responds to nitroglycerin (NTG), which he has taken sublingually (SL) about 8 to 10 times over the past week. During the week, he has also experienced increased fatigue. He states, "I just feel crappy all the time." A cardiac catheterization done several years ago revealed 50% stenosis of the right coronary artery (RCA) and 50% stenosis of the left anterior descending (LAD) coronary artery. He tells you that both his mother and father had coronary artery disease (CAD). He is currently taking amlodipine (Norvasc), metoprolol (Lopressor), atorvastatin (Lipitor), and aspirin 81 mg/day.

1. What other information are you going to ask about his episodes of chest pain?

2. What are common sites for radiation of ischemic cardiac pain?

3. You know that G.P. has atherosclerosis of the coronary arteries. You need to know his risk factors for CAD in order to plan teaching for lifestyle modifications. What will you ask him about?

1 Cardiovascular

4. Although he has been taking sublingual nitroglycerin (SL NTG) for a long time, you want to be certain he is using it correctly. Which actions are correct when taking SL NTG for chest pain? (Select all that apply.)
   a. Stop the activity and lie or sit down.
   b. Call 911 immediately.
   c. Call 911 if the pain is not relieved after taking one SL tablet.
   d. Call 911 if the pain is not relieved after taking three SL tablets, 5 minutes apart.
   e. Chew the tablet slowly then swallow.
   f. Place the NTG tablet under the tongue.

5. What other information would you need to make certain he understands the side effects and storage of SL NTG?

CASE STUDY PROGRESS

When you first admitted G.P., you placed him on telemetry and observed his cardiac rhythm.

6. Identify the rhythm:

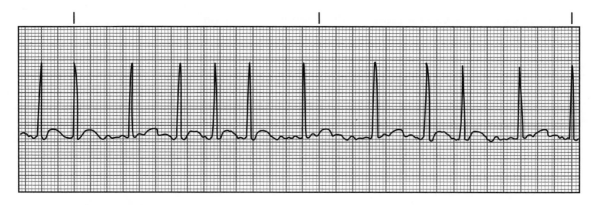

CASE STUDY PROGRESS

As you check his chart, you note that his vital signs (VS) and all of his lab tests were within normal range, including troponin and creatinine phosphokinase (CPK) levels; potassium (K) was 4.7 mEq/L. Within the hour, he spontaneously converted with medication (diltiazem [Cardizem]) to sick sinus syndrome with long sinus pauses that caused lightheadedness and hypotension.

7. What risks does the new rhythm pose for G.P.?

CASE STUDY PROGRESS

Because G.P.'s dysrhythmia is causing unacceptable symptoms, he is taken to surgery and a permanent DDDR pacemaker is placed and set at a rate of 70 beats/min.

8. What does the code *DDDR* mean?

9. The pacemaker insertion surgery places G.P. at risk for several serious complications. List three potential problems that you will monitor for as you care for him.

10. G.P. will need some education regarding his new pacemaker. What information will you give him before he leaves the hospital?

11. G.P.'s wife approaches you and anxiously inquires, "My neighbor saw this science fiction movie about this guy who got a pacemaker and then he couldn't die. Is that for real?" How are you going to respond to her?

12. G.P. and his wife tell you they have heard that people with pacemakers can have their hearts stop because of theft and security sensors in stores and airports. Where can you help them find more information?

CASE STUDY OUTCOME

After discharge, G.P. is referred to a cardiac rehabilitation center to start an exercise program. He will be exercise tested, and an individualized exercise prescription will be developed for him, based on the exercise test.

13. What information will be obtained from the graded exercise (stress) test (GXT), and what is included in an exercise prescription?

1 Cardiovascular

Case Study 8

Name _____ Class/Group _____ Date _____

Group Members _____

INSTRUCTIONS All questions apply to this case study. Your responses should be brief and to the point. When asked to provide several answers, list them in order of priority or significance. Do not assume information that is not provided. Please print or write clearly. If your response is not legible, it will be marked as ? and you will need to rewrite it.

▶ Scenario

You are assigned to care for L.J., a 70-year-old retired bus driver who has just been admitted to your medical floor with right leg deep vein thrombosis (DVT). L.J. has a 48-pack-year smoking history, although he states he quit 2 years ago. He has had pneumonia several times and frequent episodes of atrial flutter/fibrillation. He has had two previous episodes of DVT and was diagnosed with rheumatoid arthritis 3 years ago. Two months ago he began experiencing shortness of breath on exertion and noticed swelling of his right lower leg that became progressively worse until it extended up to his groin. His wife brought him to the hospital when he complained of increasingly severe pain in his leg. When a Doppler study indicated a probable thrombus of the external iliac vein extending distally to the lower leg, he was admitted for bed rest and to initiate heparin therapy. His basic metabolic panel was normal; other laboratory results are listed as follows:

■ Chart View

Laboratory Testing

PT	12.4 sec
INR	1.11
aPTT	25 sec
Hgb	13.3 g/dL
Hct	38.9%
Cholesterol	206 mg/dL

1. List six risk factors for DVT.

2. Identify at least five problems from L.J.'s history that represent his personal risk factors.

3. Something is missing from the scenario. Based on his history, L.J. should have been taking an important medication. What is it, and why should he be taking it?

4. Keeping in mind L.J.'s health history and admitting diagnosis, what are the most important assessments you will make during your physical examination and assessment?

5. What is the most serious complication of DVT?

CASE STUDY PROGRESS

Your assessment of L.J. reveals bibasilar crackles with moist cough; normal heart sounds; blood pressure (BP) 138/88 mm Hg; pulse 104 beats/min; 3+ pitting edema of right lower extremity; mild erythema of right foot and calf; and severe right calf pain. He is awake, alert, and oriented but a little restless. His Sao_2 is 92% on room air. He denies chest pain but does have shortness of breath with exertion.

6. List at least eight assessment findings you should monitor closely for in the development of the complication identified in Question 5.

CASE STUDY PROGRESS

L.J. is placed on 72-hour bed rest with bathroom privileges and given acetaminophen (Tylenol) for pain. The physician also writes orders for enoxaparin (Lovenox) injections.

7. L.J. asks, "Why do I have to get these shots? Why can't I just get a Coumadin pill to thin my blood?" What would be your response?
   a. "Good idea! I will call to ask the physician to switch medications."
   b. "It would take the Coumadin pills several days to be effective."
   c. "Your physician prefers the injections over the pills."
   d. "The enoxaparin will work to dissolve the blood clot in your leg."

8. The order for the enoxaparin reads: Enoxaparin 70 mg every 12 hours subcut. L.J. is 5 ft, 6 in. and weighs 156 lb. Is this dose appropriate?

9. What special techniques do you use when giving the subcutaneous injection of enoxaparin? (Select all that apply.)
   a. Rotate injection sites.
   b. Give the injection near the umbilicus.
   c. Expel the bubble from the prefilled syringe before giving the injection.
   d. After inserting the needle, do not aspirate before giving the injection.
   e. Massage the injection site gently after the injection is given.

10. True or False: Enoxaparin dosage is directed by monitoring activated partial thromboplastin time (aPTT) levels. Explain your answer.

11. What instructions will you give L.J. about his activity?

12. What pertinent laboratory values or test results would you expect the physician to order and you to monitor? Explain the reason for each test.

13. You identify pain as a key issue in the care of L.J. List four interventions you will choose for L.J. to address his pain.

14. You evaluate L.J.'s ECG strip. Name this rhythm, and explain what consequences it could have for L.J.

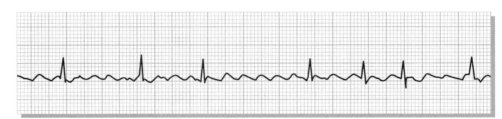

CASE STUDY PROGRESS

A week has passed. L.J. responded to heparin therapy, was started on warfarin therapy, and is being discharged to home with home care follow-up. "Good," he says, "just in time to fly out West for my grandson's wedding." His wife, who has come to pick him up, rolls her eyes and looks at the ceiling. You almost drop the discharge papers in disbelief. (You thought you had done such a good job of discharge teaching!)

15. What are you going to tell him?

CASE STUDY OUTCOME

L.J. listens to you, and Mrs. J. is quite relieved. L.J.'s son arranges to record the wedding ceremony, and guests at the reception record special greetings for him. It's been 2 weeks, and he seems quite pleased. He watches the recording daily and points out his favorite parts to the home care nurse every time she visits.

Case Study 9

Name _____ Class/Group _____ Date _____

Group Members _____

INSTRUCTIONS All questions apply to this case study. Your responses should be brief and to the point. When asked to provide several answers, list them in order of priority or significance. Do not assume information that is not provided. Please print or write clearly. If your response is not legible, it will be marked as ? and you will need to rewrite it.

▶ Scenario

A.H. is a 70-year-old retired construction worker who has experienced lumbosacral pain, nausea, and upset stomach for the past 6 months. He has a history of heart failure, high cholesterol, hypertension (HTN), sleep apnea, and depression. His chronic medical problems have been managed over the years with oral medications: benazepril (Lotensin) 5 mg/day, fluoxetine (Prozac) 40 mg/day, furosemide (Lasix) 20 mg/day, KCl 20 mEq bid, and lovastatin (Mevacor) 40 mg with the evening meal.

A.H. has just been admitted to the hospital for surgical repair of a 6.2-cm abdominal aortic aneurysm (AAA) that is now causing him constant pain. On arrival on your floor, his vital signs are 109/81, 61, 16, and 98.3° F (36.8° C). When you perform your assessment, you find that his apical heart rhythm is regular and his peripheral pulses are strong. His lungs are clear, and he is awake, alert, and oriented. There are no abnormal physical findings; however, he hasn't had a bowel movement for 3 days. His electrolytes, blood chemistries, and clotting studies are within normal range, except his hematocrit is 30.1%, and hemoglobin is 9 g/dL.

1. A.H. has several common risk factors for AAA, which are evident from his health history. Identify and explain three factors.

CASE STUDY PROGRESS

While A.H. awaits his surgery, it is important that you monitor him carefully for decreased tissue perfusion.

2. Identify five things you would assess for, and state your rationale for each.

1 Cardiovascular

3. What is the most serious, life-threatening complication of AAA, and why?

4. What single problem mentioned in the first paragraph of this case study presents a risk for AAA rupture? Why?

5. During your assessment, you notice a pulsation in A.H.'s upper abdomen, slightly left of the midline, between the umbilicus and the xiphoid process. True or False: You will need to palpate this mass as part of your physical assessment. Explain your answer.

CASE STUDY PROGRESS

The resection of A.H.'s aneurysm was successful, but, for the first 3 postoperative days, he was delirious and required one-to-one nursing care before he became coherent and oriented again. He was still somewhat confused when he was transferred back to your floor.

6. What assessments should be made specific to his postoperative care?

7. List five problems that are high priorities in A.H.'s postoperative care.

8. During the postoperative period after an aneurysmectomy, the nurse will implement which actions? (Select all that apply.)
   a. Keep the head of bed (HOB) elevated at 60 degrees.
   b. Keep firm pressure on the abdominal incision during coughing exercises.
   c. Change dressings as ordered with aseptic technique.
   d. Monitor peripheral pulses on both lower extremities.
   e. Use the bed's knee gatch to allow for knee flexion during bed rest.

CASE STUDY PROGRESS

When A.H. is being prepared for discharge, you talk to him about health promotion and lifestyle change issues that are pertinent to his health problems.

9. Identify four health-related issues you might appropriately address with him and what you would teach in each area.

10. A.H. will be receiving follow-up visits from the home health care nurse to change his dressing and evaluate his incision. What can you discuss with A.H. before discharge that will help him understand what the nurse will be doing?

Case Study **10**

Name _____ Class/Group _____ Date _____

Group Members _____

INSTRUCTIONS All questions apply to this case study. Your responses should be brief and to the point. When asked to provide several answers, list them in order of priority or significance. Do not assume information that is not provided. Please print or write clearly. If your response is not legible, it will be marked as ? and you will need to rewrite it.

▶ Scenario

R.K. is an 85-year-old woman who lives with her husband, who is 87. Two nights before her admission to your cardiac unit, she awoke with heavy substernal pressure accompanied by epigastric distress. The pain was reduced somewhat when she rolled onto her side but did not completely subside for about 6 hours. The next night, she experienced the same chest pressure. The following morning, R.K.'s husband took her to the physician, and she was subsequently hospitalized to rule out myocardial infarction (MI). Labs were drawn in the emergency department. She was started on oxygen (O_2) at 2 L via nasal cannula and given nonenteric-coated aspirin 325 mg to be chewed and swallowed. An IV was started.

You obtain the following information from your history and physical examination: R.K. has no history of smoking or alcohol use, and she has been in good general health, with the exception of osteoarthritis of her hands and knees and some osteoarthritis of the spine. Her only medications are simvastatin (Zocor), ibuprofen as needed for bone and joint pain, and "herbs." Her admission vital signs (VS) are 132/84, 88, 18, and 99° F (37.2° C). Her weight is 114 lb and height is 5 ft, 4 in. Moderate edema of both ankles is present, but capillary refill is brisk, and peripheral pulses are 1+. You hear a soft systolic murmur. You place her on telemetry, which shows the rhythm in the figure, as follows. She denies any discomfort at present.

1. Identify her cardiac rhythm.

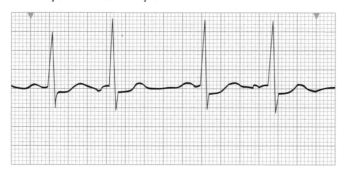

2. Give at least two reasons an IV would be inserted.

3. Explain the purpose of the aspirin tablet. Why is "nonenteric-coated" aspirin specified? What would be a contraindication to administering aspirin?

4. What additional history and physical information should you obtain related to her admitting diagnosis?

5. List seven laboratory or diagnostic tests you would expect to be performed; suggest what each might contribute.

6. What other source, besides cardiac ischemia, might be responsible for her chest and abdominal discomfort? (Specify.)

7. Define the concept of differential diagnosis, and explain how the concept applies to R.K.'s symptoms.

CASE STUDY PROGRESS

After some rest, R.K.'s chest pain has subsided, and she tells you that she feels much better now. You review her laboratory results.

■ Chart View

Laboratory Results

12-lead ECG: Light left-axis deviation, normal sinus rhythm with no ventricular ectopy
Serial CPK tests are 30 units/L (admission), 32 units/L (4 hours after admission)
Cardiac troponin T is less than 0.01 ng/mL (admission) and same result 4 hours after admission
Cardiac troponin T is less than 0.03 ng/mL (admission) and same result 4 hours after admission
D-dimer test less than 250 ng/mL

8. On the basis of the information presented so far, do you believe she had an MI? What is your rationale?

9. While you care for R.K., you carefully observe her. Identify two possible complications of coronary artery disease (CAD) and the signs and symptoms associated with each.

10. R.K. rings her call bell. When you arrive, she has her hand placed over her heart and tells you she is "having that heavy feeling again." She is not diaphoretic or nauseated but states she is short of breath. What else do you assess, and what can you do to make her more comfortable?

CASE STUDY PROGRESS

R.K.'s husband is upset. He tells you they have been married for 62 years and he doesn't know what he would do without his wife. One way to help people deal with their anxieties is to help them focus on concrete issues.

11. What information would be useful to get from him? What other health care professional might be able to help with some of these issues?

CASE STUDY PROGRESS

R.K. has no further episodes of chest pain, and she is discharged to home the next day. As you present the discharge instructions, you review the proper technique for taking sublingual nitroglycerin for chest pain.

12. Which statement by R.K. indicates that further teaching is needed?
    a. "At the first sign of chest discomfort, I will stop what I'm doing and sit down."
    b. "I will place one nitroglycerin tablet under my tongue."
    c. "If the chest pain does not stop, I can take another tablet in 5 minutes."
    d. "My husband will need to call 911 if the chest pain does not stop after 3 nitroglycerin tablets."

1 Cardiovascular

Case Study **11**

Name _____ Class/Group _____ Date _____

Group Members _____

INSTRUCTIONS All questions apply to this case study. Your responses should be brief and to the point. When asked to provide several answers, list them in order of priority or significance. Do not assume information that is not provided. Please print or write clearly. If your response is not legible, it will be marked as ? and you will need to rewrite it.

▶ Scenario

The time is 1900. You are working in a small, rural hospital. It has been snowing heavily all day, and the medical helicopters at the large regional medical center, 4 hours away by car (in good weather), have been grounded by the weather until morning. The roads are barely passable. W.R., a 48-year-old plumber with a 36-pack-year smoking history, is admitted to your floor with a diagnosis of rule out myocardial infarction (R/O MI). He has significant male-pattern obesity ("beer belly," large waist circumference) and a barrel chest, and he reports a dietary history of high-fat food. His wife brought him to the emergency department after he complained of unrelieved "indigestion." His admission vital signs (VS) were 202/124, 106, 18, and 98.2° F (36.8° C). W.R. was put on oxygen (O_2) by nasal cannula (NC) titrated to maintain Sao_2 (arterial oxygen saturation) over 90% and started on an IV of nitroglycerin (NTG). He was given aspirin 325 mg to chew and swallow and was admitted to Dr. A.'s service. There are plans to transfer him by helicopter to the regional medical center for a cardiac catheterization in the morning when the weather clears. Meanwhile, you have to deal with limited laboratory and pharmacy resources. The minute W.R. comes through the door of your unit, he announces he's just fine in a loud and angry voice and demands a cigarette. He also says he has no time to fool around with hospitals.

1. From the perspective of basic human needs, what is the first priority in his care?

2. Are these VS reasonable for a man of his age? If not, which one(s) concern(s) you? Explain why or why not.

3. Identify five priority problems associated with the care of a patient like W.R.

4. Which laboratory tests might be ordered to investigate W.R.'s condition? If the order is appropriate, place an "A" in the space provided. If inappropriate, mark with an "I," and provide rationales for your decisions.
   1. ____ CBC
   2. ____ EEG in the morning
   3. ____ Chem 7 (electrolytes)
   4. ____ PT/PTT
   5. ____ Bilirubin
   6. ____ Urinalysis (UA)
   7. ____ STAT 12-lead ECG
   8. ____ Type and crossmatch for 2 units of packed RBCs (PRBCs)

5. What significant lab tests are missing from the previous list?

6. How are you going to respond to W.R.'s angry demands for a cigarette? He also demands something for his "heartburn." How will you respond?

CASE STUDY PROGRESS

You phone Dr. A.'s partner, who is on call. She prescribes morphine sulfate 4 to 10 mg IV push (IVP) q1h prn for pain (burning, pressure, angina).

7. Explain two reasons for this order.

8. What special precautions should you follow when administering morphine sulfate IVP?

9. The pharmacy supplies morphine for injection in vials of 5 mg/mL only. For the first dose, you will be giving 4 mg of morphine. How many milliliters will you give for this dose? Mark the syringe with your answer.

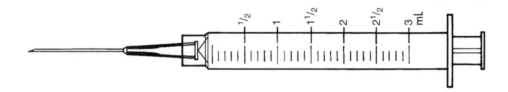

10. What will you do with the rest of the morphine in the vial?
   a. Discard it.
   b. Save it for the next dose.
   c. Return it to the pharmacy.
   d. Discard it with a second witness.

11. Angina is not always experienced as "pain" as many people understand pain. How would you describe symptoms you want him to warn you about? Why is this important?

12. What safety measures or instructions would you give W.R. before you leave his room?

13. Mrs. R. asks you, "If he can't smoke, why can't you give him one of those nicotine patches?" How will you respond?

14. Are there any alternatives to help him with his nicotine cravings? Would they be helpful now?

15. Before leaving for the night, Mrs. R. approaches you and asks, "Did my husband have a heart attack? I'm really scared. His father died of one when he was 51." How are you going to respond to her question?

16. When you come into W.R.'s room at 2200 hours to answer his call light, you see he is holding his left arm and complaining about aching in his left shoulder and arm. What information will you gather? What questions will you ask him?

17. You give him one sublingual NTG tablet, per protocol, but his pain is not relieved. Based on your assessment findings, you decide to call the physician. Using SBAR (**S**ituation, **B**ackground, **A**ssessment, **R**ecommendation), what information would you provide to the physician when you call?

CASE STUDY OUTCOME

In the morning, W.R. is transferred by helicopter to the medical center, and a cardiac catheterization is performed. It is determined that W.R. has coronary artery disease (CAD). The cardiologist suggests it would be best to treat him medically for now, with follow-up counseling on risk factor modification, especially smoking cessation. He is discharged with a referral for a follow-up visit to his local internist in 1 week.

18. What does it mean to treat him "medically" (conservatively)? What other approaches might be used to treat CAD?

Case Study 12

Name _____ Class/Group _____ Date _____

Group Members _____

INSTRUCTIONS All questions apply to this case study. Your responses should be brief and to the point. When asked to provide several answers, list them in order of priority or significance. Do not assume information that is not provided. Please print or write clearly. If your response is not legible, it will be marked as ? and you will need to rewrite it.

▶ **Scenario**

You are working at the local cardiac rehabilitation center, and R.M. is walking around the track. He summons you and asks if you could help him understand his recent lab report. He admits to being confused by the overwhelming data on the test and doesn't understand how the results relate to his recent heart attack and need for a stent. You take a moment to locate his lab reports and review his history. The findings are as follows:

R.M. is an active 61-year-old man who works full time for the postal service. He walks 3 miles every other day and admits he doesn't eat a "perfect diet." He enjoys two or three beers every night, uses stick margarine, eats red meat two or three times per week, and is a self-professed "sweet eater." He has tried to quit smoking and is down to one pack per day. His cardiac history includes a recent inferior myocardial infarction (MI) and a heart catheterization revealing three-vessel disease: in the left anterior descending (LAD) coronary artery, a proximal 60% lesion; in the right coronary artery (RCA), proximal 100% occlusion with thrombus; and a circumflex with 40% to 60% diffuse ecstatic (dilated) lesions. A stent was deployed to the RCA and reduced the lesion to 0% residual stenosis. He has had no need for sublingual nitroglycerin (NTG). He was discharged on enteric-coated aspirin 325 mg daily, clopidogrel (Plavix) 75 mg daily, atorvastatin (Lipitor) 10 mg at bedtime, and ramipril (Altace) 10 mg/day. Six weeks after his MI and stent placement, he had a fasting advanced lipid profile with other blood work.

■ Chart View

Six-Week Post Procedure Laboratory Work (Fasting)

Total cholesterol	188 mg/dL
High density lipoprotein (HDL)	34 mg/dL
Low density lipoprotein (LDL)	98 mg/dL
Triglycerides	176 mg/dL
Homocysteine	18 mmol/dL
Highly-sensitive C-reactive protein (hsCRP)	12 mg/dL
Fasting blood glucose (FBG)	99 mg/dL
Thyroid-stimulating hormone (TSH)	1.04 mU/L

1. Given the previous information, what assessment questions are important to ask R.M.?

2. When you start to discuss R.M.'s laboratory values with him, he is pleased about his results. "My cholesterol level is below 200!—and my 'bad cholesterol' is good! That's good news, right?" What would you say to him?

3. R.M.'s physician adds niacin, a vitamin preparation (folic acid, vitamin B_6, and vitamin B_{12} [Foltyx]) daily with food, and omega-3 fatty acids to his list of medications. How do these medications affect lipids? R.M. states, "But I already take Lipitor. What do all these medications do?" How do you answer him?

4. Discuss the significance of R.M.'s highly sensitive C-reactive protein (hsCRP) level.

5. Discuss the significance of the homocysteine test and R.M.'s results.

6. What else in R.M.'s history might be contributing to his elevated homocysteine levels?

7. You are teaching R.M. about the side effects of niacin. Which effects will you include in your teaching? (Select all that apply.)
   a. Flushed skin
   b. Headache
   c. Gastrointestinal (GI) distress
   d. Pruritus
   e. Dizziness

1 Cardiovascular

8. You have reviewed his other medications, including atorvastatin (Lipitor). Which statement by R.M. indicates a need for further teaching?
   a. "I will take this medication at night."
   b. "I will try to exercise more each week."
   c. "I like to take my medicines with grapefruit juice."
   d. "I will call the doctor right away if I experience muscle pain."

CASE STUDY PROGRESS

You enter R.M.'s room and hear the physician say, "There are many options for changing your LDL and triglyceride levels. You need to continue modifying your diet and exercise to enhance your medication regimen." The physician asks R.M. whether he has any questions, and the patient responds, "No."

9. After the physician leaves the room, R.M. tells you he really didn't understand what the physician said. Explain the necessary lifestyle changes to R.M.

Case Study **13**

Name _____ Class/Group _____ Date _____

Group Members _____

▶ Scenario

Your patient, 58-year-old K.Z., has a significant cardiac history. He has long-standing coronary artery disease (CAD) with occasional episodes of heart failure (HF). One year ago, he had an anterior wall myocardial infarction (MI). In addition, he has chronic anemia, hypertension, chronic renal insufficiency, and a recently diagnosed 4-cm suprarenal abdominal aortic aneurysm. Because of his severe CAD, he had to retire from his job as a railroad engineer about 6 months ago. This morning, he is being admitted to your telemetry unit for a same-day cardiac catheterization. As you take his health history, you note that his wife died a year ago (about the same time that he had his MI) and that he does not have any children. He is a current cigarette smoker with a 50-pack-year smoking history. His vital signs (VS) are 158/94, 88, 20, and 97.2° F (36.2° C). As you talk with him, you realize that he has only minimal understanding of the catheterization procedure.

1. Before he leaves for the catheterization laboratory, you briefly teach him the important things he needs to know before having the procedure. List five priority topics you will address.

2. Look at his past history. What other factors are present that could contribute to his risk for cardiac ischemia?

CASE STUDY PROGRESS

Several hours later, K.Z. returns from his catheterization. The catheterization report shows 90% occlusion of the proximal left anterior descending (LAD) coronary artery, 90% occlusion of the distal LAD, 70% to 80% occlusion of the distal right coronary artery (RCA), an old apical infarct, and an ejection fraction (EF) of 37%. About an hour after the procedure was finished, you perform a brief physical assessment and note a grade III/VI systolic ejection murmur at the cardiac apex, crackles bilaterally in the lung bases, and trace pitting edema of his feet and ankles. Except for the soft systolic murmur, these findings were not present before the catheterization.

3. Using the following diagram, identify the superior vena cava, the aorta, and the left and right ventricles. Identify the main coronary arteries, and circle the areas of the LAD and RCA that have significant occlusion, as identified in the previous report. Lightly shade the area of the heart where K.Z. had the earlier infarct.

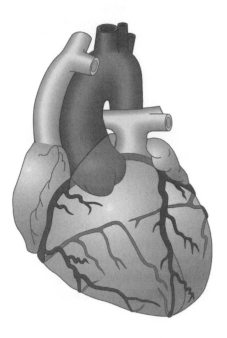

4. What is your evaluation of the catheterization results?

5. Explain the significance of having an ejection fraction of 37%.

6. What problem do the changes in assessment findings suggest to you? What led you to your conclusion?

7. List five actions you should take as a result of your evaluation of the assessment, and state your rationales.

CASE STUDY PROGRESS

After assessing K.Z., the physician admits him (with a diagnosis of CAD and HF) for CABG surgery. Significant laboratory results drawn at this time are Hct 25.3%, Hgb 8.8 g/dL, BUN 33 mg/dL, and creatinine 3.1 mg/dL. K.Z. is given furosemide (Lasix) and 2 units of packed RBCs (PRBCs).

8. Review K.Z.'s health history. Can you identify a probable explanation for his chronic renal insufficiency and anemia?

9. Why did he receive 2 units of PRBCs instead of whole blood? What was the purpose of the furosemide?

CASE STUDY PROGRESS

Five days later, after his condition is stabilized, K.Z. is taken to surgery for a three-vessel coronary artery bypass graft (CABG × 3 V). When he arrives in the surgical intensive care unit (SICU), he has a Swan-Ganz catheter in place for hemodynamic monitoring and is intubated. He is put on a ventilator at Fio_2 0.70 and positive end-expiratory pressure (PEEP) at 5 cm H_2O. His latest hemoglobin (Hgb) is 10.3 mg/dL. You review his first hemodynamic readings and arterial blood gases.

■ Chart View

Hemodynamic Readings

Pulmonary artery pressure (PAP)	38/23 mm Hg
Central venous pressure (CVP)	16 mm Hg
Pulmonary capillary wedge pressure (PCWP)	18 mm Hg
Cardiac index (CI)	1.88 L/min/mm^2

Arterial Blood Gases

pH	7.37
Pa_{CO_2}	46 mm Hg
Pa_{O_2}	61 mm Hg
Sa_{O_2}	85%

10. Why are arterial blood gases necessary in the case of K.Z.? Explain why it would be inappropriate to use pulse oximetry to assess his O_2 saturation status.

11. What is your interpretation of his arterial blood gases on 70% oxygen?

12. What is your evaluation of K.Z.'s hemodynamic status, based on the results displayed?

13. K.Z. is receiving continuous IV infusions of nitroprusside (Nitropress) and dobutamine. Do you think the hemodynamic values reported previously reflect poor left ventricular function or fluid overload, and why?

14. Why is K.Z. receiving the nitroprusside and dobutamine?

15. What is your responsibility when administering nitroprusside and dobutamine to your patient?

CASE STUDY PROGRESS

After 3 days in the SICU, K.Z.'s condition is stable, and he is returned to your telemetry floor. Now, 5 days later, he is ready to go home, and you are preparing him for discharge.

16. List at least four general areas related to his CABG surgery in which he should receive instruction before he goes home.

Case Study **14**

Name _____ Class/Group _____ Date _____

Group Members _____

INSTRUCTIONS All questions apply to this case study. Your responses should be brief and to the point. When asked to provide several answers, list them in order of priority or significance. Do not assume information that is not provided. Please print or write clearly. If your response is not legible, it will be marked as ? and you will need to rewrite it.

▶ **Scenario**

The wife of C.W., a 70-year-old man, brought him to the emergency department (ED) at 4:30 this morning. She told the ED triage nurse that he had had dysentery for the past 3 days, and, last night, he had a lot of "dark red" diarrhea. When he became very dizzy, disoriented, and weak this morning, she decided to bring him to the hospital. C.W.'s vital signs (VS) were 70/- (systolic blood pressure [BP] 70 mm Hg, diastolic BP inaudible), 110, 20, 99.1° F (37.3° C). A 16-gauge IV catheter was inserted, and a lactated Ringer's (LR) infusion was started. The triage nurse obtained the following history from the patient and his wife. C.W. has had idiopathic dilated cardiomyopathy for several years. The onset was insidious, but the cardiomyopathy is now severe, as evidenced by an ejection fraction (EF) of 13% found during a recent cardiac catheterization. He experiences frequent problems with heart failure (HF) because of the cardiomyopathy. Two years ago, he had a cardiac arrest that was attributed to hypokalemia. He also has a long history of hypertension (HTN) and arthritis. He has also had atrial fibrillation in the past but it has been under control recently. Fifteen years ago he had a peptic ulcer.

An endoscopy showed a 25 × 15 mm duodenal ulcer with adherent clot. The ulcer was cauterized, and C.W. was admitted to the medical intensive care unit (MICU) for treatment of his volume deficit. You are his admitting nurse. As you are making him comfortable, Mrs. W. gives you a paper sack filled with the bottles of medications he has been taking: enalapril (Vasotec) 5 mg PO bid, warfarin (Coumadin) 5 mg/day PO, digoxin (Lanoxin) 0.125 mg/day, PO, potassium chloride 20 mEq PO bid, and diclofenac sodium (Voltaren) 50 mg PO tid. As you connect him to the cardiac monitor, you note that he is in sinus tachycardia. Doing a quick assessment, you find a pale man who is sleepy but arousable and oriented. He is still dizzy, hypotensive, and tachycardic. You hear S3 and S4 heart sounds and a grade II/VI systolic murmur. Peripheral pulses are all 2+, and trace pedal edema is present. Lungs are clear. Bowel sounds are present, midepigastric tenderness is noted, and the liver margin is 4 cm below the costal margin. A Swan-Ganz catheter and an arterial line are inserted.

1. What may have precipitated C.W.'s gastrointestinal (GI) bleeding?

2. From his history and assessment, identify five signs and symptoms (S/S) of GI bleeding and loss of blood volume.

3. What is the most serious potential complication of C.W.'s bleeding?

4. What is the effect of C.W.'s blood pressure on his kidneys?

CASE STUDY PROGRESS

C.W. receives a total of 4 units of packed red blood cells (PRBCs), 5 units of fresh frozen plasma (FFP), and several liters of crystalloids to keep his mean BP above 60 mm Hg. On the second day in the MICU, his total fluid intake is 8.498 L and output is 3.66 L for a positive fluid balance of 4.838 L. His hemodynamic parameters after fluid resuscitation are pulmonary capillary wedge pressure (PCWP) 30 mm Hg and cardiac output (CO) 4.5 L/min.

5. Why will you want to monitor his fluid status very carefully?

6. List at least six things you will monitor to assess C.W.'s fluid balance.

7. Explain the purpose of the FFP for C.W.

CASE STUDY PROGRESS

As soon as you get a chance, you review C.W.'s admission laboratory results. These were drawn before he received the PRBCs.

■ Chart View

Lab Work

Sodium	138 mEq/L
Potassium	6.9 mEq/L
BUN	90 mg/dL
Creatinine	2.1 mg/dL
WBC	16,000/mm³
Hgb	8.4 g/dL
Hct	25%
PT	23.4 seconds
INR	4.2

8. After examining the lab results, are there any concerns with C.W.'s electrolyte levels? Explain your answer.

9. In view of the previous lab results, what diagnostic test will be performed and why?

10. Evaluate this ECG strip, and note the effect of any electrolyte imbalances.

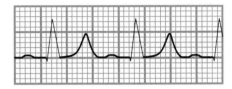

11. Why do you think BUN and creatinine are elevated?

12. What do the low hemoglobin (Hgb) and hematocrit (Hct) levels indicate about the rapidity of C.W.'s blood loss?

13. What is the explanation for the prolonged prothrombin time/international normalized ratio (PT/INR)?

14. What will be your response to the prolonged PT/INR? (Select all that apply.)
   a. Prepare to administer a STAT dose of protamine sulfate.
   b. Hold the warfarin.
   c. Monitor C.W. for signs and symptoms of bleeding.
   d. Obtain an order for aspirin if needed for pain.
   e. Avoid injections as much as possible.

15. What safety precautions should be considered in light of his prolonged PT/INR?

16. How do you account for the elevated white blood cell count?

CASE STUDY PROGRESS

Mrs. W. has been with her husband since he arrived at the emergency department and is worried about his condition and his care.

17. List four things you might do to make her more comfortable while her husband is in the MICU.

Case Study **15**

Name _____ Class/Group _____ Date _____

Group Members _____

INSTRUCTIONS All questions apply to this case study. Your responses should be brief and to the point. When asked to provide several answers, list them in order of priority or significance. Do not assume information that is not provided. Please print or write clearly. If your response is not legible, it will be marked as ? and you will need to rewrite it.

▶ Scenario

J.F. is a 50-year-old married homemaker with a genetic autoimmune deficiency; she has suffered from recurrent infective endocarditis. The most recent episodes were a *Staphylococcus aureus* infection of the mitral valve 16 months ago and a *Streptococcus viridans* infection of the aortic valve 1 month ago. During this latter hospitalization, an echocardiogram showed moderate aortic stenosis, moderate aortic insufficiency, chronic valvular vegetations, and moderate left atrial enlargement. Two years ago, J.F. received an 18-month course of parenteral nutrition for malnutrition caused by idiopathic, relentless nausea and vomiting (N/V). She has also had coronary artery disease for several years and, 2 years ago, suffered an acute anterior wall myocardial infarction (MI). In addition, she has a history of chronic joint pain.

Now, after being home for only a week, J.F. has been readmitted to your floor with endocarditis, N/V, and renal failure. Since yesterday, she has been vomiting and retching constantly; she also has had chills, fever, fatigue, joint pain, and headache. As you go through the admission process with her, you note that she wears glasses and has a dental bridge. Intravenous access is obtained with a double lumen peripherally inserted central catheter (PICC) line, and other orders are written below. Your assessment is also documented.

■ Chart View

Admission Orders

STAT blood cultures (aerobic and anaerobic) × 2
STAT electrolytes & CBC
Begin parenteral nutrition (PN) at 85 mL/hr
Penicillin 2 million units IV piggyback q4h
Furosemide (Lasix) 80 mg/day PO
Amlodipine (Norvasc) 5 mg/day PO
Potassium chloride (K-Dur) 40 mEq/day PO
Metoprolol (Lopressor) 25 mg PO bid
Prochlorperazine (Compazine) 5 mg IV push prn for N/V
Transesophageal echocardiogram ASAP

Admission Assessment

Blood pressure	152/48 (supine) and 100/40 (sitting)
Pulse rate	116 beats/min
Respiratory rate	22 breaths/min
Temperature	100.2° F (37.9° C)

Oriented × 3 but drowsy
Grade II/VI holosystolic murmur and a grade III/VI diastolic murmur noted on auscultation
Lungs clear bilaterally
Abdomen soft with slight left upper quadrant (LUQ) tenderness
Multiple petechiae on skin of arms, legs, and chest; and splinter hemorrhages under the fingernails
Hematuria noted in voided urine

1. What is the significance of the orthostatic hypotension and the tachycardia?

2. What is the significance of the abdominal tenderness, hematuria, joint pain, and petechiae?

3. What are splinter hemorrhages, and what is their significance?

4. As you monitor J.F. throughout the day, what other signs and symptoms (S/S) of embolization will you watch for?

5. Explain the diagnostic criteria for infectious endocarditis.

CASE STUDY PROGRESS

The next day, you review J.F.'s laboratory test results:

■ Chart View

Laboratory Test Results

Na	138 mEq/L
K	3.9 mEq/L
Cl	103 mEq/L
BUN	85 mg/dL
Creatinine	3.9 mg/dL
Glucose	165 mg/dL
WBC	6700/mm³
Hct	27%
Hgb	9.0 g/dL

6. Identify the values that are not within normal ranges, and explain the reason for each abnormality.

7. You note that a new intern writes an order for "Fasting blood glucose levels daily." Is this order appropriate for J.F.? Explain.

8. What is the greatest risk for J.F. during the process of rehydration, and what would you monitor to detect its development?

CASE STUDY PROGRESS

As you admitted J.F., you were aware that as soon as she became stable, she would be going home in a few days on PN and IV antibiotics. The home care agency that will be supervising her care is contacted to coordinate discharge preparations and teaching.

9. List five important questions in assessing her home health care needs.

CASE STUDY PROGRESS

Fortunately, J.F. has a supportive husband and two daughters who live nearby who can function as caregivers when J.F. is discharged. They, along with the patient, will need teaching about endocarditis. Although J.F. has been ill for several years, you discover that she and her family have received little education about the disease. You prepare a teaching plan for the family. The home care agency has a parenteral-enteral nutrition team to address her nutritional needs, which will also include vitamins, minerals, and lipids. PN formulations require complex calculations. The parenteral-enteral nutrition team takes care of the formulation of the PN through the pharmacy or dietary staff (depending on local arrangements).

10. List three things you will teach J.F. and her family.

11. After teaching J.F. about oral hygiene, which statement by J.F. reflects a need for further education?
  a. "I will remove my bridge after every meal and clean it thoroughly before replacing it."
  b. "I will use a water irrigation device to clean my teeth and gums."
  c. "I will use a soft toothbrush to brush my teeth."
  d. "I will rinse my mouth thoroughly with water after brushing my teeth."

CASE STUDY PROGRESS

Your hospital discharge planner facilitates J.F.'s transition to home care.

12. During the initial home visit, the home health nurse evaluates J.F.'s IV site for implementation of the IV therapy program. The nurse interviews the family members to determine their willingness to be caregivers and their level of understanding and enlists the patient's and family's assistance to identify 10 teaching goals. What topics would be included on this list?

13. The home health nurse also writes short- and long-term goals for J.F. and her family. Identify two short-term and three long-term goals.

CASE STUDY OUTCOME

Mr. F. and his two daughters learned to administer J.F.'s PN during the 8-month treatment. J.F.'s endocarditis resolves with no worsening of her cardiac condition.

Case Study 16

Name _____ Class/Group _____ Date _____

Group Members _____

INSTRUCTIONS All questions apply to this case study. Your responses should be brief and to the point. When asked to provide several answers, list them in order of priority or significance. Do not assume information that is not provided. Please print or write clearly. If your response is not legible, it will be marked as ? and you will need to rewrite it.

▶ Scenario

You are just getting caught up with your work when you receive the following phone call: "Hi, this is Deb in the emergency department. We're sending you M.M., a 63-year-old Hispanic woman with a past medical history of coronary artery disease (CAD). Her daughter reports that her mom has become increasingly weak over the past couple of weeks and has been unable to do her housework. Apparently, she has had complaints of swelling in her ankles and feet by late afternoon ("she can't wear her shoes") and has nocturnal diuresis × 4. Her daughter brought her in because she has had heaviness in her chest off and on over the past few days but denies any discomfort at this time. The daughter took her to see her family physician, who immediately sent her here. Vital signs are 146/92, 96, 24, 99° F (37.2° C). She has an IV of D_5W at 10 mL/hr in her right forearm. Her lab results are as follows: Na 134 mEq/L, K 3.5 mEq/L, Cl 103 mEq/L, HCO_3 23 mEq/L, BUN 13 mg/dL, creatinine 1.3 mg/dL, glucose 153 mg/dL, WBC 8300/mm³, Hct 33.9%, Hgb 11.7 g/dL, platelets 162,000/mm³. PT/INR, PTT, and urinalysis are pending. She has had her chest x-ray and ECG, and her orders have been written."

1. What additional information do you need from the emergency department (ED) nurse?

2. How are you going to prepare for this patient?

3. M.M. arrives by wheelchair. As she transfers to the bed, what observations will you make? Why?

4. Given the previous information, you can anticipate orders for this patient. Carefully review each order to determine whether it is appropriate or inappropriate as written. If the order is appropriate, mark it as "A"; if the order is inappropriate, mark it as "I" and change the order to make it appropriate. Provide any other orders that might be appropriate for this patient.

_____ 1. Routine VS

_____ 2. Serum magnesium (Mg) STAT

_____ 3. Up ad lib

_____ 4. 10 g sodium (Na), low-fat diet

_____ 5. Change IV to normal saline (NS) at 100 mL/hr

_____ 6. Cardiac enzymes on admission and q8h × 24 hr, then daily every morning

_____ 7. CBC, chem 7, and fasting lipid profile in morning

_____ 8. Schedule for abdominal CT scan for AM

_____ 9. Heparin 10,000 units subcut q8h

_____10. Docusate sodium (Colace) 100 mg/day PO

_____11. Ampicillin 250 mg IV piggyback q6h

_____12. Furosemide (Lasix) 200 mg IV push STAT

_____13. Nitroglycerin (NTG) 0.4 mg 1 SL q4h prn for chest pain

_____14. Schedule echocardiogram

5. Which interventions are appropriate for administering subcutaneous heparin? (Select all that apply.)
  a. Rotate injection sites with each dose.
  b. Monitor aPTT levels daily.
  c. Massage the area after the injection.
  d. Give the injection at least 2 inches away from the umbilicus.
  e. Do not aspirate the syringe before injecting the heparin.

6. When you respond to M.M.'s call light, you observe she is talking rapidly in Spanish and pointing to the bathroom. Her speech pattern indicates she is short of breath; she is having trouble completing a sentence without taking a labored breath. You assist her to use a bedpan and note that her skin feels clammy. While sitting on the bedpan, she vomits. On a scale of 0 to 10 (0 being no problem, 10 being a code-level emergency), how would you rate this situation, and why?

7. Identify at least four actions you should take next, and state your rationale.

8. M.M.'s physician calls your unit to find out what is happening. Using SBAR, what information would you need to convey at this time?

9. The hospital's staff physician is coming to the floor immediately to evaluate the patient. In the meantime she orders furosemide (Lasix) 40 mg IV push STAT. You have only 20 mg in stock. Should you give the 20 mg now, and then give the additional 20 mg when it comes up from the pharmacy? Explain your answer.

10. M.M. continues to experience vomiting and diaphoresis that are unrelieved by medication and comfort measures. A STAT 12-lead ECG reveals ischemic changes. The patient is transferred to the coronary care unit (CCU). As you give the report to the receiving registered nurse, what laboratory value is the most important to report, and why?

11. While recovering in the CCU, M.M. tried to get up out of the bed, fell, and fractured her right humerus. Because of the surgical risks involved, M.M. was treated conservatively and put in a full arm cast. She is again transferred to your floor. A case manager has been asked to evaluate M.M.'s home to see whether she can be discharged to her own home or will need to stay in a long-term care facility. Identify at least eight things that the CM would assess.

12. M.M.'s nutritional intake over the past few weeks has been poor. She also has increased nutritional needs because of her fractured arm. What are some of the nutritional needs that should be met? What would you recommend to help her with this?

1 Cardiovascular

CASE STUDY OUTCOME

Because the case manager determined that M.M. lived in an apartment with poor access, M.M. elects to stay with her daughter and five grandchildren in their small home. A home care nurse comes three times a week to check on her. M.M. is easily fatigued, and the children are quite lively. School is out for the summer.

13. Suggest some ways the daughter can ensure that her mother isn't overwhelmed and doesn't become exhausted in this situation.

Case Study **17**

Name _____ Class/Group _____ Date _____

Group Members _____

INSTRUCTIONS All questions apply to this case study. Your responses should be brief and to the point. When asked to provide several answers, list them in order of priority or significance. Do not assume information that is not provided. Please print or write clearly. If your response is not legible, it will be marked as? and you will need to rewrite it.

▶ **Scenario**

You are in the middle of your shift in the coronary care unit (CCU) of a large urban medical center. Your new admission, C.B., a 47-year-old woman, was just flown to your institution from a small rural community more than 100 miles away. She had an acute anterior wall myocardial infarction (MI) last evening. Her current vital signs (VS) are 100/60, 86, 14. After you make C.B. comfortable, you receive this report from the flight nurse:"C.B. is a full-time homemaker with four children. She has had episodes of 'chest tightness' with exertion for the past year, but this is her first known MI. She has a history of hyperlipidemia and has smoked one pack of cigarettes daily for more than 30 years. Surgical history consists of total abdominal hysterectomy 10 years ago after the birth of her last child. She has no other known medical problems. Yesterday at 8 PM, she began to have severe substernal chest pain that referred into her neck and down both arms. She rated the pain as 9 or 10 on a 0-to-10 scale. She thought it was severe indigestion and began taking Maalox with no relief. Her husband then took her to the local emergency department (ED), where a 12-lead ECG showed hyperacute ST elevation in the inferior leads II, III, and aVF and V5 to V6. Before tissue plasminogen activator (TPA) could be given, she went into ventricular fibrillation (V-fib) and was successfully defibrillated after two shocks. She then was given TPA and started on nitroglycerin (NTG), heparin, and lidocaine drips. She also was given IV metoprolol and aspirin 325 mg to chew and swallow. This morning, her systolic pressure dropped into the 80s, and she was placed on a dopamine drip and urgently flown to your institution for coronary angiography and possible percutaneous coronary angioplasty (PTCA). Currently, she has lidocaine infusing at 2 mg/min, heparin at 1200 units/hr, and dopamine at 5 mcg/kg/min. The NTG has been stopped because of low blood pressure. Lab work that was done yesterday showed Na 145 mEq/L, K 3.6 mEq/L, HCo_3 19 mEq/L, BUN 9 mg/dL, creatinine 0.8 mg/dL, WBC 14,500/mm³, Hct 44.3%, and Hgb 14.5 g/dL."

1. Because the 12-lead ECG can tell you the location of the infarction, evaluate the leads that showed ST elevation. What areas of C.B.'s heart have been damaged?

2. Given the diagnosis of acute MI, what other lab results are you going to look at?

■ Chart View

Laboratory Test Results

Creatine Phosphokinase (CK) Levels

On ED admission	95 units/L
4 hours	1931 units/L
8 hours	4175 units/L

CK-MB Isoenzymes

On ED admission	5%
4 hours	79%
8 hours	216%
LDL	160 mg/dL
PT	11.9 sec
INR	1.02
aPTT (before heparin)	26.9 sec.
Mg	2.2 mg/dL
K	3.3 mEq/L

3. You review the lab work on her chart. For each laboratory value listed previously, interpret the result, and evaluate the meaning for C.B.

4. You note that C.B.'s Sao_2 on oxygen (O_2) at 6 L/min by nasal cannula is 92%. How do you interpret this result?

5. You are working with a nursing student, who asks you about the tissue plasminogen activator (TPA) therapy. Which of these statements about TPA is true? (Select all that apply.)
   a. TPA is a thrombolytic agent used to dissolve the clot in the coronary artery.
   b. Treatment with TPA must start within 4 hours after the onset of chest pain.
   c. TPA, when given properly, is able to reverse cardiac tissue infarction.
   d. The use of TPA might cause internal, intercranial, and superficial bleeding.
   e. Monitor the patient closely for cardiac dysrhythmias and anaphylactoid reactions while on TPA.

6. You are working with a nursing student. The student asks you, "If C.B. has received TPA, then why is she also receiving heparin at this time? Isn't she in danger of bleeding to death?" How will you respond?

7. An hour after her admission, you are preparing C.B. for her coronary intervention. Evaluate her readiness for teaching and her learning needs. What would you tell her?

CASE STUDY PROGRESS

The following day, you care for C.B. again. She is still on the lidocaine and heparin drips. The dopamine has been discontinued. VS are stable. Pulmonary capillary wedge pressure (PCWP) is 14 mm Hg, and cardiac output (CO) is 6 L/min. You check her lab results for lidocaine and aPTT levels.

8. The lidocaine level is 2.5 mg/mL, and the aPTT is 40 seconds. Analyze the results, and state any actions you would take.

CASE STUDY PROGRESS

As you work with C.B., you notice that she is extremely anxious. You had observed some anxiety yesterday, which you had attributed to the strange CCU environment, pain, and anticipation of the stenting procedure. You know that the stent was successful and that she is physically stable. You wonder what is wrong. She tells you that her MI occurred right in the middle of a move with her family from her rural community to an even smaller and unfamiliar town some 500 miles away in a neighboring state. She is dreading the move. Her husband "becomes angry easily and starts lashing out" toward her and the children. She is afraid to move to a community where she will have no friends and family to support her.

9. How can you help your patient? Evaluate the situation and describe possible interventions.

10. C.B.'s husband comes to visit. He is a handsome, well-dressed man who appears to be loving and attentive toward C.B. He brought a bouquet of roses for her and a box of chocolates for the nurses, "because I appreciate how good you girls have been to my wife." One of your younger colleagues comments to you, "Why, what a nice guy! What is her problem? Every woman would love to be married to a man like that!" How are you going to respond?

Respiratory Disorders

Case Study 18

Name _____ Class/Group _____ Date _____

Group Members _____

INSTRUCTIONS All questions apply to this case study. Your responses should be brief and to the point. When asked to provide several answers, list them in order of priority or significance. Do not assume information that is not provided. Please print or write clearly. If your response is not legible, it will be marked as ? and you will need to rewrite it.

▶ Scenario

You are a public health nurse working at a county immunization and tuberculosis (TB) clinic. B.A. is a 61-year-old woman who wishes to obtain a food handler's license and is required to show proof of a negative Mantoux (purified protein derivative [PPD]) test before being hired. She came to your clinic 2 days ago to obtain a PPD test for TB. She has returned to have you evaluate her reaction.

1. What is TB, and what microorganism causes it?

2. What is the route of transmission for TB?

3. The Centers for Disease Control and Prevention (CDC) recommends screening people at high risk for TB. List five populations at high risk for developing active disease.

4. Describe the two methods for TB screening.

2 Respiratory

5. How do you determine whether a Mantoux test is positive or negative?

B.A. consumes 3 to 4 ounces of alcohol (ETOH) per day and has smoked 1.5 packs of cigarettes per day for 40 years. She is a natural-born American, has no risk factors according to the CDC guidelines, lives with her daughter, and becomes angry at the suggestion that she might have TB. She admits that her mother had TB when she was a child but says she herself has never tested positive. She says, "I feel just fine and I don't think all this is necessary."

6. What additional information would you want to obtain from B.A. before interpreting her skin test result as positive or negative?

7. Determine whether B.A.'s skin test is positive or negative.

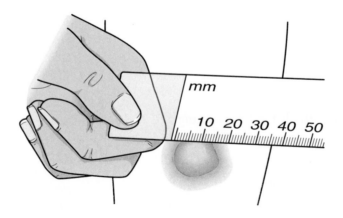

8. B.A. asks you what a positive PPD result means. How will you respond?

9. What steps will need to be done to determine whether B.A. has an active TB infection?

CASE STUDY PROGRESS

The physician orders a chest x-ray (CXR) and informs B.A. that her CXR is clear (shows no signs of TB). He tells her that she has a latent TB infection and that he will report her condition to the local public health department. The health department will monitor her over time and initiate treatment if she gets TB.

10. What is a latent TB infection (LTBI)?

11. What parameters are used to determine whether treatment should be initiated for LTBI?

2 Respiratory

12. According to the most current CDC guidelines, what constitutes usual preventive therapy for LTBI?

13. Different medications are associated with different side effects. Identify the test used to monitor each possible side effect listed as follows:

____A. Peripheral neuropathy
____B. Clinical hepatitis
____C. Fever and bleeding problems
____D. Nephrotoxicity/renal failure
____E. Hyperuricemia
____F. Optic neuritis
____G. Hearing neuritis

1. Audiogram
2. CBC (WBC and platelets)
3. Cr/BUN, Cr Cl (creatinine clearance)
4. AST/ALT
5. Physical exam and monofilament testing
6. Red-green discrimination and visual acuity
7. Uric acid

14. Nonadherence to drug therapy is a major problem that leads to treatment failure, drug resistance, and continued spread of TB. The CDC recommends two methods to ensure compliance with medication for all patients who have drug-resistant TB and for those who take medication two or three times every week. Identify one of those methods.

15. What information should B.A. receive before leaving the clinic?

CASE STUDY OUTCOME

B.A. is hired under the condition that she must immediately report any signs and symptoms of active disease to the county health department or her physician and have a yearly CXR.

Case Study 19

Name _____ Class/Group _____ Date _____

Group Members _____

INSTRUCTIONS All questions apply to this case study. Your responses should be brief and to the point. When asked to provide several answers, list them in order of priority or significance. Do not assume information that is not provided. Please print or write clearly. If your response is not legible, it will be marked as ? and you will need to rewrite it.

▶ **Scenario**

M.N., age 40, was admitted with acute cholecystitis. After undergoing an open cholecystectomy, she is being admitted to your surgical floor. She has a nasogastric tube to continuous low wall suction, one peripheral IV, and a large abdominal dressing. Her orders are as follows:

■ **Chart View**

Physician's Orders

    Progress diet to low-fat diet as tolerated
    D5 ½ NS with 40 mEq KCl at 125 mL/hr
    Turn, cough, and deep breathe q2h
    Incentive spirometer q2h while awake
    Dangle in AM, ambulate in PM
    Morphine sulfate 10 mg IM q4h prn for pain
    Ampicillin (Omnipen) 2 g IVPB q6h
    Chest x-ray in AM

1. Are these orders appropriate for M.N.? State your rationale.

2. What gastrointestinal complication might result from one of the medications listed in M.N.'s orders?

CASE STUDY PROGRESS

Four hours after admission, the nursing assistive personnel (NAP) reports to you the following:

■ Chart View

Vital Signs

Blood pressure	148/82 mm Hg
Heart rate	118 beats/min
Respiratory rate	24 breaths/min
Temperature	101° F (38.3°C)
Sao_2	88%

3. Based on her vital signs, what do you think could be happening with M.N., and why?

4. You know M.N. is at risk for postoperative pneumonia and atelectasis. What is atelectasis, and why is M.N. at risk?

5. Describe the assessment you would need to perform to differentiate what might be occurring with M.N.

CASE STUDY PROGRESS

Knowing M.N.'s vital signs, you do an assessment and auscultate decreased breath sounds and crackles in the right base posteriorly. Her right middle and lower lobes percuss slightly dull. She splints her right side when attempting to take a deep breath. She does not have a productive cough, chest pain, or any anxiety. You suspect that she is developing atelectasis.

6. Describe four actions you would take next in the next few hours.

7. Outline nursing interventions that are used to prevent pulmonary complications in patients undergoing abdominal surgery.

8. To promote optimal oxygenation with M.N., which action(s) could you delegate to the NAP? (Select all that apply.)
   a. Reminding the patient to cough and deep breathe
   b. Instructing the patient on the use of IS
   c. Assisting the patient in getting up to the chair
   d. Taking the patient's temperature and reporting elevations
   e. Encouraging the patient to splint the incision
   f. Auscultating the patient's lung sounds

9. Identify three outcomes that you expect for M.N. as a result of your interventions.

10. M.N.'s sister questions you, saying, "I don't understand. She came in here with a bad gallbladder. What has happened to her lungs?" How would you respond?

11. Despite your interventions, 4 hours later M.N. is not improved. Using SBAR, what would you report to the physician?

12. The physician orders a CXR. Radiology calls with a report, confirming that M.N. has atelectasis. Will that change anything that you have already planned for M.N.? Explain what you would do differently if M.N. had pneumonia.

2 Respiratory

Case Study **20**

Name _____ Class/Group _____ Date _____

Group Members _____

INSTRUCTIONS All questions apply to this case study. Your responses should be brief and to the point. When asked to provide several answers, list them in order of priority or significance. Do not assume information that is not provided. Please print or write clearly. If your response is not legible, it will be marked as ? and you will need to rewrite it.

▶ Scenario

S.R. is a 69-year-old man who presents to the clinic because his "wife complains that his snoring is difficult to live with."

1. As the clinic nurse, what routine information would you want to obtain from S.R.?

CASE STUDY PROGRESS

After interviewing S.R., you note the following: S.R. is under considerable stress. He owns his own business. The stress of overseeing his employees, meeting deadlines, and carrying out negotiations has led to poor sleep habits. He sleeps 3 to 4 hours per night. He keeps himself going by drinking 2 quarts of coffee and smoking three to four packs of cigarettes per day. He has gained 50 pounds over the past year, leading to a current weight of 280 pounds. He complains of difficulty staying awake, wakes up with headaches on most mornings, and has midmorning somnolence. He states that he is depressed and irritable most of the time and reports difficulty concentrating and learning new things. He has been involved in three auto accidents in the past year.

S.R.'s vital signs are BP of 164/90, pulse of 92 beats/min, 18 breaths/min with Sao_2 90% on room air. His examination is normal, except for multiple bruises over the right ribcage. You inquire about the bruises, and S.R. reports that his wife jabs him with her elbow several times every night. In her own defense, the wife states, "Well, he stops breathing and I get worried, so I jab him to make him start breathing again. If I don't jab him, I find myself listening for his next breath and I can't go to sleep." You suspect sleep apnea.

2. Identify two of the main types of apnea, and explain the pathology of each.

3. Identify at least five signs or symptoms of obstructive sleep apnea (OSA), and star those symptoms that S.R. is experiencing.

4. What tests help the provider diagnose OSA?

5. S.R. and his wife ask why it is so important to determine whether or not S.R. has OSA. You would tell them that properly diagnosing OSA is important because effective treatment is necessary to prevent which common complications of OSA? (Select all that apply.)
a. Stroke
b. Early onset of chronic obstructive pulmonary disease (COPD)
c. Hypotension
d. Right-sided heart failure
e. Cardiac dysrhythmias

CASE STUDY PROGRESS

The primary care provider (PCP) examined S.R. and documented a long soft palate, recessed mandible, and medium-sized tonsils. S.R.'s overnight screening oximetry study showed 143 episodes of desaturation ranging from 68% to 76%; episodes of apnea were also documented. He was diagnosed with OSA with hypoxemia, and a full sleep study is ordered.

6. S.R. and his wife ask about a full sleep study. How would you explain a polysomnogram to them?

7. The PCP asks you to counsel S.R. about lifestyle changes that he could make immediately to help with his situation. Name four topics you would address with S.R.

CASE STUDY PROGRESS

S.R. returns for a follow-up visit after being diagnosed with OSA. He reports that he has lost 10 pounds, but there has been little improvement in his symptoms. He states that he fell asleep while driving to work and wrecked his car. He wants to discuss further treatment options.

8. What are the treatment options for OSA? Describe each.

CASE STUDY PROGRESS

S.R. and the PCP decide on the least invasive treatment—continuous positive airway pressure (CPAP). The provider writes a prescription for CPAP. The patient has a choice of which durable medical equipment company he wants to get his equipment from. You help him by giving him the names of three reputable companies and advise him to call his insurance company to find out how much they will pay and how much he will be responsible for.

9. S.R. calls in 2 weeks with complaints of dry nasal membranes, nosebleeds, and sores behind his ears. What advice would you give S.R.?

2 Respiratory

Case Study 21

Name _____ Class/Group _____ Date _____

Group Members _____

▶ Scenario

B.T., a 22-year-old man who lives in a small mountain town in Colorado, is highly allergic to dust and pollen. B.T.'s wife drove him to the clinic when his wheezing was unresponsive to fluticasone/salmeterol (Advair) and ipratropium bromide (Atrovent) inhalers, he was unable to lie down, and he began to use accessory muscles to breathe. B.T. is started on 4 L oxygen by nasal cannula and an IV of D5W at 15 mL/hr. He appears anxious and says that he is short of breath.

■ Chart View

Vital Signs

Blood pressure	152/84 mm Hg
Pulse rate	124 beats/min
Respiratory rate	42 breaths/min
Temperature	100.4° F (38.4° C)

1. Are B.T.'s vital signs (VS) acceptable? State your rationale.

2. What is the pathophysiology of asthma?

3. How is asthma categorized? Describe the characteristics of each classification.

■ Chart View

Arterial Blood Gases

pH	7.31
$Paco_2$	48 mm Hg
HCO_3	26 mmol/L
Pao_2	55 mm Hg
Sao_2	88%

4. Interpret B.T.'s arterial blood gas results.

5. What is the rationale for immediately starting B.T. on O_2?

6. You will need to monitor B.T. closely for the next few hours. Identify four signs and symptoms of impending respiratory failure that you will be assessing for.

■ **Chart View**

Medication Orders

Albuterol 2.5 mg plus ipratropium 250 mcg nebulizer treatment STAT

Albuterol (Ventolin) inhaler 2 puffs q4h

Metaproterenol sulfate (Alupent) 0.4% nebulizer treatment q3h

Fluticasone (Flovent) 250 mcg by MDI twice daily

7. What is the rationale for the albuterol 2.5 mg plus ipratropium 250 mcg nebulizer treatment STAT (immediately)?

8. Identify the drug classification and expected outcomes B.T. should experience through using metaproterenol sulfate (Alupent) and Fluticasone (Flovent).

9. B.T. stated he had taken his Advair that morning, then again when he started to feel short of breath. Is fluticasone/salmeterol (Advair) appropriate for use during an acute asthma attack? Explain.

10. What are your responsibilities while administering aerosol therapy?

11. When combination inhalation aerosols are prescribed without specific instructions for the sequence of administration, you need to be aware of the proper recommendations for drug administration. What is the correct sequence for administering B.T.'s treatments?

12. List five independent nursing interventions that may help relieve B.T.'s symptoms.

CASE STUDY PROGRESS

After several hours of IV and PO rehydration and aerosol treatments, B.T.'s wheezing and chest tightness resolve, and he is able to expectorate his secretions. The physician discusses B.T.'s asthma management with him; B.T. says he has had several asthma attacks over the last few weeks. The physician discharges B.T. with a prescription for oral steroid "burst" (prednisone 40 mg/day × 5 days), fluticasone/salmeterol (Advair) 100/50 mcg two puffs twice daily, albuterol (Proventil) metered-dose inhaler (MDI) two puffs q6h as needed using a spacer, and montelukast (Singulair) 10 mg daily each evening. He recommends that B.T. call the pulmonary clinic for follow-up with a pulmonary specialist.

13. What is the rationale for B.T. being on the oral steroid "burst"?

14. What issues will you address in discharge teaching with B.T.?

CASE STUDY PROGRESS

You ask B.T. to demonstrate the use of his MDI. He vigorously shakes the canister, holds the aerosolizer at an angle (pointing toward his cheek) in front of his mouth, and squeezes the canister as he takes a quick, deep breath.

15. What common mistakes has B.T. made when using the inhaler?

16. What would you teach B.T. about the use of his MDI?

17. B.T.'s wife asks about the possibility of B.T. having another attack. How would you respond?

18. B.T. states he would like to read more about asthma on the Internet. List three credible websites you could give him.

Case Study 22

Name _____ Class/Group _____ Date _____

Group Members _____

INSTRUCTIONS All questions apply to this case study. Your responses should be brief and to the point. When asked to provide several answers, list them in order of priority or significance. Do not assume information that is not provided. Please print or write clearly. If your response is not legible, it will be marked as ? and you will need to rewrite it.

▶ Scenario

L.B. is a 30-year-old secretary who is being seen in the clinic with 6 weeks of a dry, hacking cough after recovering from bronchitis this winter. The cough is worse at night and associated with shortness of breath. In the past, she has experienced coughing spells after running a 5 K race. She has hay fever that seems to be year-round and has eczema in the winter. Both of her children and her maternal grandmother have asthma.

1. As the intake nurse, what routine information do you want to obtain from L.B.?

2. L.B.'s chief complaint is a cough. What are the main causes of chronic cough, and what questions should you ask to elicit information about each cause?

CASE STUDY PROGRESS

L.B. denies symptoms in answers to all of your questions except those given in the initial interview. She is not taking any medication other than a multiple vitamin.

3. What would you include in your physical examination, and why?

CASE STUDY PROGRESS

L.B. was not in acute distress. Vital signs were 110/60, 55, 18. She had no sinus tenderness, ears were negative, nasal mucosa was pale and boggy, mouth was negative, there was no cervical adenopathy, and lungs were clear to auscultation. Forced expiration using the peak flow meter (PFM) generated a cough. Her peak flow was 350 L/min with good effort. Expected peak flow for her height and age is 512 L/min, giving a response of 68% of predicted.

4. The provider orders a predilator and postdilator pulmonary function test (PFT). What is the purpose of completing the PFTs predilator and postdilator?

5. The diagnosis of asthma is confirmed, and L.B. returns to the clinic for asthma education. What topics will you address?

6. What is a PFM? Give L.B. precise instructions to perform the PFM maneuver.

7. L.B. asks why she has to use the PFM. Explain the purpose of the peak expiratory flow rate (PEFR) measurement and what role it plays in L.B.'s self-management of her asthma.

8. The provider ordered triamcinolone (Azmacort) two puffs bid and albuterol (Ventolin) two puffs q6h prn. What points will you include when teaching L.B. about her medications?

9. L.B. asks, "Why do I have to use this inhaler? Can't I just take some different pills?" Your response to L.B. is based on the knowledge that the inhalation route is:
  a. Safer and more effective than pills
  b. Less expensive than combination therapy
  c. Easier to master than oral therapy
  d. More likely to assist in curing her asthma

10. You instruct L.B. in the proper use of the metered-dose inhaler (MDI) using a spacer. How would you explain proper MDI use?

11. Because L.B. is taking two puffs twice daily of triamcinolone (Azmacort), how long should the inhaler last? The canister label states that it contains 200 inhalations.

12. What will you teach L.B. to do if her PEFR value falls?

13. You would recognize the need for additional teaching if L.B. says: (Select all that apply.)
   a. "I will use the albuterol inhaler thirty minutes before exercising."
   b. "My husband needs to know what to do in case I have an attack."
   c. "I will keep a diary of all of my PEFR measures."
   d. "I will place a plastic cover on our mattress and my pillows."
   e. "The bed linens need to be washed in cold water to reduce dust mites."

CASE STUDY OUTCOME

During a follow-up visit, L.B.'s asthma is listed as mild persistent asthma. Her peak flow on the albuterol (Ventolin) and triamcinolone (Azmacort) has increased to 450 L/min, which is 88% of the predicted; her cough has subsided, and she can again participate in sports without problems. There is no nighttime awakening, no loss of work, and no emergency department visits. She can demonstrate appropriate inhaler technique and has her completed peak flow diary with her.

Case Study 23

Name _____ Class/Group _____ Date _____

Group Members _____

INSTRUCTIONS All questions apply to this case study. Your responses should be brief and to the point. When asked to provide several answers, list them in order of priority or significance. Do not assume information that is not provided. Please print or write clearly. If your response is not legible, it will be marked as ? and you will need to rewrite it.

▶ **Scenario**

The sister of C.K. brought her 71-year-old brother to the primary care clinic after he came down with a fever 2 days ago. She said he has shaking chills, a productive cough, and he can't lie down to sleep because "he can't stop coughing." After C.K. is examined, he is diagnosed with community-acquired pneumonia (CAP) and admitted to your floor. The intern is busy and asks you to complete your routine admission assessment and call her with your findings.

1. Identify the four most important things to include in your assessment.

CASE STUDY PROGRESS

Your assessment findings are as follows: C.K.'s vital signs are 154/82, 105, 32, 103° F (39.4° C), Sao$_2$ 84% on room air. You auscultate decreased breath sounds in the left lower lobe anteriorly and posteriorly and hear coarse crackles in the left upper lobe. His nail beds are dusky on fingers and toes. He has cough productive of rust-colored sputum and complains of pain in the left side of his chest when he coughs. C.K. seems to be well nourished and adequately hydrated. He is a lifetime nonsmoker. Past medical history includes coronary artery disease and myocardial infarction (MI) with a stent; he is currently on metoprolol (Lopressor), amlodipine (Norvasc), lisinopril (Zestril), and furosemide (Lasix); for his type 2 diabetes mellitus, he is also taking metformin (Glucophage) and rosiglitazone (Avandia). He has never gotten the Pneumovax or flu shot. He does report getting "hives" when he took "an antibiotic pill" a few years ago but doesn't remember the name of the antibiotic.

2. Which of these assessment findings concern you? State your rationale.

■ Chart View

Physician's Orders

2100-Calorie ADA diet
VS with temperature q2h
IV of D5 ½ NS at 125 mL/hr
Ceftriaxone (Rocephin) 1 g IV bid
Metaproterenol sulfate (Alupent) 0.4% nebulizer treatment q3h
Titrate O_2 to maintain Sao_2 over 90%
Obtain sputum for C&S
Blood cultures for temperature over 102° F (38.9° C)
CBC with differential and basic metabolic panel
Urinalysis (UA) with C&S
Chest x-ray (CXR) now and in the morning

3. Review the orders and outline a plan of what you need to do in the next 2 to 3 hours.

4. Is the IV fluid of D5 ½ NS appropriate for C.K.? State your rationale.

5. What is the rationale for ordering O_2 to maintain Sao_2 over 90%?

6. What is a C&S test, and why is it important?

7. Why were blood cultures ordered to be drawn?

8. Why are blood cultures drawn from two different sites?

9. What would you expect the CXR results to reveal?

10. The pharmacy sends the ceftriaxone (Rocephin) IV 1 g in 100 mL 0.9% NaCl with instructions to infuse over 40 minutes. At how many milliliters per hour will you regulate the IV infusion pump?

11. Which of the following assessment findings would best indicate that C.K. is responding to therapy?
   a. Complaints of dyspnea; respiratory rate of 26 on 2 L oxygen; clear lung sounds
   b. Cough productive of white sputum; temperature of 100.0° F (37.8° C); Sao_2 98% on 2 L NC
   c. Coarse crackles in posterior lower lobes; respiratory rate 22; no complaints of chills
   d. Cough productive of yellow sputum; lung sounds clear; Sao_2 96% on room air

CASE STUDY PROGRESS

C.K. recovers from his pneumonia and is preparing for discharge. You know that C.K. is at increased risk for contracting CAP infections.

12. Discuss four strategies for prevention.

13. C.K. confides in you, "You know, my wife died a year ago, and I live alone now. I've been thinking … this pneumonia stuff has been a little scary." How will you respond?

2 Respiratory

2 Respiratory

Case Study 24

Name_____ Class/Group _____ Date _____

Group Members _____

INSTRUCTIONS All questions apply to this case study. Your responses should be brief and to the point. When asked to provide several answers, list them in order of priority or significance. Do not assume information that is not provided. Please print or write clearly. If your response is not legible, it will be marked as ? and you will need to rewrite it.

▶ Scenario

A.B., a 40-year-old man, is admitted to your medical floor with a diagnosis of pleural effusion. He complains of shortness of breath; pain in his chest; weakness; and a dry, irritating cough. His vital signs (VS) are 142/82, 118, respirations are 38 and labored and shallow, 102.1° F (38.9° C). His chest x-ray shows a large pleural effusion and pulmonary infiltrates in the right lower lobe consistent with pneumonitis.

1. Given his diagnosis, are A.B.'s admission VS expected? Explain.

2. What is pleural effusion?

3. What is the difference between transudate and exudate?

4. List three common causes of pleural effusion.

5. Review the pathophysiology and consequences of pleural effusion and pulmonary infiltrates.

6. How does the underlying pathophysiology give rise to A.B.'s presenting signs and symptoms?

7. How do you differentiate between cardiac and pleural pain?

8. How does A.B.'s increased metabolic rate affect his nutritional needs?

CASE STUDY PROGRESS

The physician performs a thoracentesis and drains 1500 mL of fluid. A specimen for culture and sensitivity (C&S) is sent to the laboratory, and A.B. is started on cefuroxime (Ceftin) 1 g IV piggyback q8h.

9. What is a thoracentesis?

10. The order for the cefuroxime (Ceftin) reads to infuse 1 g in 100 mL 0.9% NaCl over 30 minutes. You have IV tubing that supplies 20 gtt/mL. At how many gtt per minute will you regulate the infusion?

11. What maneuvers would promote the clearance of pulmonary secretions?

12. The pleural C&S results indicate a large amount of *Klebsiella* organism growth that is not sensitive to cefuroxime (Ceftin). What action will you take next?

13. Because fluid continues to collect in the pleural space, the physician decides to insert a pleural chest tube under nonemergent conditions. What is your responsibility as A.B.'s nurse?

14. Evaluate each of the following statements about chest tube drainage systems. Enter "T" for true or "F" for false. Discuss why the false statements are incorrect.

_____ 1. It is the height of the column of water in the suction control mechanism, not the setting of the suction source, that actually limits the amount of suction transmitted to the pleural cavity.

_____ 2. A suction pressure of +20 cm H_2O is commonly recommended for adults.

_____ 3. Bubbling in the water-seal chamber usually means that air is leaking from the lungs, the tubing, or the insertion site.

_____ 4. The rise and fall of the water level with the patient's respirations reflect normal pressure changes in the pleural cavity with respirations.

_____ 5. The chamber is a closed system; therefore, water cannot evaporate.

_____ 6. To declot the drainage tubing, put lotion on your hands, compress the tubing, and vigorously strip long segments of the tubing before releasing.

_____ 7. You lower the bed on top of the drainage system and break it. You immediately clamp the chest tube, leaving it clamped until you can reestablish the drainage system.

_____ 8. The chest tube becomes disconnected from the drainage system. Because you noted an air leak from the lung during your initial assessment, you can submerge the chest tube 1 to 2 inches below the surface of a 250 mL bottle of sterile saline or water.

_____ 9. The collection chamber is full, so you need to connect a new drainage system to the chest tube. It is appropriate to momentarily clamp the chest tube while you disconnect the old system and reconnect the new.

_____10. The drainage system falls over, spilling the chest drainage into the other drainage columns. The total amount of drainage can be obtained by adding the amount of drainage in each of the columns.

15. How will you appropriately maintain A.B.'s chest tube system?

CASE STUDY PROGRESS

After 7 days of aggressive antibiotic and pulmonary therapy, the chest tube is discontinued and A.B. is ready to be discharged.

16. What type of discharge instructions do you need to give to A.B.?

Case Study 25

Name _____ Class/Group _____ Date _____

Group Members _____

INSTRUCTIONS All questions apply to this case study. Your responses should be brief and to the point. When asked to provide several answers, list them in order of priority or significance. Do not assume information that is not provided. Please print or write clearly. If your response is not legible, it will be marked as ? and you will need to rewrite it.

▶ Scenario

A.W., a 52-year-old woman disabled from severe emphysema, was walking at a mall when she suddenly grabbed her right side and gasped, "Oh, something just popped." A.W. whispered to her walking companion, "I can't get any air." Her companion yelled for someone to call 911 and helped her to the nearest bench. By the time the rescue unit arrived, A.W. was stuporous and in severe respiratory distress. She was intubated, an IV of lactated Ringer's (LR) to KVO (keep vein open) was started, and she was transported to the nearest emergency department (ED).

On arrival at the ED, the physician auscultates muffled heart tones, no breath sounds on the right, and faint sounds on the left. A.W. is stuporous, tachycardic, and cyanotic. The paramedics inform the physician that it was difficult to ventilate A.W. A portable chest x-ray (CXR) shows an 80% pneumothorax on the right.

■ Chart View

Arterial Blood Gases (100% O_2)

pH	7.25
Pa_{CO_2}	92 mm Hg
Pa_{O_2}	32 mm Hg
HCO_3	27 mmol/L
Sa_{O_2}	53%

1. Given the diagnosis of pneumothorax, explain why the paramedics had difficulty ventilating A.W.

2. Interpret A.W.'s arterial blood gases (ABGs).

3. What is the reason for A.W.'s ABG results?

4. The physician needs to insert a chest tube. What are your responsibilities as A.W.'s nurse?

5. As the nurse, it is your responsibility to ensure pain control. In A.W.'s case, would you administer pain medication before the chest tube insertion?

6. The ED physician inserts a size 32 F chest tube in the sixth intercostal space, midaxillary line. Would you expect to observe an air leak when A.W.'s chest drainage system is in place and functioning?

7. Would you expect A.W.'s lung to reexpand immediately after the chest tube insertion and initiation of underwater suction? Explain.

8. Part of your responsibilities after the chest tube is inserted is to assess for fluctuation in the water-seal chamber and bubbling in the suction-control chamber. Label the areas on the chest drainage system that you would be monitoring.

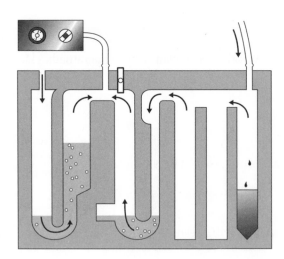

9. What do you need to document regarding A.W.'s chest drainage system?

10. What instructions do you need to give to the nursing assistive personnel (NAP) who is working with A.W.?

11. The clerk tells you A.W.'s husband has just arrived; A.W. will be admitted to the hospital. How would you address this issue with her husband?

12. You approach A.W.'s bedside and ask about what looks like two healed chest tube sites on her right chest. A.W.'s husband informs you that this is the third time she has had a collapsed lung. He asks whether this trend will continue. How will you respond?

CASE STUDY PROGRESS

Because A.W. has a history of spontaneous pneumothoraces on the right side, the physician elects to perform chemical pleurodesis.

13. A.W. asks what a pleurodesis is. How would you describe this procedure and what will happen?

CASE STUDY PROGRESS

A.W. recovers and is discharged to her home 4 days later with a chest tube and Heimlich valve. The physician connects the one-way (Heimlich) valve between the distal end of the chest tube and a drainage pouch.

14. Discuss the purpose of this device. *air in valve closed prevents air escape.*

inhale - ⊖ pressure.

15. You teach A.W. and her husband about the care of the chest tube and Heimlich valve. Which of these statements would indicate that further teaching is necessary? (Select all that apply.)
   a. "I will maintain an occlusive dressing around the chest tube site."
   b. "I can shower if the device is completely covered in plastic."
   c. "When moving around, the collection system must be kept below the insertion site."
   d. "I will notify the physician if there is a change in the color or amount of drainage."
   e. "The arrow on the flutter valve should always point toward me."
   f. "I will check the insertion site twice daily for swelling, redness, and drainage."

Case Study **26**

Name _____ Class/Group _____ Date _____

Group Members _____

INSTRUCTIONS All questions apply to this case study. Your responses should be brief and to the point. When asked to provide several answers, list them in order of priority or significance. Do not assume information that is not provided. Please print or write clearly. If your response is not legible, it will be marked as ? and you will need to rewrite it.

▶ **Scenario**

P.R., a 61-year-old woman who has no history of respiratory disease, is being admitted to your unit with a diagnosis of pneumonia and acute respiratory failure. She was endotracheally intubated orally in the emergency room and placed on mechanical ventilation. Her vital signs are 112/68, 134, 101° F (38.3° C) with an Sao_2 of 53%. Her ventilator settings are synchronized intermittent mandatory ventilation of 12 breaths/min (BPM), tidal volume (V_T) 700 mL, Fio_2 0.50, positive end-expiratory pressure (PEEP) 5 cm H_2O.

1. Describe the pathophysiology of acute respiratory failure (ARF).

2. What assessment findings would you expect P.R. to exhibit?

■ **Chart View**

Arterial Blood Gases	
pH	7.28
$Paco_2$	62 mm Hg
HCO_3	26 mmol/L
Pao_2	48 mm Hg
Sao_2	53%

2 Respiratory

3. The arterial blood gas (ABG) results drawn in the emergency room before intubation are sent to you. Interpret P.R.'s ABG results.

4. List eight interventions that would be implemented for P.R. and the rationale for each.

5. After the insertion of the endotracheal tube (ETT), how is correct placement verified?

6. Describe each of P.R.'s ventilator settings and the rationale for the selection of each.

2 Respiratory

■ Chart View

Arterial Blood Gases

pH	7.30
$Paco_2$	52 mm Hg
HCO_3	22 mmol/L
Pao_2	70 mm Hg
Sao_2	88%

7. ABGs are redrawn after P.R. is on mechanical ventilation for 1 hour. What ventilator changes do you anticipate, based on your interpretation of these values? (Select all that apply, and explain your rationale.)
   a. Increasing the PEEP to 10 cm
   b. Increasing the rate on the ventilator to 16 breaths/min
   c. Increasing the tidal volume to 850 mL
   d. Changing to continuous mandatory ventilation

8. Evaluate each of the following statements about caring for P.R. or a similar patient receiving mechanical ventilation with an ETT. Enter "T" for true or "F" for false. Discuss why the false statements are incorrect.
   ____ 1. Administer mandatory muscle-paralyzing agents to keep the patient from "fighting the vent."
   ____ 2. Check ventilator settings at the beginning of each shift and then hourly.
   ____ 3. When suctioning the ETT, each pass should not exceed 15 seconds.
   ____ 4. Assign an experienced NAP to take vital signs every 2 to 4 hours.
   ____ 5. Perform a respiratory assessment once per shift.
   ____ 6. Empty excess water as it collects in the ventilation tubing back into the humidifier.
   ____ 7. Keep a resuscitation bag at the bedside.
   ____ 8. Monitor the cuff pressure of the ETT every 8 hours.
   ____ 9. Keep ventilator alarms silenced when in the room to maintain a quiet environment.
   ____10. Change the ventilator tubing every 12 hours.

9. You hear the high pressure alarm sounding on the mechanical ventilator and see that P.R.'s Sao_2 is 80%. What are the potential causes of this problem?

CASE STUDY PROGRESS

As P.R.'s nurse, you are concerned about meeting her needs for fluids, nutrition, oral hygiene, and skin integrity.

10. Discuss five indicators that would help you assess fluid status.

11. What are your nutritional goals for P.R.?

12. Describe interventions that you could use to assist in meeting P.R.'s nutrition goals.

13. The goal related to P.R.'s mouth care is to preserve the oral mucosa and dentition. Identify three strategies for providing oral hygiene with an ETT in place.

14. What is the rationale for not taking an oral temperature near an ETT?

15. You assess P.R.'s skin every 4 hours. Identify three treatment goals in relation to skin and positioning.

16. What four strategies will facilitate the expected outcome of maintaining skin integrity?

17. That afternoon, a powerful storm causes a power failure. What do you do?

Case Study 27

Name _____ Class/Group _____ Date _____

Group Members _____

INSTRUCTIONS All questions apply to this case study. Your responses should be brief and to the point. When asked to provide several answers, list them in order of priority or significance. Do not assume information that is not provided. Please print or write clearly. If your response is not legible, it will be marked as ? and you will need to rewrite it.

▶ Scenario

P.W., a 33-year-old woman diagnosed with Guillain-Barré syndrome (GBS), is being cared for on a special ventilator unit of an extended care facility because she requires 24-hour-a-day nursing coverage. She has been intubated and mechanically ventilated for 3 weeks and has shown no signs of improvement in respiratory muscle strength. Her ventilator settings are assist-control (A/C) of 12 breaths/min, tidal volume (V_T) 700 mL, Fio_2 0.50, and positive end-expiratory pressure (PEEP) 5 cm H_2O. Her vital signs are 108/64, 118, 12, 100.6° F (38.1° C). She is receiving enteral nutrition by PEG (percutaneous endoscopic gastrostomy [with a transjejunal limb]) tube (2800 kcal/24 hr).

1. Why is P.W.'s ventilator mode on A/C?

2. P.W. is receiving lorazepam (Ativan) 1 mg slow IV push (IVP) q4h to reduce her anxiety. Identify two factors that should be considered when choosing lorazepam for P.W.

3. Identify nine nonpharmacologic strategies that you could use to reduce P.W.'s anxiety, increase her comfort, and reduce the need for lorazepam. Be creative!

4. You note that 2800 kcal/24 hr is a higher than expected caloric requirement for a woman who is 5′4″ and 123 pounds. Offer a possible explanation for her caloric needs.

5. You give P.W. a bath and note that her cheeks billow outward each time the ventilator delivers a breath. What could cause this phenomenon?

6. You try repositioning P.W., place a stopcock in the inflation valve, auscultate the lungs, check the length of the tube at the lip (the tube had not moved), check the cuff, and note the air pressure is low. You insert more air in the cuff to seal the leak. Over the next 24 hours, the leak becomes worse, and the ventilator's low exhaled volume alarm repeatedly sounds. What action will you take?

7. The physician elects to insert a no. 8 Shiley tracheostomy (trach) tube with a disposable inner cannula. P.W. becomes increasingly anxious after receiving the news. How would you prepare P.W. and her husband for the tracheostomy?

8. P.W. undergoes the tracheostomy procedure without complications. When you return in the morning and assess the new tracheostomy, you note that the trach tape looks tight. You are unable to insert one finger between P.W.'s neck and the trach tape. Discuss whether this is problematic.

9. What should be your next actions?

10. You note that the tissue surrounding the incision is edematous. As you palpate the area, your fingers sink into the skin, and you auscultate a popping sound through your stethoscope. What does this mean?

11. What will be your next actions?

12. After lunch, you evaluate P.W.'s activity tolerance and note that she desaturates when turned to her right side. You auscultate posteriorly tubular breath sounds in the entire right lung. Based on your knowledge of pathophysiology, explain the probable cause of the desaturation.

CASE STUDY PROGRESS

You notify the physician of the change in P.W.'s breath sounds. The paramedic unit transports P.W. to the hospital, where she is readmitted for recurring pneumonia.

13. P.W.'s husband arrives shortly after the paramedics transport P.W. to the hospital. He collapses into the nearest chair, tears begin to roll down his cheeks, and he says, "It has been almost a month now. Are you sure she will recover?" How would you respond?

CASE STUDY PROGRESS

P.W. undergoes aggressive antibiotic therapy and returns to the extended care facility 7 days later. Over the several weeks, she progressively regains neurological functioning.

2 Respiratory

14. What factors would be considered in determining whether P.W. is ready to be weaned from mechanical ventilation?

15. What are your responsibilities during the weaning process?

2 Respiratory

Case Study 28

Name _____ Class/Group _____ Date _____

Group Members _____

INSTRUCTIONS All questions apply to this case study. Your responses should be brief and to the point. When asked to provide several answers, list them in order of priority or significance. Do not assume information that is not provided. Please print or write clearly. If your response is not legible, it will be marked as ? and you will need to rewrite it.

▶ Scenario

C.E., a 73-year-old married man and retired railroad engineer, visits his internist, complaining: "Whenever I try to do anything, I get so out of breath I can't go on. I think I'm just getting older, but my wife told me I had to come see you about it." His resting Sao_2 registers 83%. He is sent to the local hospital for a chest x-ray and arterial blood gases to be drawn after resting 20 minutes on room air. C.E. returns to the office, and after obtaining the results, the physician tells him that he has severe emphysema and must start on continuous oxygen (O_2) therapy at 2 L flow rate.

1. How should C.E.'s chief complaint be recorded?

2. What is emphysema?

3. What is the most common cause of emphysema?

4. Based on this information, what questions will you ask about health behaviors?

5. What is the rationale for starting C.E. on oxygen at only 2 L flow rate?

CASE STUDY PROGRESS

The physician tells C.E. that his office will have a home health equipment company call him to make arrangements to deliver liquid O_2 equipment and educate him in its use. As a registered nurse (RN) working for the company, you are assigned to make the initial home visit.

2 Respiratory

6. What general criteria need to be fulfilled for Medicare to pay for C.E.'s home oxygen therapy?

7. How would you prepare for the first visit?

8. What issues would you address with C.E. and his wife?

9. The next time you visit, C.E. complains of sores behind his ears. He explains, "That long oxygen tubing seems to take on a life of its own. It twists around and gets caught under doors, chairs, everything. It darn near rips the ears off my head." What can you tell him that could help?

10. You auscultate C.E.'s breath sounds and detect the odor of Vicks VapoRub. When you question C.E. about the use of Vicks, he tells you that he started to apply it in and around his nose to prevent his nose from becoming dry and sore. How would you counsel C.E. and his wife regarding safety issues with oxygen use?

CASE STUDY PROGRESS

At your next visit 3 weeks later, C.E. tells you that the previous evening he walked to the kitchen for a snack and became increasingly short of breath. As per your instructions, C.E. removed the nasal cannula, tested the flow against his check, and felt no O_2 flowing from the catheter. He lacked the force and volume required to yell for help and was too short of breath to return to the living room to check his O_2 tank. He bent forward with his elbows on the countertop and struggled to breathe. He became more frightened with each passing second, and his breathing became increasingly more difficult. A minute later, C.E.'s wife found him and reconnected his O_2 tubing. C.E. sat at the table for 20 minutes before he could walk back to the living room.

11. Why did C.E. assume the peculiar position at the countertop?

12. A week later you receive a call from C.E.'s wife. Since the incident, C.E. "doesn't want her out of his sight." She asks you to come to the house and "talk some sense into him." What teaching strategies will you use with C.E. and his wife?

2 Respiratory

13. C.E.'s wife asks you what her husband can do to help her around the house. She says, "The doctor told him to go home and take it easy. He sits in a chair all day. He won't even get up to get himself a glass of water. I've got a bad hip and this has been very hard on me." How would you address her issue?

14. What referrals could you consider at this time?

15. C.E. states, "You seem to know what you are talking about, so let me ask you something. I wake up with a headache almost every morning. My wife says it's because I snore so loud and don't breathe right when I sleep. Do you know anything about that?" After asking several questions, you inform C.E. that it sounds like he might not be getting enough O_2 at night. Explain the connection between hypoxemia and morning headaches.

CASE STUDY PROGRESS

C.E. seems impressed by your explanation. He asks whether there is anything that can be done for his problem. He asks whether there is anything that can be done for his problem. You inform him that the first step is to identify the problem. You report to the covering health care provider, and an oximetry study is ordered. You comment that C.E. sounds like he has a cold. He replies, "Oh, our great-grandchildren were over to visit several days ago and they all had snotty noses. I suspect that I'll get it pretty soon. The problem is, every time I get a cold it goes straight to my lungs."

16. What information would you want to review with C.E. and his wife about the signs and symptoms of infection and when to seek treatment?

17. What basic hygiene measures can C.E. and his wife take to prevent his developing an infection? (List at least four.)

18. Why is it important for people with lung disease to seek early intervention for infection?

19. C.E.'s wife says she would like to read more about emphysema on the Internet. List an authoritative Internet resource of professional and patient or family information on lung disease.

2 Respiratory

Case Study 29

Name _____ Class/Group _____ Date _____

Group Members _____

INSTRUCTIONS All questions apply to this case study. Your responses should be brief and to the point. When asked to provide several answers, list them in order of priority or significance. Do not assume information that is not provided. Please print or write clearly. If your response is not legible, it will be marked as ? and you will need to rewrite it.

▶ Scenario

D.Z., a 65-year-old man, is admitted to a medical floor for exacerbation of his chronic obstructive pulmonary disease (COPD; emphysema). He has a past medical history of hypertension, which has been well controlled by enalapril (Vasotec) for the past 6 years, has had pneumonia yearly for the past 3 years, and has been a 2-pack-a-day smoker for 38 years. He appears as a cachectic man who is experiencing difficulty breathing at rest. He reports cough productive of thick yellow-green sputum. D.Z. seems irritable and anxious; he complains of sleeping poorly and states that lately feels tired most of the time. His vital signs (VS) are 162/84, 124, 36, 102°F, Sao_2 88%. His admitting diagnosis is an acute exacerbation of chronic emphysema.

■ Chart View

Physician's Orders

Diet as tolerated
Out of bed with assistance
Oxygen (O_2) to maintain Sao_2 of 90%
IV of D5W at 50 ml/hr
ECG monitoring
Arterial blood gases (ABGs) in AM
CBC with differential now
Basic metabolic panel (BMP) now
Chest x-ray (CXR) q24h
Sputum culture
Albuterol 2.5 mg plus ipratropium 250 mcg nebulizer treatment STAT

---

1. Explain the pathophysiology of emphysema.

2. Are D.Z.'s vital signs and Sao_2 appropriate? If not, explain why.

3. Describe a plan for implementing these physician's orders.

4. Identify three independent nursing actions you would try to improve D.Z.'s oxygenation.

■ Chart View

Medication Administration Record

Methylprednisolone (Solu-Medrol) 125 mg IVP q8h
Doxycycline (Doryx) 100 mg PO q12h × 10 days
Azithromycin (Zithromax) 500 mg IVPB q24h × 2 days then 500 mg PO × 7 days
Fluticasone/salmeterol (Advair) 100/50 mcg 2 puffs bid
Heparin 4000 units subcut q12h
Enalapril (Vasotec) 10 mg PO q AM
Albuterol 2.5 mg/ipratropium 250 mcg nebulizer treatment q6h

5. Indicate the expected outcome for D.Z. that is associated with each of the medications he is receiving.

6. Since D.Z. is on azithromycin (Zithromax), what nursing actions need to be added to the plan of care? Select all that apply.
   a. Monitor IV site for inflammation or extravasation
   b. Assess liver function studies and bilirubin levels
   c. Obtain a hearing test prior to initiating therapy
   d. Carefully dilute the medication in the proper amount of solution
   e. Place D.Z. on intake and output
   f. Administer the medication over one-half hour

7. D.Z is ordered heparin 4000 units subcutaneous q12 hr. The following vial is available. How many milliliters will D.Z. receive? Shade in the dose on the tuberculin syringe.

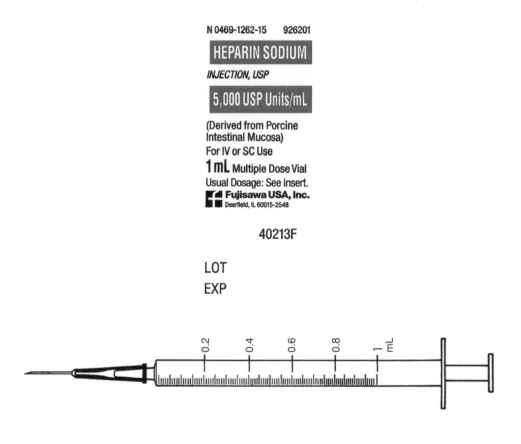

8. What are two of the most common side effects of bronchodilators?

9. Identify three outcomes that you expect for D.Z. as a result of your interventions.

10. You deliver D.Z.'s dietary tray, and he comments how hungry he is. As you leave the room, he is rapidly consuming the mashed potatoes. When you pick up the tray, you notice that he hasn't touched anything else. When you question him, he states, "I don't understand it. I can be so hungry, but when I start to eat, I have trouble breathing and I have to stop." One theory for the increased work of breathing is based on carbohydrate (CHO) loading. Explain this phenomenon based on your knowledge of the breakdown of CHO.

11. Identify four strategies that might improve his caloric intake.

12. You notice a box of dark chocolate on D.Z.'s overbed table. He tells you that he wakes at night and eats 4 or 5 pieces of chocolate. Several of your COPD patients have identified a craving for chocolate in the past. What is the basis for this craving?

13. What would you do to address dietary and nutritional teaching needs with D.Z. and his wife?

14. List six other educational topics that you need to explore with D.Z.

15. What other health care professional would probably be involved in D.Z.'s treatments and how? What is the licensure or certification status of that profession in the state in which you are practicing?

CASE STUDY PROGRESS

D.Z.'s wife approaches you in the hallway and says, "I don't know what to do. My husband used to be so active before he retired 6 months ago. Since then he's lost 35 pounds. He is afraid to take a bath, and it takes him hours to dress—that's if he gets dressed at all. He has gone downhill so fast that it scares me. He's afraid to do anything for himself. He wants me in the room with him all the time, but if I try to talk with him, he snarls and does things to irritate me. I have to keep working. His medical bills are draining all of our savings, and I have to be able to support myself when he's gone. You know, sometimes I go to work just to get away from the house and his constant demands. He calls me several times a day asking me to come home, but I can't go home. You may not think I'm much of a wife, but quite honestly, I don't want to come home anymore. I just don't know what to do."

16. How would you respond to her statement?

Case Study 30

Name_____ Class/Group _____ Date _____

Group Members _____

▶ Scenario

The intensive care unit (ICU) nurse calls to give you the following report: "D.S. is a 56-year-old man with a past medical history of chronic bronchitis. He quit smoking 12 years ago and exercises regularly. He went to see his physician with complaints of increasing exertional dyspnea; a large mass was found in his right lung. Three days ago he underwent an right middle lobe (RML) and right lower lobe (RLL) lobectomy; the pathology report showed adenocarcinoma. He has no neurologic deficits, and his VS run 120/70, 110, about 30, and he has been running a fever of 100.2° F. His heart tones are clear, all peripheral pulses are palpable, and he has an IV of D 5½ NS at 50 mL/hr in his right forearm. He has a right midaxillary chest tube to Pleur-evac drain; there's no air leak, and it's draining small amounts of serosanguineous fluid. He has C/O pain at the insertion site, but the site looks good, and the dressing is dry and intact. He's on 5 L oxygen by nasal cannula. He refuses pain medication. He's a real nervous guy and hasn't slept since surgery. He'll be there in about 20 minutes."

1. What additional information would you ask the nurse to provide at this time?

CASE STUDY PROGRESS

D.S. is transported by wheelchair past the nurses' station to a room at the far end of the hall. You enter his room for the first time to find him sitting on the edge of the bed with his left leg in bed and his right foot on the floor. You introduce yourself and tell him that you are going to be his nurse for the rest of the shift. You note that he keeps rubbing his left hand over the right side of his chest.

2. What issues or problems can you already identify?

3. List four things you will do for D.S.

CASE STUDY PROGRESS

D.S. states, "I have a nephew who rolled his Jeep and busted himself up real bad. He got hooked on those drugs, and I don't want any part of them."

4. How would you respond to D.S.'s statement?

5. Why is D.S. experiencing difficulty using his right arm? Given the type of surgery he underwent, is this expected?

6. You administer morphine sulfate 4 mg IV and tell D.S. that you will return in 30 minutes; 15 minutes later he turns on his call light. When you enter the room, D.S. says, "I think I'm going to throw up." What are the next three things you would do?

7. D.S. states, "I started to feel sick a couple minutes ago. It just kept getting worse until I knew I was going to throw up." Given this information, what do you think is responsible for the sudden onset of nausea?

8. Would it be appropriate to give D.S. a second dose of morphine before reporting his reaction to the physician? State your rationale. Describe your next steps.

9. D.S.'s pain and nausea are under control an hour later. You remove the chest tube dressing and note that the area around the insertion site looks slightly inflamed, the tissue immediately around the tube looks white and moist, and there is scant amount of brown drainage. What action would you take next?

CASE STUDY PROGRESS

The next day, the nurse giving you D.S.'s report says that he has been driving her crazy all day long. She tells you that he is fine but has been paranoid and demanding. You enter D.S.'s room to see how he is doing and to tell him you are going to be his nurse again today. You note that his head bobs up and his mouth opens, like a fish taking in water, every time he inhales. He says, "I just can't [breath] seem to [breath] get enough [breath] air."

10. Identify six possible problems that D.S. could have that would account for his behavior.

11. What actions will you take next? Give your rationale.

CASE STUDY PROGRESS

D.S.'s respiratory rate is 46 breaths/min; you auscultate slight air movement over the large airways and no breath sounds distal to the third intercostal space. He's sitting on the side of the bed with his arms hunched up on the overbed table. His gown is in his lap, he is diaphoretic, you note intercostal retractions with inspiration, and all muscles of the upper torso are engaged in respiration.

12. What will you do next?

13. After D.S. is successfully resuscitated, you accompany him during transfer to the ICU. Why would you do this, and what information would you provide to the ICU nurse?

2 Respiratory

CASE STUDY PROGRESS

After stabilizing D.S. in the ICU, the physician returns to your floor and compliments you on your clear thinking and fast action. The nurse who gave you his report comes up to you to apologize. She is relatively new and asks you to explain how you know when a patient is in the early and late stages of respiratory difficulty. She states that she wants to learn from her mistakes so that she doesn't put another patient through what D.S. experienced.

14. How would you distinguish between early and late stages of respiratory failure?

CASE STUDY OUTCOME

D.S. is completely recovered 5 months following the lobectomy. He receives 6 months of external beam radiation therapy to the chest. His chest x-ray at 5 years shows no recurrence.

Case Study 31

Name _____ Class/Group _____ Date _____

Group Members _____

INSTRUCTIONS All questions apply to this case study. Your responses should be brief and to the point. When asked to provide several answers, list them in order of priority or significance. Do not assume information that is not provided. Please print or write clearly. If your response is not legible, it will be marked as ? and you will need to rewrite it.

▶ Scenario

G.S., a 36-year-old secretary, was involved in a motor vehicle accident; a car drifted left of the center line and struck G.S. head-on, pinning her behind the steering wheel. She was intubated immediately after extrication and flown to your trauma center. Her injuries were found to be extensive: bilateral flail chest, torn innominate artery, right hemothorax and pneumothorax, fractured spleen, multiple small liver lacerations, compound fractures of both legs, and probable cardiac contusion. She was taken to the operating room for repair of her injuries. In OR, she received 36 units of packed RBCs, 20 units of platelets, 20 units of cryoprecipitate, 12 units fresh frozen plasma, and 18 L of lactated Ringer's solution. G.S. was admitted to the ICU postop, where she developed adult respiratory distress syndrome (ARDS).

1. What is ARDS?

2. What are the risk factors for developing ARDS? Which does G.S. have?

CASE STUDY PROGRESS

G.S. has been in ICU for 6 weeks, and her ARDS has almost resolved. She is transferred to your unit. You receive the following report: She is awake, alert, and oriented to person and place and can move both of her arms and wiggle her toes on both feet. Heart tones are clear, vital signs are 138/90, 88, 26, 99.3° F (37.4° C); bilateral radial pulse 3+, and foot pulses by Doppler only. All of her incisions and lacerations have healed. She has bilateral chest tubes to water suction with closed drainage, both dressings are dry and intact. She has a duodenal feeding tube, a Foley catheter to down drain, and a double lumen PICC line.

3. What additional information will you require during this report?

CASE STUDY PROGRESS

You complete your assessment of G.S. You note shortness of breath (SOB), fine crackles throughout all lung fields posteriorly and in both lower lobes anteriorly, and coarse crackles over the large airways.

4. What is the significance of the fine and coarse crackles in G.S.'s case?

5. The nurse from the previous shift charted the following statement: "Fine and coarse crackles that clear with vigorous coughing." Based on your knowledge of pathophysiology, determine the accuracy of this statement.

6. It is time to administer furosemide (Lasix) 40 mg IV push (IVP). What effect, if any, will furosemide have on G.S.'s breath sounds?

7. What action should you take before giving the furosemide (Lasix)?

■ Chart View

Laboratory Test Results at 0500

Sodium	129 mmol/L
Potassium	3.0 mmol/L
Chloride	92 mmol/L
HCO_3	26 mmol/L
BUN	37 mg/dL
Creatinine	2 mg/dL
Glucose	128 mg/dL
Calcium	7.1 mg/dL

8. Keeping in mind that you are about to administer furosemide (Lasix), which laboratory values concern you, and why?

9. Given the laboratory values listed, what action would you take before administering the furosemide (Lasix), and why?

CASE STUDY PROGRESS

The physician prescribes the following:

■ **Chart View**

Physician's Orders

STAT magnesium (Mg) level

KCl 40 mEq IVPB over 4 hours now

Calcium gluconate 2 g in 100 mL NS intravenous piggyback (IVPB) over 3 hours

10. G.S. has one available port to use on the PICC line. Describe your plan for administering the potassium chloride and the calcium gluconate.

11. You open G.S.'s medication drawer, prepare the furosemide (Lasix) for administration, and find one 20-mg ampule. The pharmacist tells you that it will be at least an hour before he can send the drug to you. You realize it is illegal to take medication dispensed by a pharmacist for one patient and use it for another patient. What should you do?

12. While you administer the furosemide (Lasix) and hang the IVPB medication, G.S. says, "This is so weird. A couple times this morning, I felt like my heart flipped upside down in my chest, but now I feel like there's a bird flopping around in there." What are the first two actions you should take next? Give your rationale.

13. G.S.'s pulse is 66 beats/min and irregular. Her BP is 92/70 and respirations are 26. She admits to being "a little lightheaded" but denies having pain or nausea. Your co-worker connects G.S. to the code cart monitor for a "quick look." This is what you see. What do you think is happening with G.S.?

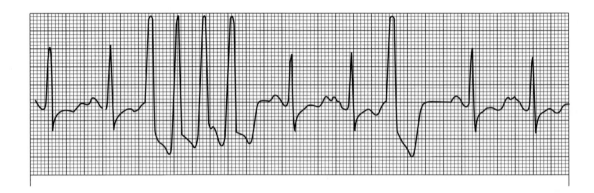

14. What will your next actions be?

15. What are the most likely causes of G.S. having abnormal beats?

■ Chart View

Arterial Blood Gases on 6 L O$_2$ by NC

pH	7.30
Paco$_2$	59 mm Hg
Pao$_2$	82 mm Hg
HCO$_3$	36 mmol/L
Sao$_2$	91%

16. How would you interpret G.S.'s ABGs?

17. You notice that G.S. looks frightened and is lying stiff as a board. How would you respond to this situation?

CASE STUDY OUTCOME

G.S. responded well to treatment. Unfortunately, 1 week later she threw a large embolus. All attempts at resuscitation failed.

Musculoskeletal Disorders

3

Case Study 32

Name _____ Class/Group _____ Date _____

Group Members _____

INSTRUCTIONS All questions apply to this case study. Your responses should be brief and to the point. When asked to provide several answers, list them in order of priority or significance. Do not assume information that is not provided. Please print or write clearly. If your response is not legible, it will be marked as ? and you will need to rewrite it.

▶ Scenario

M.S., a 72-year-old white woman, comes to your clinic for a complete physical examination. She has not been to a provider for 11 years because "I don't like doctors." Her only complaint today is "pain in my upper back." She describes the pain as sharp and knifelike. The pain began approximately 3 weeks ago when she was getting out of bed in the morning and hasn't changed at all. M.S. rates her pain as 6 on a 0- to 10-point pain scale and says the pain decreases to 3 or 4 after taking "a couple of ibuprofen." She denies recent falls or trauma.

M.S. admits she needs to quit smoking and start exercising but states, "I don't have the energy to exercise, and besides, I've always been thin." She has smoked one to two packs of cigarettes per day since she was 17 years old. Her last blood work was 11 years ago, and she can't remember the results. She went through menopause at the age of 47 and has never taken hormone replacement therapy. The physical exam was unremarkable other than moderate tenderness to deep palpation over the spinous process at T7. No masses or tenderness to the tissue surrounded the tender spot. No visible masses, skin changes, or erythema were noted. Her neurologic exam is intact, and no muscle wasting is noted.

1. An x-ray examination of the thoracic spine reveals osteopenic changes at T7. What does this result mean?

2. The physician suspects osteoporosis. List seven risk factors associated with osteoporosis.

3. Place a star or asterisk next to those risk factors specific to M.S.

CASE STUDY PROGRESS

M.S. has never had an osteoporosis screening. She confides that her mother and grandmother were diagnosed with osteoporosis when they were in their early 50s.

4. What diagnostic test is most commonly used to diagnose osteoporosis?

5. M.S.'s diagnostic test revealed a bone density T-score of –2.7. How will this be interpreted?

6. M.S. receives a prescription for alendronate (Fosamax) 70 mg/week. Which instructions are appropriate as you provide patient teaching to M.S. about this drug? (Select all that apply.)
   a. "Take the medication with 8 ounces of water immediately upon arising."
   b. "You can take this medication with your morning coffee or orange juice."
   c. "You can eat your breakfast along with this medication."
   d. "You need to sit or stand upright for at least 30 minutes after taking the medication."
   e. "If you experience any severe abdominal pain, vomiting, or jaw pain, notify your doctor immediately."

7. M.S. is also instructed to take a calcium plus vitamin D supplement. She asks, "If I am taking the osteoporosis pill, won't that be enough?" How do you answer her?

8. What nonpharmacologic interventions will you teach M.S. to prevent further bone loss?

Case Study **33**

Name _____ Class/Group _____ Date _____

Group Members _____

INSTRUCTIONS All questions apply to this case study. Your responses should be brief and to the point. When asked to provide several answers, list them in order of priority or significance. Do not assume information that is not provided. Please print or write clearly. If your response is not legible, it will be marked as ? and you will need to rewrite it.

▶ **Scenario**

J.C. is a 41-year-old man who comes to the emergency department with complaints of acute low back pain. He states that he did some heavy lifting yesterday, went to bed with a mild backache, and awoke this morning with terrible back pain, which he rates as a "10" on a 1 to 10 scale. He admits to having had a similar episode of back pain years ago "after I lifted something heavy at work." J.C. has a past medical history of peptic ulcer disease (PUD) related to nonsteroidal anti-inflammatory drug (NSAID) use. He is 6 feet tall, weighs 265 pounds, and has a prominent "potbelly."

1. What questions would be appropriate to ask J.C. in evaluating the extent of his back pain and injury?

2. What observable characteristic does J.C. have that makes him highly susceptible to low back injury?

3. J.C. used to take piroxicam (Feldene) 20 mg until he developed his duodenal ulcer. What is the relationship between the two? What signs and symptoms would you expect if an ulcer developed?

CASE STUDY PROGRESS

All serious medical conditions are ruled out, and J.C. is diagnosed with lumbar strain. The nurse practitioner (NP) orders a physical therapy consult to develop a home stretching and back-strengthening exercise program and a dietary consult for weight reduction. J.C. is given prescriptions for cyclobenzaprine (Flexeril) 10 mg tid × 3 days only, and celecoxib (Celebrex) 100 mg/day for 3 months. He receives the following instructions: heat applications to the lower back for 20 to 30 minutes four times a day (using moist heat from heat packs or hot towels), no twisting or unnecessary bending, and no lifting more than 10 pounds. J.C. is instructed to rest his back for 1 or 2 days, getting up only now and then to move around to relieve muscle spasms in his back and strengthen his back muscles. He is given a written excuse to stay off work for 5 days and, when he returns to work, specifying the limitation of lifting no more than 10 pounds for 3 months. He is instructed to contact his primary care provider if the pain gets worse.

4. J.C. looks at the prescription for cyclobenzaprine (Flexeril) and states, "I'm glad you didn't give me that Valium. They gave me Valium last time and that stuff knocked me out." How would you respond to J.C.?

3 Musculoskeletal

5. Why do you think that cyclobenzaprine was prescribed instead of diazepam (Valium)?

6. J.C. states, "Well, I'm glad I'll still be able to take my sleeping pill." True or False? Explain.

CASE STUDY PROGRESS

J.C. asks, "What is Celebrex? I hope it won't do what that Feldene did to me years ago."

7. Why do you think it was prescribed for J.C., considering his GI history?

8. You know that it has been over 5 years since his last episode of GI bleeding. Are there any other conditions that you need to assess for before J.C. begins to take the celecoxib? Explain.

9. Why would the NP prescribe an NSAID rather than acetaminophen for J.C.'s pain?

10. A physical therapist teaches J.C. maintenance exercises he can do on his own to promote back health. Identify two common exercises that would be included.

Case Study **34**

Name _____ Class/Group _____ Date _____

Group Members _____

INSTRUCTIONS All questions apply to this case study. Your responses should be brief and to the point. When asked to provide several answers, list them in order of priority or significance. Do not assume information that is not provided. Please print or write clearly. If your response is not legible, it will be marked as ? and you will need to rewrite it.

▶ Scenario

D.M., a 25-year-old man, hops into the emergency department (ED) with complaints of right ankle pain. He states that he was playing basketball and stepped on another player's foot, inverting his ankle. You note swelling over the lateral malleolus down to the area of the fourth and fifth metatarsals, and pedal pulses are 3+ bilaterally. His vital signs are 124/76, 82, 18. He has no allergies and takes no medication. He states he has had no prior surgeries or medical problems.

1. When assessing D.M.'s injured ankle, what should be evaluated?

2. What will initial management of the ankle involve to prevent further swelling and injury?

3. You note significant swelling over the fourth and fifth metatarsals. How would you further evaluate this finding?

CASE STUDY PROGRESS

X-ray results are negative for fracture, and a second-degree sprain is diagnosed. The physician orders immobilization with an elastic bandage and an air stirrup brace, with instructions for crutches. The physician instructs D.M. not to bear weight on his ankle for 2 days, then to use only partial weight-bearing until the ankle heals.

4. Describe the technique for applying an elastic wrap. Give the rationale.

5. When instructing D.M. to use crutches, D.M. states that he "likes it better" when the crutches rest under his arms while walking with the crutches. Is this correct? Explain.

6. You instruct D.M. on using the three-point gait with the crutches. Which would be the correct first step for the three-point gait?
   a. Step first with the affected leg.
   b. Step first with the unaffected leg.
   c. Step first with both crutches and the affected leg.
   d. Step first with the affected leg and the crutch opposite of the affected leg.

7. You are to instruct D.M. on application of cold, activity, and care of the ankle. What would be appropriate instructions in these areas?

8. D.M. is given a prescription for Lortab 2.5/500. Explain the meaning of the numbers.

9. What instructions concerning the Lortab are needed?

10. Four days later, D.M. hobbles into the ED and boldly informs you that he "did it again, only this time it was touch football." He states that the pain pills worked so well, he thought it would be OK. You detect the odor of beer on his breath. What are you going to do?

11. You remove his sock and find a large hematoma forming on the lateral aspect of an already swollen ankle. The ankle also shows the color of a bruise that is several days old. You inquire about D.M.'s pain perception. He states, "It doesn't feel too bad now, but I sure saw stars when it popped." What is the significance of his statement?

Case Study **35**

Name _____ Class/Group _____ Date _____

Group Members _____

INSTRUCTIONS All questions apply to this case study. Your responses should be brief and to the point. When asked to provide several answers, list them in order of priority or significance. Do not assume information that is not provided. Please print or write clearly. If your response is not legible, it will be marked as ? and you will need to rewrite it.

▶ Scenario

S.P. is admitted to the orthopedic ward. She has fallen at home and has sustained an intracapsular fracture of the hip at the femoral neck. The following history is obtained from her: She is a 75-year-old widow with three children living nearby. Her father died of cancer at age 62; mother died of heart failure at age 79. Her height is 5 feet 3 inches; weight is 118 pounds. She has a 50-pack-year smoking history and denies alcohol use. She has severe rheumatoid arthritis (RA), had an upper gastrointestinal bleed in 1993, and had coronary artery disease with a coronary artery bypass graft 9 months ago. Since that time she has engaged in "very mild exercises at home." Vital signs (VS) are 128/60, 98, 14, 99° F (37.2° C), Sao$_2$ 94% on 2 L oxygen by nasal cannula. Her oral medications are rabeprazole (Aciphex) 20 mg/day, prednisone (Deltasone) 5 mg/day, and methotrexate (Amethopterin) 2.5 mg/wk.

1. List at least four risk factors for hip fractures.

2. Place a star or asterisk next to each of the responses in question 1 that represent S.P.'s risk factors.

CASE STUDY PROGRESS

S.P. is taken to surgery for a total hip replacement. Because of the intracapsular location of the fracture, the surgeon chooses to perform an arthroplasty rather than internal fixation. The postoperative orders include:

■ Chart View

Physician's Orders

- Cefazolin (Kefzol) 1000 mg IV q8h × 3 doses
- Enoxaparin (Lovenox) 30 mg subcut q12h
- Warfarin (Coumadin) 2.5 mg × 3 days, starting postoperative day 1, then titrated to INR
- Docusate and senna (Peri-Colace) 1 capsule PO bid
- Multivitamin with iron (Trinsicon) 1 capsule/day PO with meals

- CBC in morning after blood reinfusion
- Hydromorphone (Dilaudid) by IV patient-controlled analgesia, intermittent with 0.1 mg dosing, lockout 10 minutes
- PT and OT to evaluate on postoperative day 1 and start therapy
- Ketorolac (Toradol) 15 mg IV q6h prn pain × 5 days only
- Hip precautions per protocol
- Ondansetron (Zofran) 4 mg IV q6h prn for nausea
- Toilet seat extension
- Straight catheterization if no void by 8 hours postoperatively

3. Why is the patient receiving enoxaparin (Lovenox) and warfarin (Coumadin)?

4. S.P. had an arthroplasty. For each characteristic listed, mark A for *arthroplasty* and O for *open reduction and internal fixation (ORIF) of the hip*.
_____a. Also known as *total hip replacement*.
_____b. Metal pins, screws, rods, and plates are used to immobilize the fracture.
_____c. Replacement of the entire hip joint with a prosthetic (artificial) joint system.

5. S.P. received blood as an intraoperative blood salvage. Which statements about this procedure are true? (Select all that apply.)
a. The blood that is lost from surgery is immediately re-administered to the patient.
b. The blood lost from surgery is collected into a cell saver.
c. One hundred percent of the red blood cells are saved for reinfusion.
d. This procedure has the same risks as blood transfusions from donors.
e. The salvaged blood must be reinfused within 6 hours of collection.

6. List four critical potential postoperative problems for S.P.

7. How will you monitor for excessive postoperative blood loss?

8. According to the lateral traditional surgical approach, there are two main goals for maintaining proper alignment of S.P.'s operative leg. What are they, and how are they achieved?

9. Postoperative wound infection is a concern for S.P. Describe what you would do to monitor her for a wound infection.

10. Taking S.P.'s RA into consideration, what interventions should be implemented to prevent complications secondary to immobility?

3 Musculoskeletal

11. What predisposing factor, identified in S.P.'s medical history, places her at risk for infection, bleeding, and anemia?

12. Briefly discuss S.P.'s nutritional needs.

13. Explain four techniques you can teach S.P. to help her protect herself from infection related to medication-induced immunosuppression.

CASE STUDY PROGRESS

Discharge planning should begin when the patient is admitted. The case manager or social worker will work with the family to initiate placement in a rehabilitation facility.

14. What factors need to be taken into consideration when choosing a rehabilitation facility?

CASE STUDY OUTCOME

S.P. is admitted to the rehabilitation facility close to one daughter's home; she completed rehab and is discharged to home. Her daughter still checks on her every day.

Case Study 36

Name _____ Class/Group _____ Date _____

Group Members _____

INSTRUCTIONS All questions apply to this case study. Your responses should be brief and to the point. When asked to provide several answers, list them in order of priority or significance. Do not assume information that is not provided. Please print or write clearly. If your response is not legible, it will be marked as ? and you will need to rewrite it.

▶ Scenario

H.K. is a 26-year-old man who tried to light a cigarette while driving and lost control of his truck. The truck flipped and landed on the passenger side. H.K. was transported to the emergency department with a deformed, edematous right lower leg and a deep puncture wound approximately 5 cm long over the deformity. Blood continues to ooze from the wound.

1. What further assessment will you make of the leg injury, and what precautions will you take in making this assessment?

2. What is the most appropriate method for controlling bleeding at this wound site?

3. From the above information, it is clear that H.K. is a smoker. List at least three issues related to his smoking that can complicate his care and recovery. What interventions could be instituted to counter these complications? Would using a nicotine patch eliminate these problems?

4. What is the best way to immobilize the leg injury before surgery?

3 Musculoskeletal

H.K. is taken to surgery for open reduction and internal fixation (ORIF) of the tibia and fibula fractures. He returns with a full-leg fiberglass cast with windows over the areas of surgery.

5. Describe the assessment of a patient with a long leg cast involving trauma and surgery.

6. In assessing H.K.'s cast on the third day postoperatively, you notice a strong foul odor. Drainage on the cast is extending, and H.K. is complaining of pain more often and seems considerably more uncomfortable. Vital signs are 123/78, 102, 18, 102.2° F (39° C). What is your analysis of these findings?

H.K. returns to surgery. The wound over H.K.'s fracture site has become necrotic with purulent drainage. The wound is debrided and cultured; then a posterior splint is applied. H.K. returns to his room with orders for wet-to-moist dressing changes. The physician suspects osteomyelitis and orders nafcillin (Unipen) and ciprofloxacin (Cipro). Contact precautions are implemented.

7. Why are two antibiotics ordered?

8. H.K. asks you about the isolation precautions. "Does this mean I have something bad?" What is your best answer?
   a. "These are precautions that we use for every patient who has surgery."
   b. "These precautions prevent the spread of the infection to other patients and to health care personnel."
   c. "These are precautions we are taking to help your infection get better."
   d. "This is an extremely serious infection; these precautions will keep the infection from getting worse."

9. As you continue to assess H.K. over the following days, what evidence will you look for that antibiotics are effectively treating the infection?

10. What will H.K. be taught concerning the care of his cast?

11. What nutritional needs will H.K. have, and why?

12. To ensure pain management, H.K. is given a fentanyl (Duragesic) 75 mcg/hr transdermal patch. To which therapeutic category does this drug belong? What signs and symptoms would you see if he were to have a toxic or overdose reaction?

13. What is the first thing you will need to do if you note a toxic or overdose reaction to the fentanyl transdermal patch?

14. What is the antidote to toxic opioid reactions, and how is it administered?

15. What issues would the discharge planner need to address with H.K.?

CASE STUDY OUTCOME

H.K. stayed in his apartment with a loan from his parents. Friends drove him to physical therapy on their way to class at the university and took him back on their way home. He managed well and went back to work while still in his cast.

Case Study **37**

Name _____ Class/Group _____ Date _____

Group Members _____

INSTRUCTIONS All questions apply to this case study. Your responses should be brief and to the point. When asked to provide several answers, list them in order of priority or significance. Do not assume information that is not provided. Please print or write clearly. If your response is not legible, it will be marked as? and you will need to rewrite it.

▶ **Scenario**

M.M., a 76-year-old retired schoolteacher, underwent open reduction and internal fixation (ORIF) for a fracture of his right femur. His preoperative control prothrombin time (PT/INR) was 11 sec/1.0 and his aPTT was 35 seconds. He has been on bed rest for the first 2 days postoperatively. At 0600, his vital signs were 132/84, 80 with regular rhythm, 18 unlabored, and 99° F (37.2° C). He is awake, alert, and oriented with no adventitious heart sounds. Breath sounds are clear but diminished in the bases bilaterally. Bowel sounds are present, and he is taking sips of clear liquids. An IV of D5 ½ NS is infusing 75 mL/hr in his left hand and orders are to change it to a saline lock in the morning if he is able to maintain adequate PO fluid intake. He has orders for oxygen (O_2) to maintain Sao_2 over 92%. His lab work shows Hct, 34%; Hgb, 11.3 mg/dL; K, 4.1 mEq/L; aPTT, 44 sec. Pain is controlled with morphine sulfate 4 mg IV as needed every 4 hours, and he has promethazine (Phenergan) 25 mg IV q3h if needed for nausea. He is also receiving heparin 5000 units subcutaneously bid, taking docusate sodium (Colace) PO once daily, and wearing a nitroglycerin patch.

At 2330 on the second postoperative day, you answer M.M.'s call light and find him lying in bed breathing rapidly and rubbing the right side of his chest. He is complaining of right-sided chest pain and appears to be restless.

1. What will you do?

CASE STUDY PROGRESS

You check his vital signs, with these results: BP 98/60; P 120; R 24. In addition, you note that he is restless and slightly confused. The pulse oximeter reads 86%, so you start him on 6 L O_2 by nasal cannula. You identify faint crackles in the posterior bases bilaterally; you recall that the lungs were clear this morning. The heart monitor on lead II shows nonspecific T-wave changes.

2. Using SBAR, what information, based on the findings, would you provide to the physician when you call?

3. The physician orders that the patient be transferred to ICU and have blood coagulation studies, arterial blood gases (ABGs) on room air, continuous pulse oximetry, STAT chest x-ray (CXR), and STAT 12-lead ECG. What information will the physician gain from each of the above?

4. Why would the physician order ABGs on room air as opposed to with supplemental O_2?

CASE STUDY PROGRESS

You evaluate the room air ABG results:

■ Chart View

Arterial Blood Gases

pH	7.55
$Paco_2$	24 mm Hg
HCO_3	24 mEq/L
Pao_2	56 mm Hg
Sao_2	86% (room air)

Vital Signs

Blood pressure	150/92 mm Hg
Heart rate	110 beats/min
Respiratory rate	28 breaths/min
Temperature	99° F (37.2° C)

5. What is your interpretation of the ABGs, and what do you think the physician will order next?

CASE STUDY PROGRESS

The chest x-ray showed a small right infiltrate. The physician suspects an embolism, either fat or pulmonary, and orders a STAT ventilation/perfusion ($\dot{V}/\dot{Q}$) lung scan. The interpretation of the results reads "strongly suggestive of a pulmonary embolus (PE)."

6. What are the most likely sources of the embolus?

7. For each characteristic listed in the following, note whether it is a characteristic of a fat embolus (F), a blood clot embolus (BC) in the lungs, or both (B).
___a. Altered mental status
___b. Decreased Sao_2
___c. Petechiae
___d. Chest pain
___e. Crackles
___f. Increased respirations and pulse

8. Before the latest PTT/INR results are back, the physician orders a heparin bolus of 5000 units IV followed by an infusion of 1200 units/hr. The lab calls with a critical value—the aPTT is 120 seconds. Based on these results, what action will you take?

9. The physician is considering administering an antidote to the heparin. Which generic drug is considered an antidote to heparin therapy?
a. Potassium chloride
b. Vitamin K
c. Protamine sulfate
d. Atropine

CASE STUDY PROGRESS

The physician decides not to administer an antidote, and M.M. is monitored closely. Four hours later, the aPTT is 40 seconds.

10. The next day the physician's orders read, "Warfarin (Coumadin) 2.5 mg PO, PT/INR in AM; D/C heparin." What is wrong with these orders?

11. Some thrombolytics, such as alteplase (Activase), have been beneficial in the treatment of PE. Would M.M. be a candidate for treatment with thrombolytics? Why or why not?

12. List three priority problems related to the care of M.M. in his current situation.

13. Several days later you hear M.M. asking his son to bring in a "decent razor" because he is tired of the stubble left by the unit's shaver. How would you address this issue?

Case Study 38

Name _____ Class/Group _____ Date _____

Group Members _____

▶ **Scenario**

J.F., a 67-year-old woman, was involved in an auto accident and is flown by emergency helicopter to your facility. She sustained a ruptured spleen, fractured pelvis, and compound fractures of the left femur. On admission (5 days ago) she underwent a splenectomy. Her pelvis was stabilized with an external fixation device 3 days ago, and, yesterday, her left femur was stabilized using balanced suspension with skeletal traction. She has a Thomas splint with a Pearson attachment on her left leg. She has 20 pounds of skeletal traction and 5 pounds applied to the balanced suspension. Her left femur is elevated off of the bed at approximately 45 degrees. The lower leg is parallel to the bed and lies in a sling that the nurse adjusts on the frame, and the foot hangs freely. This morning, J.F. was transferred to your orthopedic unit for specialized care. You are the nurse assigned to care for her on the night shift.

1. You enter J.F.'s room for the first time. What aspects of the traction will you inspect?

2. When inspecting the skeletal pin sites, you note that the skin is reddened for an inch around the pin on both the medial and lateral left leg. What does this finding indicate, and what action will you take?

3. What key points of the assessment will you document in the patient's record?

4. You find J.F.'s body in the lower 75% of the bed, and her left upper leg is at an exaggerated angle (more than 45 degrees). The knot at the end of the bed is caught in the pulley, and the 20-pound weight is dangling just above the floor. What are you going to do?

5. When you lift J.F., you notice that her sheets are wet. You decide to change J.F.'s linen. How would you accomplish this task?

6. J.F. tells you that she feels like she needs to have a bowel movement (BM), but it is too painful to sit on the bedpan. How would you respond?

7. J.F. expels a few small, hard, round pieces of stool. What could be done to promote normal elimination?

CASE STUDY PROGRESS

You ask J.F. whether she is ready for her bath, and she responds positively. You let her bathe the parts she can reach and engage her in a conversation as you attend to the rest of her body. While performing perineal care, you notice that the folds of skin around her perineal area are reddened and excoriated.

8. Given that J.F. has been on antibiotics for the past 5 days, what is the likely cause of the problem, and what needs to be done to encourage healing?

9. You ask J.F. what she is doing to exercise while she is confined to the bed. She looks surprised and states that she isn't doing anything. What activities can J.F. engage in while on bed rest?

10. You realize that maintaining skin integrity is a challenge in J.F.'s case. What measures will you take to prevent skin breakdown?

11. Although J.F. is recovering nicely, she is becoming increasingly withdrawn. You enter her room and find her crying. She tells you that she is all alone here, that she misses her family terribly. You know that her son is flying into town tomorrow but will only be able to stay a few days. What can be done so that J.F. benefits from her family support system?

Case Study **39**

Name _____ Class/Group _____ Date _____

Group Members _____

INSTRUCTIONS All questions apply to this case study. Your responses should be brief and to the point. When asked to provide several answers, list them in order of priority or significance. Do not assume information that is not provided. Please print or write clearly. If your response is not legible, it will be marked as ? and you will need to rewrite it.

▶ Scenario

You are working in the emergency department when M.C., an 82-year-old widow, arrives by ambulance. Because M.C. had not answered her phone since noon yesterday, her daughter went to her home to check on her. She found M.C. lying on the kitchen floor, incontinent of urine and stool, with complaints of pain in her right hip. Her daughter reports a past medical history of hypertension, angina, and osteoporosis. M.C. takes propranolol (Inderal), a nitroglycerin patch, indapamide (Lozol), and conjugated estrogen (Premarin) daily. The daughter reports that her mother is normally very alert and lives independently. On examination, you see an elderly woman, approximately 100 pounds, holding her right thigh. You note shortening of the right leg with external rotation and a large amount of swelling at the proximal thigh and right hip. M.C. is oriented to person only and is confused about place and time, but she is able to say that her "leg hurts so bad." M.C.'s vital signs (VS) are 90/65, 120, 24, 97.5° F (36.4° C); her Spo₂ is 89%. She is profoundly dehydrated. Preliminary diagnosis is a fracture of the right hip.

1. Considering her medical history and that she has been without her medications for at least 24 hours, explain her current VS.

2. Based on her history and your initial assessment, what three priority interventions would you expect to be initiated?

3. M.C.'s daughter states, "Mother is always so clear and alert. I have never seen her act so confused. What's wrong with her?" What are three possible causes for M.C.'s disorientation that should be considered and evaluated?

3 Musculoskeletal

CASE STUDY PROGRESS

X-ray films confirm the diagnosis of intertrochanteric femoral fracture. Knowing that M.C. is going to be admitted, you draw admission labs and call for the orthopedic consult.

4. What laboratory and diagnostic studies will be ordered to evaluate M.C.'s condition, and what critical information will each give you?

5. What are the five P's that should guide the assessment of M.C.'s right leg before and after surgery?

6. In evaluating M.C.'s pulses, you find her posterior tibial pulse and dorsalis pedis pulse to be weaker on her right foot than on her left. What could be a possible cause of this finding?

7. In planning further care for M.C., list four potential complications for which M.C. should be monitored.

8. M.C. keeps asking about "Peaches." No one seems to be paying attention. You ask her what she means. She says Peaches is her little dog, and she's worried about who is taking care of it. How will you answer?

CASE STUDY PROGRESS

M.C. is placed in Buck's traction and sent to the orthopedic unit until an open reduction and internal fixation (ORIF) can be scheduled. Hydrocodone-acetaminophen (Lortab 2.2/500) q4h prn is ordered for severe pain with orders for acetaminophen (Tylenol) 650 mg q4h prn, and tramadol (Ultram) 100 mg q6h prn, for mild and moderate pain, respectively. M.C.'s cardiovascular, pulmonary, and renal status is closely monitored.

9. As you assess the Buck's traction, you check the setup and M.C.'s comfort. Which of these are characteristics of Buck's traction? (Select all that apply.)
   a. The weights can be lifted manually as needed for comfort.
   b. Weights need to be freely hanging at all times.
   c. Pin site care is an essential part of nursing management of Buck's traction.
   d. A Velcro boot is used to immobilize the affected leg and connect to the weights.
   e. Weights used for Buck's traction are limited to 5 to 10 pounds.

10. Ultram and Lortab are both constipating. What will you do to prevent constipation?

11. Between her admission at 1500 and the next day, she has received five doses of the Lortab and two doses of the acetaminophen (Tylenol). At 1300, she develops a fever of 101° F (38.3° C), and the physician writes an order to give acetaminophen (Tylenol), 650 mg PO every 4 hours for temperature over 100.5° F (38.1° C). Is there a concern with this order?

CASE STUDY OUTCOME

After an uneventful postoperative course, M.C. is transferred to a long-term care facility for physical and occupational therapy rehabilitation. She is placed on prophylactic warfarin (Coumadin).

Case Study **40**

Name _____ Class/Group _____ Date _____

Group Members _____

INSTRUCTIONS All questions apply to this case study. Your responses should be brief and to the point. When asked to provide several answers, list them in order of priority or significance. Do not assume information that is not provided. Please print or write clearly. If your response is not legible, it will be marked as ? and you will need to rewrite it.

▶ Scenario

E.B., a 69-year-old man with type 1 diabetes mellitus (DM), is admitted to a large regional medical center complaining of severe pain in his right foot and lower leg. The right foot and lower leg are cool and without pulses (absent by Doppler). Arteriogram demonstrates severe atherosclerosis of the right popliteal artery with complete obstruction of blood flow. Despite attempts at endarterectomy and administration of intravascular alteplase (tissue plasminogen activator [TPA]) over several days, the foot and lower leg become necrotic. Finally, the decision is made to perform an above-the-knee amputation (AKA) on E.B.'s right leg. E.B. is recently widowed and has a son and daughter who live nearby. In preparation for E.B.'s surgery, the surgeons wish to spare as much viable tissue as possible. Hence, an order is written for E.B. to undergo 5 days of hyperbaric therapy for 20 minutes bid.

1. What is the purpose of hyperbaric therapy?

CASE STUDY PROGRESS

As you prepare E.B. for surgery, he is quiet and withdrawn. He follows instructions quietly and slowly without asking questions. His son and daughter are at his bedside, and they also are very quiet. Finally, E.B. tells his family, "I don't want to go like your mother did. She lingered on and had so much pain. I don't want them to bring me back."

2. You look at his chart and find no advance directives. What is your responsibility?

3. What is your assessment of E.B.'s behavior at this time?

4. What are some appropriate interventions and responses to E.B.'s anticipatory grief?

CASE STUDY PROGRESS

E.B. returns from surgery with the right stump dressed with gauze and an elastic wrap. The dressing is dry and intact, without drainage. He is drowsy with the following vital signs (VS): 142/80, 96, 14, 97.9° F (36.6°C), Spo_2 92%. He has a maintenance IV of D5NS infusing at 125 mL/hr in his right forearm.

5. The surgeon has written to keep E.B.'s stump elevated on pillows for 48 hours; after that, have him lie in a prone position for 15 minutes, four times a day. In teaching E.B. about his care, how will you explain the rationale for these orders?

6. In reviewing E.B.'s medical history, what factors do you notice that might affect the condition of his stump and ultimate rehabilitation potential?

CASE STUDY PROGRESS

You have just returned from a 2-day workshop on guidelines for the care of surgical patients with type 1 DM. You notice that E.B.'s daily fasting blood glucose has been running between 130 and 180 mg/dL. The sliding-scale insulin intervention does not begin until blood glucose values equal to or greater than 200 mg/dL are reported. You recognize that patients with blood glucose values even slightly above normal suffer from impaired wound healing.

7. Identify four interventions that would facilitate timely healing of E.B.'s stump.

8. What should the postoperative assessment of E.B.'s stump dressing include?

9. You are reviewing the plan of care for E.B. Which of these care activities can be safely delegated to the nursing assistive personnel (NAP)? (Select all that apply.)
   a. Rewrapping the stump bandage
   b. Checking E.B.'s vital signs
   c. Assessing E.B.'s IV insertion site
   d. Assisting E.B. with repositioning in the bed
   e. Asking E.B. to report his level of pain on a 1-to-10 scale

10. On the evening of the first postoperative day, E.B. becomes more awake and begins to complaining of (C/O) pain. He states, "My right leg is really hurting; how can it hurt so bad if it's gone?" What is your best response?
   a. "That is a side effect of the medication."
   b. "You can't be feeling that because your leg was amputated."
   c. "Don't worry, that sensation will go away in a few days."
   d. "Are you able to rate that pain on a scale of 1 to 10?"

11. What is causing E.B.'s pain?

CASE STUDY PROGRESS

The case manager is contacted for discharge planning. E.B. will be discharged to an extended care facility for strength training. Once the patient receives his prosthesis, he will receive balance training. After that, he will be discharged to his daughter's home. A physical therapy and occupational therapy home evaluation should be ordered.

12. What instructions should be given to E.B.'s daughter concerning safety around the home?

3 Musculoskeletal

3 Musculoskeletal

CASE STUDY OUTCOME

E.B. makes a smooth transition from the hospital to the rehab facility and then to the daughter's home. He was never able to adapt to independent living, so he eventually moved into his daughter's home.

Case Study 41

Name _____ Class/Group _____ Date _____

Group Members _____

INSTRUCTIONS All questions apply to this case study. Your responses should be brief and to the point. When asked to provide several answers, list them in order of priority or significance. Do not assume information that is not provided. Please print or write clearly. If your response is not legible, it will be marked as ? and you will need to rewrite it.

▶ Scenario

J.T. has injured his hand at work and is accompanied to the emergency department (ED) by a co-worker. You examine his left hand and find a piece of a drill bit sticking out of the skin between the third and fourth knuckles. There is another puncture site about an inch below and toward the center of the hand. Bleeding is minimal. J.T. is 41 years old, has no significant medical history, and has no known drug allergies. He states the accident occurred when a mill at work malfunctioned and knocked his hand onto a rack of drill bits. His last tetanus booster was 12 years ago. It is your job to provide the initial care for J.T.'s injury.

1. You examine J.T.'s hand. What is the priority action? What should you include in your initial assessment, and why?

CASE STUDY PROGRESS

You record that J.T.'s fingers are warm with capillary refill in less than 2 seconds. Sensory perception is intact. He is able to flex and extend the distal joints but not the proximal joints of the third and fourth fingers.

2. You notice J.T.'s wedding band and promptly ask him to remove it. Why is this important?

3. J.T. asks you why the doctor can't just pull the bit out and then he can go home. How should you respond to his question?

4. What common diagnostic test will identify fractures and the location of metal fragments in J.T.'s hand?

CASE STUDY PROGRESS

The drill bit is impaled ½ inch below the surface of the skin, and there are no fractures. Because the hand contains so many blood vessels, nerves, ligaments, and tendons, the ED physician decides to consult a surgical hand specialist. A neurologic consult says there is no nerve damage. The surgeon suspects tendon damage and decides to operate immediately.

5. You accompany the surgeon to J.T.'s bedside and listen to the explanation of the surgery, and then you witness J.T. signing the surgical consent form. What do you need to do to prepare J.T. for immediate surgery?

6. How will you verify that he understands about the surgical procedure?

7. You record that J.T. has had no food "since 8:00 PM yesterday" and drank "some water" this morning. Based on this information, do you anticipate problems during surgery, and why?

8. Does J.T. need a tetanus booster? If so, will he receive a Td or Tdap? Explain your answer, based on the latest Centers for Disease Control and Prevention (CDC) guidelines.

CASE STUDY PROGRESS

The surgeon repairs two partially severed tendons and wraps the hand in a large padded dressing. The distal ½ inch of each digit protrudes from the bulky dressing.

9. While in the short-stay recovery area, J.T. asks the nurse why his fingers look yellowish brown. How should she respond to his question?

CASE STUDY PROGRESS

The surgeon tells J.T. that he had to repair tendons in his third and fourth fingers and instructs J.T. that he is not to work until approval is given after being reevaluated. He gives J.T. prescriptions for ceftazidime (Ceptaz) and naproxen (Naprosyn). He instructs J.T. to make an appointment to see him in the surgery clinic in 2 days. The nurse provides patient teaching about the purpose of these medications, as well as how to take them, and possible side effects.

10. Which statement by J.T. indicates that further teaching about the medications is needed?
   a. "I need to take these pills on an empty stomach."
   b. "I won't stop taking these until the prescription is finished."
   c. "I will not drink alcohol or take over-the-counter medicines while on these drugs."
   d. "I will call my doctor if I notice a rash, diarrhea, or increased bruising."

11. What additional instructions should the nurse in the short-stay area discuss with J.T. and his wife before releasing him?

12. J.T. says, "How in the world is the ice supposed to keep my hand cold with this big bandage on it?" How will the nurse reply?

13. J.T. says, "I'll be able to keep my hand up when I'm awake, but what about when I go to sleep?" What suggestion can the nurse make to help J.T. comply with the instructions?

CASE STUDY OUTCOME

J.T.'s recovery was uncomplicated; he received follow-up occupational therapy and regained the full use of his hand.

Gastrointestinal Disorders

Case Study 42

Name _____ Class/Group _____ Date _____

Group Members _____

INSTRUCTIONS All questions apply to this case study. Your responses should be brief and to the point. When asked to provide several answers, list them in order of priority or significance. Do not assume information that is not provided. Please print or write clearly. If your response is not legible, it will be marked as ? and you will need to rewrite it.

▶ Scenario

T.H., a 57-year-old stockbroker, has come to the gastroenterologist for treatment of recurrent mild to severe cramping in his abdomen and blood-streaked stool. You are the registered nurse doing his initial workup. Your findings include a mildly obese man who demonstrates moderate guarding of his abdomen with both direct and rebound tenderness, especially in the left lower quadrant (LLQ). His vital signs are 168/98, 110, 24, 100.4° F (38° C), and he is slightly diaphoretic. T.H. reports that he has periodic constipation. He has had previous episodes of abdominal cramping, but this time the pain is getting worse.

Past medical history reveals that T.H. has a "sedentary job with lots of emotional moments," he has smoked a pack of cigarettes a day for 30 years, and he has had "2 or 3 mixed drinks in the evening" until 2 months ago. He states, "I haven't had anything to drink in two months." He denies having regular exercise: "just no time." His diet consists mostly of "white bread, meat, potatoes, and ice cream with fruit and nuts over it." He denies having a history of cardiac or pulmonary problems and no personal history of cancer, although his father and older brother died of colon cancer. He takes no medications and denies the use of any other drugs or herbal products.

1. Identify four general health risk problems that T.H. exhibits.

2. Identify a key factor in his family history that might have profound implications for his health and present state of mind.

3. Identify three key findings on his physical exam, and indicate their significance.

CASE STUDY PROGRESS

The physician ordered a KUB (x-ray of the kidneys, ureters, and bladder), CBC, and complete metabolic profile. Based on x-ray and lab findings, physical examination, and history, the physician diagnoses T.H. as having acute diverticulitis and discusses an outpatient treatment plan with him.

4. What is diverticulitis? What are the consequences of untreated diverticulitis?

5. While the patient is experiencing the severe crampy pain of acute diverticulitis, what interventions would you perform to help him feel more comfortable?

6. What is the rationale for ordering bed rest?

CASE STUDY PROGRESS

T.H. is being sent home with prescriptions for metronidazole (Flagyl) 500 mg PO q6h, ciprofloxacin (Cipro) 500 mg PO q12h, and dicyclomine (Bentyl) 20 mg qid PO × 5 days.

7. For each medication, state the drug class and the purpose for T.H.

8. Given his history, what questions must you ask T.H. before he takes the initial dose of metronidazole? State your rationale.

9. What is a disulfiram reaction?

4 Gastrointestinal

10. When teaching T.H. about the metronidazole prescription, which instructions need to be included? (Select all that apply.)
   a. Avoid all alcohol-containing products while on this medication.
   b. If his urine turns reddish brown, notify his doctor immediately.
   c. Take the medication exactly as scheduled, without skipping doses.
   d. He might feel some tingling or numbness in his hands, which is an expected effect.
   e. Take the medication with or after meals.
   f. This medication might cause a metallic taste.

11. What specific information would you want to know before T.H. starts the antibiotics?

12. What are the signs and symptoms of an allergic reaction?

13. T.H. asks you if he can take a laxative for his occasional constipation. What is your answer?

14. T.H. asks you about his diet. "I'm confused. I was always told that I needed to be eating a high-fiber diet, which is difficult for me. But the doctor just told me that I need to be on a low-fiber diet for now, so now I'm confused. Which is it supposed to be?" How will you answer his question?

CASE STUDY PROGRESS

To help T.H. work through his dietary concerns, you obtain a referral to a registered dietitian.

15. What measures do you think the dietitian will discuss with T.H. to avoid recurrent diverticulitis once his acute symptoms are resolved?

CASE STUDY OUTCOME

T.H. returns for a checkup 14 days later; all signs and symptoms of diverticulitis are gone. He is working on his lifestyle changes and reports he is walking 30 minutes every day.

Case Study 43

Name _____ Class/Group _____ Date _____

Group Members _____

INSTRUCTIONS All questions apply to this case study. Your responses should be brief and to the point. When asked to provide several answers, list them in order of priority or significance. Do not assume information that is not provided. Please print or write clearly. If your response is not legible, it will be marked as ? and you will need to rewrite it.

▶ Scenario

T.B. is a 65-year-old retiree who is admitted to your unit from the emergency department (ED). On arrival, you note that he is trembling and nearly doubled over with severe abdominal pain. T.B. indicates that he has severe pain in the right upper quadrant (RUQ) of his abdomen that radiates through to his mid-back as a deep, sharp, boring pain. He is more comfortable walking or sitting bent forward rather than lying flat in bed. He admits to having had several similar bouts of abdominal pain in the last month, but "none as bad as this." He feels nauseated but has not vomited, although he did vomit a week ago with a similar episode. T.B. experienced an acute onset of pain after eating fish and chips at a fast-food restaurant earlier today. He is not happy to be in the hospital and is grumpy that his daughter insisted on taking him to the ED for evaluation.

After orienting him to the room, you perform your physical assessment. The findings are as follows: He is awake, alert, and oriented × 3, and he moves all extremities well. He is restless, is constantly shifting his position, and complains of fatigue. Breath sounds are clear to auscultation. Heart sounds are clear and crisp, with no murmur or rub noted and with a regular rate and rhythm. Abdomen is flat, slightly rigid, and very tender to palpation throughout, especially in the RUQ; bowel sounds are present. He reports having light-colored stools for 1 week. The patient voids dark amber urine but denies dysuria. Skin and sclera are jaundiced. Admission vital signs are BP 164/100, pulse of 132 beats/min, respiration 26 breaths/min, temperature of 100° F (37.8° C), Spo$_2$ 96% on 2 L of oxygen by nasal cannula.

1. What structures are located in the RUQ of the abdomen?

2. Which of the previously mentioned organs are typically palpable in the RUQ?

3. As you palpate T.B.'s abdomen, you deeply palpate the costal margin in the RUQ, and ask him to take a deep breath. This causes T.B. to stop inspiration abruptly, midway, and exclaim, "Oh, that hurts!" What does this finding indicate?
   a. Rebound tenderness
   b. Hepatomegaly
   c. Splenomegaly
   d. Murphy's sign

CASE STUDY PROGRESS

T.B.'s abdominal ultrasound demonstrates several retained stones in the common bile duct and a stone-filled gallbladder. T.B. is admitted to your floor, NPO status, and is scheduled to undergo an endoscopic retrograde cholangiopancreatogram (ERCP) that afternoon. During an ERCP, the patient is sedated, and an ERCP scope is inserted through the mouth, past the stomach, to the outlet of the common bile duct, the ampulla of Vater. Typically, this muscle will be cut to widen the opening and outflow of the common bile duct, a procedure called a *papillotomy*. This allows the bile and stones to flow out into the small intestine. You review T.B.'s other laboratory results:

■ Chart View

Preoperative Laboratory Test Results

WBC	11,900/mm^3
Hgb	14.3 g/dL
Hct	43%
Platelets	250,000/mm^3
Alanine transaminase (ALT)	200 units/L
Aspartate transaminase (AST)	260 units/L
Alkaline phosphatase (ALP)	450 units/L
Total bilirubin	4.8 mg/dL
Prothrombin time (PT)/INR	11.5 sec/1.0
Amylase	50 units/L
Lipase	23 units/L
Urinalysis	Negative

4. Which results are abnormal, and what do they reflect?

CASE STUDY PROGRESS

The patient undergoes the ERCP, and stones and bile are released, but imaging reveals that a stone is still retained within the cystic duct, and multiple stones remain within the gallbladder itself. A surgical consult is obtained, and a laparoscopic cholecystectomy ("lap choley") is planned.

5. Identify at least four preoperative orders that will likely need to be completed before T.B. goes to surgery.

6. T.B. is medicated with morphine sulfate 2 mg IV push (IVP) q2h as needed. After the first dose, he reports that on a scale of 1 to 10, his pain has decreased from a 10 to a 4 within 30 minutes. What other methods could be used to help T.B.'s pain?

7. Which data charted in the assessment are consistent with CBD obstruction?

At 2330, T.B. spikes a temperature of 101.5° F (38.6° C) (tympanic). His Spo$_2$ on 2 L oxygen per nasal cannula is now 90%, so you immediately increase the flow rate to raise his O$_2$ saturation. You inform the on-call surgeon, and she orders a STAT chest x-ray and a broad-spectrum antibiotic—imipenem and cilastatin (Primaxin) 500 mg IV now, then q6h.

8. Before you give the antibiotic, what will you assess?

9. As you review the orders, you note that the Primaxin contains cilastatin. What is the purpose of the cilastatin?
   a. It enhances the action of the imipenem.
   b. It reduces the chance of an allergic reaction.
   c. It promotes the renal secretion of the imipenem.
   d. It causes the bacterial cell wall to become unstable.

T.B. undergoes a successful laparoscopic cholecystectomy the next morning. An intraoperative cholangiogram shows that the ducts are finally cleared of stones at the conclusion of the surgery. When he returns to the nursing unit, his stomach is soft but quite distended. His wife asks you whether anything is wrong.

10. How will you respond to her question?

11. When you remove the tape the next day to change the dressing, you note that the skin is red and blistered underneath. Otherwise, he is doing well; his vital signs are 128/72, 80, 16, 99.8° F (37.7° C), and Spo$_2$ of 95% on room air. He even tolerated a light breakfast. To protect the blistered area from further damage, you apply a hydrocolloid dressing to the damaged skin. What has T.B. experienced, and what are the benefits of this type of dressing?

The rest of the day is uneventful, and the next day T.B. is discharged to home.

12. What discharge teaching does T.B. need?

Case Study **44**

Name _____ Class/Group _____ Date _____

Group Members _____

INSTRUCTIONS All questions apply to this case study. Your responses should be brief and to the point. When asked to provide several answers, list them in order of priority or significance. Do not assume information that is not provided. Please print or write clearly. If your response is not legible, it will be marked as ? and you will need to rewrite it.

▶ Scenario

M.R. is a 56-year-old general contractor who is admitted to your telemetry unit directly from his internist's office with a diagnosis of chest pain. On report, you are informed that he has an intermittent 2-month history of chest tightness with substernal burning that radiates through to the mid-back intermittently, in a stabbing fashion. Symptoms occur after a large meal; with heavy lifting at the construction site; and in the middle of the night when he awakens from sleep with coughing, shortness of breath, and a foul, bitter taste in his mouth. Recently, he has developed nausea, without emesis, that is worse in the morning or after skipping meals. He complains of "heartburn" three or four times a day. When this happens, he takes a couple of Rolaids or Tums. He keeps a bottle at home, at the office, and in his truck. Vital signs (VS) at his physician's office were 130/80 lying, 120/72 standing, 100, 20, 98.6° F (37° C), Spo_2 92% on room air. A 12-lead ECG showed normal sinus rhythm with a rare premature ventricular contraction (PVC).

1. What are some common causes of chest pain?

2. What mnemonic can you use to help you better evaluate his pain?

3. What other history is important?

CASE STUDY PROGRESS

M.R. indicates that usually the chest pain is relieved with his antacids, but this time they had no effect. A "GI cocktail" consisting of Mylanta and viscous lidocaine given at his physician's office briefly helped decrease symptoms.

4. What tests can be done to determine the source of his problems?

CASE STUDY PROGRESS

M.R. has smoked one pack of cigarettes a day for the past 35 years, drinks two or three beers on most nights, and has noticed a 20-pound weight gain over the past 10 years. He feels "so tired and old now." M.R. has dark circles under his eyes and complains of constant daytime fatigue. His wife is even sleeping in another bedroom because he is snoring so loudly. He also reinjured his lower back a month ago at work, lifting a pile of boards, so his physician prescribed ibuprofen (Motrin) 800 mg bid or tid for 4 weeks.

5. Which factors in M.R.'s life are likely contributing to his chest pain and nausea? Explain how.

CASE STUDY PROGRESS

M.R. explains that 6 months ago his physician prescribed famotidine (Pepcid) 20 mg PO at bedtime for heartburn, and that it helped a little, but that it never really "did the job." Now he keeps a bottle of Tums or Rolaids in his truck and at his bedside, in addition to the ranitidine, "because I always seem to need them."

6. Why do you think the famotidine did not help M.R.?

CASE STUDY PROGRESS

M.R.'s 12-lead ECG was normal, and the first set of cardiac enzymes was normal. CBC showed WBC 6000/mm³, Hgb 15.0 g/dL, Hct 47%, platelets 220,000/mm³. Complete metabolic panel (CMP) revealed Na 140 mEq/L, K 3.7 mEq/L, BUN 20 mg/dL, creatinine 1.0 mg/dL, lipase 20 units/L, amylase 18 units/L, PT 12.0 sec, INR 1.0. The *H. pylori* antibody test came back as 20 units/mL. The chest x-ray showed no abnormalities. Room air Spo_2 is 94%, and breathing is unlabored. Suddenly, M.R. begins to complain of nausea; as you hand him the emesis basin, he promptly vomits coffee-ground emesis with specks of bright red blood. VS remain stable.

7. What concerns do you have about the coffee-ground emesis?

8. What is the significance of the *H. pylori* antibody test result?

CASE STUDY PROGRESS

You ask the charge nurse to contact the gastrointestinal (GI) consulting doctor to explain the recent events while you stay with M.R. The gastroenterologist gives several orders and states he will be there in 45 minutes. The orders are as follows:

■ Chart View

Physician's Orders

- NPO status for emergent esophagogastroduodenoscopy (EGD)
- STAT CBC
- Oxygen by nasal cannula; titrate oxygen to maintain Spo_2 over 92%
- Type and crossmatch (T&C) 2 units packed RBCs (PRBCs), and hold
- Start a pantoprazole (Protonix) drip at 8 mg/hr, preceded by an 80-mg bolus IV over 8 minutes.
- Insert a Salem Sump nasogastric tube (NGT) and start a gastric lavage with normal saline.
- Insert two large-bore IVs and start normal saline (NS) at 100 mL/hr.

9. List the previous orders in order of priority.

10. Explain the rationale for each of the preceding orders.

4 Gastrointestinal

CASE STUDY PROGRESS

The gastroenterologist finds erosive esophagitis LA Class B, a moderately sized hiatal hernia, diffuse erosive gastritis, and an ulcer in the antrum of the stomach that is oozing blood. The duodenal bulb yielded a normal endoscopic appearance. During the EGD, the bleeding was stopped with cautery. Biopsies were obtained of the gastric mucosa, and the biopsies are negative for *H. pylori* bacteria; his bleeding ulcer is attributed to the NSAIDs (i.e., ibuprofen). He is kept NPO until the next morning to allow good hemostasis of the cauterized site. Clear liquids are allowed at breakfast. His hematocrit (Hct) dropped to 32%, but he remained asymptomatic from the mild anemia; the drop was believed, in part, to reflect that he was dehydrated on admission, and the decrease reflected the dilution of the blood from the IV fluids added. Thus, he did not receive a transfusion of blood.

M.R. tolerated the liquid diet without any nausea and vomiting and is discharged to home the next day with the following instructions:

- Advance diet slowly, as tolerated, to mechanical soft.
- Take pantoprazole 40 mg PO q AM on an empty stomach, at least 30 minutes before eating.
- Make a follow-up appointment in 6 to 8 weeks with physician (give name and telephone number).
- Stop all aspirin and over-the-counter (OTC) or herbal pain relief medications (ibuprofen, naproxen, etc.).
- Stop or limit alcohol intake and smoking.

11. Why does the patient need to take the pantoprazole first thing in the morning?

12. After discussing lifestyle modifications for controlling acid reflux with M.R., which statement by M.R. indicates a further need for teaching?
   a. "I will try to stop smoking."
   b. "I will wait thirty minutes before lying down or sitting in my recliner after meals."
   c. "I will avoid fatty foods, caffeine, and chocolate."
   d. "I will avoid eating two to three hours before my bedtime."

Case Study 45

Name _____ Class/Group _____ Date _____

Group Members _____

INSTRUCTIONS All questions apply to this case study. Your responses should be brief and to the point. When asked to provide several answers, list them in order of priority or significance. Do not assume information that is not provided. Please print or write clearly. If your response is not legible, it will be marked as ? and you will need to rewrite it.

▶ Scenario

While you are working as a nurse on a gastrointestinal/genitourinary (GI/GU) unit, you receive a call from your affiliate outpatient clinic notifying you of a direct admission, with an estimated time of arrival of 60 minutes. She gives you the following information: A.G. is an 87-year-old woman with a 3-day history of intermittent abdominal pain, abdominal bloating, and nausea and vomiting (N/V). A.G. moved from Italy to join her grandson and his family only 2 months ago, and she speaks very little English. All information was obtained through her grandson. Past medical history includes colectomy for colon cancer 6 years ago and ventral hernia repair 2 years ago. She has no history of coronary artery disease, diabetes mellitus, or pulmonary disease. She takes only ibuprofen (Motrin) occasionally for mild arthritis. Allergies include sulfa drugs and meperidine. A.G.'s tentative diagnosis is small bowel obstruction (SBO) secondary to adhesions. A.G. is being admitted to your floor for diagnostic workup. Her vital signs (VS) are stable, she has an IV of D5½NS with 20 mEq KCl infusing at 100 mL/hr, and 3 L oxygen by nasal cannula (O₂/NC).

1. Based on the nurse's report, what signs of bowel obstruction does A.G. manifest?

2. Are there other signs and symptoms that you should observe for while A.G. is in your care?

3. While A.G. is on the way, you have secured the hospital's interpreter service on the telephone. A.G. arrives on your unit with her grandson. You admit A.G. to her room and introduce yourself as her nurse. As her grandson introduces her, she pats your hand. You know that you need to complete a physical examination and take a history. What will you do first?

4. Before you begin your examination, you ask the grandson to excuse himself, explaining the hospital's confidentiality policies. The grandson, an attorney, tells you that elderly Italian women are extremely modest and might not answer questions completely. How might you gather information, in this case?

5. What key questions must you ask this patient while you have the use of an interpreter?

6. For each characteristic listed, specify whether it is a characteristic of small-bowel obstruction (SBO), large-bowel obstruction (LBO), or both (B).
____a. Intermittent lower abdominal cramping
____b. Abdominal discomfort or pain accompanied by visible peristaltic waves in the upper and middle abdomen
____c. Upper or epigastric abdominal distention
____d. Distention in the lower abdomen
____e. Obstipation
____f. Ribbon-like stools
____g. Nausea and early, profuse vomiting, which may contain fecal material
____h. Minimal or no vomiting
____i. Severe fluid and electrolyte imbalances

7. What is obstipation?

8. With some difficulty, you insert a Salem Sump nasogastric tube (NGT) into A.G. and connect it to intermittent low wall suction. How will you check for placement of the NGT?

9. List, in order, the structures through which the NGT must pass as it is inserted.

10. A.G.'s grandson asks you, "What is that blue thing at the end of the tube? Shouldn't it be connected to something?" How do you answer?

11. What comfort measures are important for A.G. while she has an NGT?

12. You note that A.G.'s NGT has not drained in the last 3 hours. What can you do to facilitate drainage?

13. The NGT suddenly drains 575 mL; then it slows down to about 250 mL over 2 hours. Is this an expected amount?

14. You enter A.G.'s room to initiate your shift assessment. A.G. has been hospitalized for 3 days, and her abdomen seems to be more distended than yesterday. How would you determine whether A.G.'s abdominal distention has changed?

CASE STUDY PROGRESS

After 3 days of NGT suction, A.G.'s symptoms are unrelieved. She reports continued nausea, cramps, and sometimes strong abdominal pain; her hand grips are weaker; and she seems to be increasingly lethargic. You look up her latest laboratory values and compare them with the admission data.

■ **Chart View**

Laboratory Test Results

Test	Admission	Hospital Day 3
Sodium	136 mEq/L	130 mEq/L
Potassium	3.7 mEq/L	2.5 mEq/L
Chloride	108 mEq/L	97 mEq/L
Carbon dioxide	25 mEq/L	31 mEq/L
BUN	19 mg/dL	38 mg/dL
Creatinine	1 mg/dL	2.2 mg/dL
Glucose	126 mg/dL	65 mg/dL
Albumin	3.0 g/dL	3.1 g/dL
Protein	6.8 g/dL	4.9 g/dL

15. Which lab values are of concern to you? Why?

16. What measures do you anticipate to correct in each of the imbalances described in Question 15?

CASE STUDY OUTCOME

In view of A.G.'s continued slow deterioration, the surgeon met with the patient and her family, and they agreed to surgery. The surgeon released an 18-inch section of proximal ileum that had been constricted by adhesions. Several areas looked ischemic, so these were excised, and an end-to-end anastomosis was done. A.G. tolerated the procedure well. Her recovery was slow but steady. A.G. went home in the care of her grandson and his wife on the seventh postop day. Discharge plans included a home health nurse, home health aide, in-home physical therapy, and dietitian consult. The grandson was included in the plans.

Case Study **46**

Name _____ Class/Group _____ Date _____

Group Members _____

INSTRUCTIONS All questions apply to this case study. Your responses should be brief and to the point. When asked to provide several answers, list them in order of priority or significance. Do not assume information that is not provided. Please print or write clearly. If your response is not legible, it will be marked as ? and you will need to rewrite it.

▶ **Scenario**

P.M., a 24-year-old house painter, has been too ill to work for the past 3 days. When he arrives at your outpatient clinic with his girlfriend, he seems alert but acutely ill, with an average build and a deep tan over the exposed areas of skin. He reports headaches, joint pain, a low-grade fever, cough, anorexia, and nausea and vomiting (N/V), especially after eating any fatty food. P.M. describes vague abdominal pain that started about the same time as the other problems. His past medical history reveals he has no health problems, is a nonsmoker, and drinks a "few" beers each evening to relax. Vital signs (VS) are 128/84, 88, 26, 100.6° F (38.1° C); awake, alert, and oriented × 3; moves all extremities well except for aching pain in his muscles; very slight scleral jaundice present; heart tones clear and without adventitious sounds; bowel sounds clear throughout abdomen and pelvis; and abdomen soft and palpable without distinct masses. You note moderate hepatomegaly measured at the midclavicular line; liver edge is easily palpated and tender to palpation. P.M. mentions that his urine has been getting darker over the past 2 days.

P.M. is manifesting the key signs of hepatitis. Lab work is sent for identification of his precise problem, and results are shown below.

■ **Chart View**

Laboratory Test Results

Sodium	140 mEq/L
Potassium	3.9 mEq/L
Chloride	102 mEq/L
CO_2	26 mEq/L
BUN	10 mg/dL
Creatinine	1.0 mg/dL
Platelets	210,000/mm³
Indirect bilirubin	1.6 mg/dL
Total bilirubin	2.3 mg/dL
Albumin	3.8 g/dL
Total protein	6.5 g/dL
Alanine aminotransferase (ALT)	66 units/L
Aspartate aminotransferase (AST)	52 units/L
Lactic dehydrogenase (LDH)	245 units/L
Alkaline phosphatase	176 units/L
Prothrombin time (PT)/INR	12 sec/1.06
Activated partial thromboplastin time (aPTT)	32 sec
Urine urobilinogen	1.6 IU/L
Anti-HAV (hepatitis A virus) IgM	Negative
Hepatitis B surface antigen (HBsAg)	Positive

4 Gastrointestinal

1. Which key diagnostic tests will determine exactly what type of hepatitis is present?

2. Which of P.M.'s lab results, listed previously, specifically indicates liver disease?

3. What is the difference between the hepatitis B surface antigen (HBsAg) and the hepatitis B surface antibody (HBsAb)?

4. List three drugs that can cause increased ALT levels.

5. Considering the basic pathology of hepatitis, what type of diet will you strongly encourage P.M. to follow?

6. For each characteristic below, identify whether it belongs to hepatitis A (A) or hepatitis B (B).
____a. Fecal-oral transmission
____b. Transmitted by sharing needles
____c. Transmitted by blood transfusions
____d. Vaccination is a three-shot series.
____e. Illness is usually mild, similar to a flu-like infection.
____f. Symptoms of illness include anorexia, nausea, vomiting, fever, fatigue, and jaundice.

7. In P.M.'s case, the hepatitis B surface antigen (HBsAg) is positive. This result indicates that P.M. is infected with hepatitis B and is in the acute period of the disease. Is this disease contagious? What precautions would you take while he is in the hospital?

8. Pruritus is usually associated with jaundice. What will you do to ease this problem for P.M.?

9. How will you explain to P.M. the likely progression of his disease?

10. P.M. is living at home with his parents and four younger siblings. The youngest is 4 years old. His parents ask how to prevent the rest of the family from getting hepatitis. What specific instructions will you give? How will you know that these instructions are understood?

11. Given P.M.'s lifestyle, what specific patient teaching points must you emphasize?

CASE STUDY OUTCOME

P.M. is ready for discharge in a few days, and he confides in you that he feels so "guilty" about having hepatitis and endangering his girlfriend and family. He tells you that he was at a party and did not think the one-time needle use could hurt him. He has been told that he has lost his job because he is not able to go back to work, and he hopes his family is not too afraid to have him return home.

12. What action will you take?

Case Study 47

Name _____ Class/Group _____ Date _____

Group Members _____

INSTRUCTIONS All questions apply to this case study. Your responses should be brief and to the point. When asked to provide several answers, list them in order of priority or significance. Do not assume information that is not provided. Please print or write clearly. If your response is not legible, it will be marked as ? and you will need to rewrite it.

▶ **Scenario**

John Doe, approximately 50 years old, is admitted to your unit for observation from the emergency department (ED) with the diagnosis of rule out hepatic encephalopathy with acute alcohol (ETOH) intoxication. This man was sent to the ED by local police, who found him lying unresponsive along a rural road.

Examination and x-ray studies are negative for any injury, and you are awaiting the results of the blood alcohol level and toxicology tests. He has no identification and is not awake or coherent enough to give any history or to answer questions. He is lethargic, has a cachectic appearance, does not follow commands consistently, and is mildly combative when aroused. He smells strongly of ETOH and has a notably distended abdomen and edematous lower extremities. He has a Foley catheter and an IV of D5½NS with 20 mEq KCl and 1 ampule of multivitamins infusing at 75 mL/hr.

Admitting orders are listed in the following:

▪ Chart View

Admission Orders

- IV D5 ½ NS with 20 mEq KCl at 75 mL/hr; add 1 ampule multivitamins to 1 L of IV fluid per day.
- Insert Salem Sump nasogastric tube (NGT), and attach to low continuous suction (LCS).
- Insert Foley catheter to gravity drainage.
- Elevate head of bed (HOB) at 30 to 45 degrees at all times.
- Check all stools for occult blood.
- Lactulose (Cephulac) 45 mL PO qid until diarrhea
- Abdominal ultrasound (US) in AM
- Vitamin K (AquaMEPHYTON) 10 mg/day IV or PO may (when alert and able to swallow) × 3 doses
- Vitamin B_1/thiamine (generic) 100 mg/day IV; change to PO when alert and able to swallow.
- Vitamin B_9/folic acid (generic) 0.4 mg/day IM
- Vitamin B_6/pyridoxine (generic) 100 mg/day PO
- Labs: CBC with differential, basic metabolic panel (BMP), liver function tests (LFTs), PT/INR and PTT, serum ammonia (NH_3) now and in AM
- Once patient is alert and able to swallow, may have low-protein diet. Observe for any difficulty swallowing, and offer assistance with meals if needed.
- Call house officer for any sign of gastrointestinal bleed; delirium tremens (DTs); systolic blood pressure (BP) over 140 or less than 100 mm Hg; diastolic BP less than 50 mm Hg; or pulse over 120 beats/min.

1. Which of the preceding orders can be delegated to the nursing assistive personnel (NAP)?

2. Some of the lab work drawn in the ED has come back. The blood alcohol level (BAL) is 320 mg/dL, and the blood ammonia (NH_3) level is 155 mcg/dL. His total protein is 5.2 g/dL and albumin is 2.1 g/dL. What do these values indicate?

3. Which of the ordered medications might help with the elevated ammonia levels? Explain.

4. Why are so many different vitamins ordered for John Doe?

CASE STUDY PROGRESS

While you are getting John Doe settled, you continue your assessment.

Neurologic findings: PERRL (Pupils Equal, Round, Reactive to Light), moves all extremities, but patient is sluggish, pulling away during assessment, and follows commands sporadically.

Cerebrovascular findings: Pulse is regular but tachycardic without adventitious sounds. All peripheral pulses are palpable, with 3+ bilateral and 3+ pitting edema in lower extremities.

Respiratory assessment: Breath sounds decreased to all lobes, no adventitious sounds audible, patient not cooperating with cough and deep breathing, and Sao_2 at 90% on room air.

GI assessment: Tongue and gums are beefy red and swollen, abdomen is enlarged and protuberant, girth is 141 cm, and abdominal skin is taut and slightly tender to palpation. His Salem Sump NGT is patent, connected to LCS with small to moderate greenish drainage; bowel sounds positive with NGT clamped.

Genitourinary (GU) assessment: Foley to gravity drainage, with 75 mL dark amber urine since admission (2 hours).

Skin: Pale on torso and lower extremities; heavily sunburned on upper extremities and head. Skin appears thin and dry. Numerous spider angiomas are found on the upper abdomen with several dilated veins across abdomen.

Vital signs: 120/60, 104, 32, 99.1° F (37.3° C).

5. What is the significance of the spider angiomas, dilated abdominal veins, peripheral edema, and distended abdomen?

6. How would you further assess the distended abdomen, and what is the clinical name for your findings?

7. What is your concern about John Doe's nutritional status? What are your objective findings?

8. If his protein levels are so low, why isn't John Doe on a high-protein diet?

9. How might you respond to fellow staff nurses' remarks, "Why are we wasting time with this 'wino'? He isn't worth the time or money. Why don't they let him die?"

4 Gastrointestinal

10. A nursing problem relative to John Doe's care is the possibility of injury. Ensuring safety is a priority when caring for a person who might be withdrawing from alcohol. Identify two areas of injury risk, and specify actions you will take to ensure his safety.

11. You monitor John Doe for signs and symptoms of alcohol withdrawal and delirium tremens (DTs). So far he is restless, has tremors, and has a low-grade fever. Which of the symptoms listed are symptoms of the more severe DTs? (Select all that apply.)
a. GI bleeding
b. Hallucinations
c. Hypotension
d. Somnolence
e. Extreme diaphoresis
f. Tachycardia
g. Vomiting

12. Falls are particularly dangerous for someone in this patient's situation. Why?

CASE STUDY PROGRESS

During John Doe's hospitalization, a staff psychiatrist evaluates him for mental decline associated with alcohol abuse and dependence, including alcoholic dementia, or Korsakoff's psychosis.

13. What are alcoholic dementia and Korsakoff's psychosis?

CASE STUDY PROGRESS

John Doe survives a rocky course of hepatic encephalopathy and near-renal failure. After 27 days, including a week in the ICU, he is discharged to a drug and alcohol rehabilitation facility. He is employed as a longshoreman; fortunately, his insurance covers his month of in-house intense rehabilitation.

4 Gastrointestinal

Case Study **48**

Name _____ Class/Group _____ Date _____

Group Members _____

INSTRUCTIONS All questions apply to this case study. Your responses should be brief and to the point. When asked to provide several answers, list them in order of priority or significance. Do not assume information that is not provided. Please print or write clearly. If your response is not legible, it will be marked as ? and you will need to rewrite it.

▶ Scenario

C.W., a 36-year-old woman, was admitted several days ago with a diagnosis of recurrent inflammatory bowel disease (IBD) and possible small bowel obstruction (SBO). C.W. is married, and her husband and 11-year-old son are supportive, but she has no extended family in-state. She has had IBD for 15 years and has been taking mesalamine (Asacol) for 15 years and prednisone 40 mg/day for the past 5 years. She is very thin; at 5 feet 2 inches she weighs 86 pounds and has lost 40 pounds over the past 10 years. She has an average of 5 to 10 loose stools per day. C.W.'s life has gradually become dominated by her disease (anorexia; lactase deficiency; profound fatigue; frequent nausea and diarrhea; frequent hospitalizations for dehydration; and recurring, crippling abdominal pain that often strikes unexpectedly). The pain is incapacitating and relieved only by a small dose of diazepam (Valium), oral electrolyte solution (Pedialyte), and total bed rest. She confides in you that sexual activity is difficult: "It always causes diarrhea, nausea, and lots of pain. It's difficult for both of us." She is so weak she cannot stand without help. You indicate complete bed rest on the nursing care plan.

1. Identify six priority problems for C.W.

2. Considering C.W.'s weakness, chronic diarrhea, and lower-than-desired body weight, what nursing interventions need to be implemented to minimize skin breakdown?

CASE STUDY PROGRESS

C.W.'s condition deteriorates on the third day after admission; she experiences intractable abdominal pain and unrelenting nausea and vomiting. C.W. is taken to the operating room for probable SBO and is readmitted to your unit from the postanesthesia care unit. During surgery, 38 inches of her small bowel were found to be severely stenosed with two areas of visible perforation. Much of the remaining bowel is severely inflamed and friable. A total of 5 feet of distal ileum and 2 feet of colon have been removed, and a temporary ileostomy was established. She has a Jackson-Pratt (JP) drain to bulb suction in her right lower quadrant (RLQ), and her wound was packed and left open. She has two peripheral IVs, a Salem Sump nasogastric tube (NGT), and a Foley catheter. Her vital signs (VS) are 112/72, 86, 24, 100.8° F (38.2° C) (tympanic). You attach her NGT to low-continuous wall suction per the postoperative orders.

3. You begin a thorough postoperative assessment of C.W.'s abdomen. What does your assessment include? List these steps in the order in which the assessment should be completed.

4. A nursing student enters C.W.'s room and auscultates her abdomen. She looks at you and excitedly announces that she hears good bowel sounds. You take the opportunity to teach her the proper method of auscultating bowel sounds on a patient who has NGT to continuous low wall suction. How would you correct her error?

5. Four hours later, you measure the drainage from the JP tube. Look at the following figure and state how much drainage you obtained.

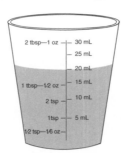

6. What else about the drainage will you note?

7. Describe the proper method for reestablishing the suction on the JP drain after you have emptied the bulb container.

8. C.W. asks you, "I know why I have the pouch. Why do I have to have this other little tube?" How will you explain the purpose of the JP drain?

CASE STUDY PROGRESS

C.W. is at 4 days postop. During the routine dressing change, you note a small pool of yellow-green drainage in the deepest part of the wound. You realize the physician will want a wound culture.

9. How will you culture C.W.'s wound?

10. What information do you need to send to the lab with the wound culture specimen?

11. You obtain a wound culture, complete the dressing change, obtain a full set of VS, note a temperature of 100.4° F (38° C), and assess increased tenderness in C.W.'s abdomen. What orders do you anticipate receiving once you notify the physician of C.W.'s condition?

12. The physician calls back and asks you to describe C.W.'s wound. What key aspects of the wound should be included?

13. As you assess C.W.'s stoma and drainage, what would indicate that they are healthy? (Select all that apply.)
   a. The stoma will be in the shape of a donut.
   b. The stoma will be level with the skin.
   c. The stoma will be a uniform medium cherry red in color.
   d. The stoma will be light pink, and an occasional dark spot might appear.
   e. The skin around the stoma should be intact.
   f. The drainage will be thick and dark brown in color.

14. Will any aspect of C.W.'s history significantly affect the wound healing process? If so, how?

15. With a fairly significant wound infection developing, why is C.W.'s temperature relatively low?

16. The physician tells you that she will be over to examine C.W. As you tell C.W. that her doctor is coming to talk to her, C.W. says that she feels something wet running down her side. You find some leakage of intestinal drainage onto the skin. What should you do?

CASE STUDY OUTCOME

You change the ileostomy appliance before the physician arrives. C.W. is evaluated, and it is determined that she needs to return to surgery for exploratory laparotomy.

Case Study 49

Name _____ Class/Group _____ Date _____

Group Members _____

INSTRUCTIONS All questions apply to this case study. Your responses should be brief and to the point. When asked to provide several answers, list them in order of priority or significance. Do not assume information that is not provided. Please print or write clearly. If your response is not legible, it will be marked as ? and you will need to rewrite it.

▶ **Scenario (Continuation of Case Study 48)**

C.W. is a 36-year-old woman admitted 7 days ago for inflammatory bowel disease (IBD) with small bowel obstruction (SBO). She underwent surgery 3 days after admission for a colectomy and ileostomy. She developed peritonitis and, 4 days later, returned to the operating room (OR) for an exploratory laparotomy, which revealed another area of perforated bowel, generalized peritonitis, and a fistula tract to the abdominal surface. Another 12 inches of ileum were resected (total of 7 feet of ileum and 2 feet of colon). The peritoneal cavity was irrigated with normal saline (NS), and three drainage tubes were placed: a Jackson-Pratt (JP) drain to bulb suction, a rubber catheter to irrigate the wound bed with NS, and a sump drain to remove the irrigation. The initial JP drain remains in place. A right subclavian triple-lumen catheter was inserted.

1. C.W. returns from the post-anesthesia recovery unit (PACU) on your shift. What do you do when she is in the bed in her room?

2. You pull the covers back to inspect the abdominal dressing and find that the original surgical dressing is saturated with fresh bloody drainage. What do you do?

3. C.W. has a total of four tubes in her abdomen, as well as a nasogastric tube (NGT). What information do you want to know about each tube?

4. The sump irrigation fluid bag is nearly empty. You close the roller clamp, thread the IV tubing through the infusion pump, check the irrigation catheter connection site to make certain it is snug, and then discover that the nearly empty liter bag infusing into C.W.'s abdomen is D5W, not NS. Does this require any action? If so, give rationale for actions, and explain the overall situation.

CASE STUDY PROGRESS

The surgeon arrives on the unit and removes C.W.'s surgical dressing. There is a small "bleeder" at the edge of the incision, so the surgeon calls for a suture and ties off the bleeder. You take the opportunity to ask her about a morphine patient-controlled analgesia (PCA) pump for C.W., and the surgeon says she will write the orders.

5. Postoperative pain will be a problem for C.W. after the anesthesia wears off. How do you plan to address this?

6. Pharmacy delivers C.W.'s first bag of total parenteral nutrition (TPN). The physician has instructed you to start the TPN at a rate of 60 mL/hr and decrease the maintenance IV rate by the same amount. What is the purpose of this order?

7. The physician did not specifically order glucose monitoring, but you know that it should be initiated. You plan to conduct a fingerstick blood test every 6 hours unless she is symptomatic, then more frequently. What is your rationale?

8. C.W.'s blood glucose increased temporarily, but, by the next day, it dropped to an average of 70 to 80 mg/dL and has remained there for 2 days. Her VS are stable, but her abdominal wound shows no signs of healing. She has lost 1 kg over the past 3 days. What do these data mean?

9. During the night shift, the TPN solution bag becomes nearly empty, and the night nurse discovers that the next bag of TPN has not been prepared. The hospital pharmacy does not prepare TPN during the night shift. What does the nurse need to do next?
   a. Convert the line to a saline lock until the TPN solution is ready.
   b. Slow the TPN rate to 10 mL/hr until the next TPN bag can be prepared.
   c. Hang a bag of D5W when the TPN is finished.
   d. Hang a bag of D10W when the TPN is finished.

CASE STUDY PROGRESS

You discuss your concerns with C.W.'s physician, and she agrees to request a consult from a registered dietitian (RD). After gathering data and making several calculations, the RD makes recommendations to the attending physician. The TPN orders are adjusted, C.W. begins to gain weight slowly, and her wound shows signs of healing. Nutritional problems in clinical populations can be complex and often require special attention.

10. You and a co-worker read the following in C.W.'s progress notes: "Wound healing by secondary closure. Formation of granular tissue with epithelialization noted around edges. Have requested dietitian consult on ongoing basis. Will continue to follow." Your co-worker turns to you and asks whether you know what that means. How would you explain?

11. Both of you start to discuss what specific digestive difficulties C.W. is likely to face in the future. What problems might C.W. be prone to develop after having so much of her bowel removed?

12. The RD consults with C.W. about dietary needs. You attend the session so that you will be able to reinforce the information. What basic information is the RD likely to discuss with C.W.?

13. After 3 days of dressing changes, C.W.'s skin is irritated, and a small skin tear has appeared where tape was removed. How can you minimize this type of skin breakdown and help this area heal?

14. What specifics of ostomy teaching do you plan to do?

4 Gastrointestinal

CASE STUDY PROGRESS

C.W. successfully battled peritonitis. Gradually, tubes were removed as she grew stronger with TPN and time. C.W. learned how to change her ostomy appliance and was discharged to home.

Case Study 50

Name _____ Class/Group _____ Date _____

Group Members _____

INSTRUCTIONS All questions apply to this case study. Your responses should be brief and to the point. When asked to provide several answers, list them in order of priority or significance. Do not assume information that is not provided. Please print or write clearly. If your response is not legible, it will be marked as ? and you will need to rewrite it.

▶ **Scenario**

You are a nurse working on a surgical unit and take the following report from the registered nurse in the emergency department. "We are sending you a direct admit with rule out small bowel obstruction (R/O SBO) and/or food blockage. Dr. N., the gastrointestinal specialist is on his way in to see the patient. D.S. is a 78-year-old obese man with complaints of sudden onset of severe abdominal cramping, distention, and nausea and vomiting; he denies passing of flatus or stool within the past 12 hours. Past medical history includes heart failure, hypertension, colon cancer, and ulcerative colitis. He underwent a total colectomy 16 years ago and had an enterocutaneous fistula 12 years ago. Lab samples have been drawn, and the results will be sent to your floor. We started an IV and placed a Salem Sump nasogastric tube (NGT). His vital signs are 143/76, 82, respirations 26 and slightly labored, and 101.1° F (38.4° C). He is on his way up."

1. Given that D.S. had had a total colectomy, would he have a colostomy or an ileostomy? Explain your answer.

2. What would you expect to see if D.S.'s ostomy had normal function?

CASE STUDY PROGRESS

After D.S. is settled into his room, the NGT and IV are functioning well, and he receives pain medication, you begin your admission assessment. His abdomen is extremely large, firm to touch, with multiple scars and an ileostomy pouching system in his RLQ.

3. What are the more common complications of an ileostomy?

4. D.S.'s past medical history of fistula, combined with the probability of blockage or obstruction, places him at an increased risk for which problems?

5. As you assess the stoma, you look for signs that it is healthy. Which of these assessment findings are the characteristics of a healthy stoma? (Select all that apply.)
   a. The stoma is cherry-red, dark pink in color.
   b. The stoma is pale pink in color.
   c. The stoma is moist.
   d. The stoma is dry.
   e. The stoma is flat against the skin.

6. What stoma changes would you report immediately to the physician?

7. Why are transparent ostomy pouches recommended postoperatively or when patients are hospitalized?

8. Will the stoma present visual clues of D.S.'s bowel blockage or obstruction?

CASE STUDY PROGRESS

D.S. continues to complain of abdominal pain and cramping and becomes increasingly restless. You notice that the abdomen behind and around his stoma and pouch appears larger when compared with the other side of his abdomen.

9. How would you assess for a possible peristomal hernia?

10. Why is a peristomal hernia a problem?

CASE STUDY PROGRESS

You note that the ostomy pouch has liquid brown effluent along the lateral edge of the wafer. You check to see that the pouch is properly attached to the wafer and discover that stool is indeed leaking from under the barrier. D.S. apologizes for not bringing any supplies with him, stating, "My ostomy nurse told me to always carry extra supplies for times like this."

D.S. does not remember what size he needs, but you note he is wearing a 2-piece system with a plastic ring-flange that attaches to the pouch with a matching ring.

11. How will you determine the correct pouching size and system?

CASE STUDY PROGRESS

You have finished with your general head-to-toe assessment and order the appropriate pouching products for D.S. You have already taken clean towels, washcloths, and underpads into his room, along with a hamper to receive dirty, used laundry. You gather scissors, skin-prep, and adhesive remover to assist with the pouching change.

12. As you return to his room, you review the steps for changing an ostomy pouch. What are the steps you will need to follow?

CASE STUDY PROGRESS

You have gathered all needed supplies, and D.S. is as comfortable as possible. You begin the pouching change. Using the adhesive remover, with the push-pull method, you gently remove the wafer. As you lift the wafer, you note that the peristomal skin has severe erythema directly encircling the stoma. There is denudation (partial-thickness breakdown) at the medial stoma-skin edge.

13. How should the skin around the stoma look?

4 Gastrointestinal

14. Generally, there are four different causes of erythema or skin breakdown. Identify two.

15. After you discover the reddened skin, how will you proceed with the ostomy care?

CASE STUDY PROGRESS

The next day, D.S.'s vital signs return to normal, and his abdomen is less distended. The ileostomy is steadily draining greenish-brown liquid stool. The NGT is removed, and D.S. is started on sips of clear liquids. When you go to check his ileostomy pouch, D.S. tells you, "I know I've had this a long time, but I still can't stand to look at this thing. My wife usually helps me with it, and I hate that."

16. What will you suggest for D.S. at this time?

Case Study 51

Name _____ Class/Group _____ Date _____

Group Members _____

INSTRUCTIONS All questions apply to this case study. Your responses should be brief and to the point. When asked to provide several answers, list them in order of priority or significance. Do not assume information that is not provided. Please print or write clearly. If your response is not legible, it will be marked as ? and you will need to rewrite it.

▶ Scenario

B.K. is a 63-year-old woman who is admitted to the medical-surgical unit from the emergency department (ED) with nausea and vomiting (N/V) and epigastric and left upper quadrant (LUQ) abdominal pain that is severe, sharp, and boring and radiates through to her mid-back. The pain started 24 hours ago and awoke her in the middle of the night. B.K. is a divorced, retired sales manager who smokes a half-pack of cigarettes daily. The ED nurse reports that B.K. is anxious and demanding. B.K. denies using alcohol. Her vital signs (VS) are as follows: 100/70, 97, 30, 100.2° F (37.9° C) (tympanic), SpO_2 88% on room air and 92% on 2 L of oxygen by nasal cannula (NC). She is in normal sinus rhythm. She will be admitted to the hospitalist service. She has no primary care provider (PCP) and hasn't seen a physician "in years."

The ED nurse giving you the report states that the admitting diagnosis is acute pancreatitis of unknown etiology. A computed tomography (CT) scan has been ordered, but, unfortunately, the CT scanner is down and won't be fixed until morning. However, an ultrasound of the abdomen was performed, and "no cholelithiasis, gallbladder wall thickening, or choledocholithiasis was seen. The pancreas was not well visualized due to overlying bowel gas." Admission labs have been drawn; a clean-catch urine specimen was sent to the lab, and the urine was dark in color.

1. What are the possible causes of pancreatitis?

2. If a CT scan is planned for the morning, what orders would you expect?

3. What other information do you need from the ED nurse before you assume responsibility for the patient?

CASE STUDY PROGRESS

You complete your admission assessment and note the following abnormalities: B.K. is restless and lying on her right side in a semifetal position. Cerebrovascular findings are: Skin is cool, diaphoretic, and pale with poor skin turgor; mucous membranes are dry. Heart rate is regular but tachycardic, without murmurs or rubs. Peripheral pulses are faintly palpable in four extremities. Respirations are rapid but unlabored on 2 L O_2/NC with Spo_2 90%. Breath sounds are absent in lower left lobe (LLL) posteriorly—otherwise, clear to auscultation throughout. She complains of nausea and is having dry heaves. Bowel sounds are hypoactive. Abdomen is distended, firm, and tender in a diffuse fashion to light palpation, with guarding noted.

■ Chart View

Admission Laboratory Test Results

Lipase	3000 units/L
Amylase	2000 units/L
Alk phos (ALP)	350 units/L
ALT (SGPT)	90 units/L
AST (SGOT)	150 units/L
Total bilirubin	2.0 mg/dL
Albumin	3.0 g/dL
BUN	24 mg/dL
Creatinine	1.4 mg/dL
WBC	17,500/mm³

4. Which specific laboratory results point to a diagnosis of pancreatitis?

5. Which labs are the most important to monitor in acute pancreatitis? Why are they significant?

6. What do the BUN and creatinine tell you about her renal function and volume status?

7. Why are the WBCs elevated?

CASE STUDY PROGRESS

During your physical exam, you noted "respirations rapid but unlabored on 2 L O_2/NC with Spo_2 90%. Breath sounds are absent in LLL posteriorly—otherwise, clear to auscultation throughout." The admission chest x-ray (CXR) report reads, "small pleural effusion in the left lower lobe (LLL)."

8. Identify three actions you could initiate to help correct this situation.

9. B.K. turns on her call light. She complains of thirst and demands something to drink. Her orders indicate "NPO, except sips and chips." What is your response to her request? What nursing action would help her complaints?

CASE STUDY PROGRESS

B.K. eventually falls asleep and seems to be sleeping peacefully. Several hours later, you hear an alarm on her pulse oximeter and enter her room to investigate. You find B.K. moaning softly; her oximeter reads 87%.

10. What will you do next?

11. Your assessment findings are as follows: lung sounds absent in the LLL and very diminished in the right lower lobe (RLL). You percuss a dull thud over the left middle lobe (LML) and LLL up to the scapula tip. On percussion, you hear resonance over the entire right lung and left upper lobe (LUL). What is the significance of your findings?

12. What actions should you take next?

CASE STUDY PROGRESS

The physician orders a STAT CXR which shows a significant pleural effusion developing in the LLL, with extension into the RLL.

13. Based on the evolving pleural effusion with evidence of decompensation (hypoxia) by the patient, what treatment would the physician likely pursue, and what preparations would you be responsible for?

CASE STUDY PROGRESS

The physician removed 200 mL of slightly cloudy serous fluid. Antibiotics were adjusted to provide broad-spectrum coverage for an upper respiratory tract infection until culture and sensitivity results return. B.K. is resting quietly with oxygen at 3 L per nasal cannula, and her respirations are unlabored and regular. Her Spo$_2$ reads 96%.

It is now 72 hours after B.K.'s admission, and her labs show improvement. An abdominal CT scan is completed and shows "a moderately severe pancreatitis, but no local fluid collection or pseudocysts. No ileus or evidence of neoplasia was noted." BUN is 9.0 mg/dL, and creatinine is 1.0 mg/dL. She has adequate urinary output. Her IV fluids are decreased to 75 mL/hr. Her amylase and lipase levels are decreasing toward normal levels. The physician writes an order to advance B.K.'s diet to full liquids.

14. How would you know whether B.K. was not able to tolerate the advancement in diet?

15. If B.K. does not tolerate the advancement in diet, what physiologic need should be addressed at 72 hours?

CASE STUDY PROGRESS

The afternoon of the third day of B.K.'s hospitalization, she becomes agitated with tremors, some disorientation, and auditory hallucinations. Her pulse and blood pressure (BP) are elevated, although her pain has not increased, and the pain medication schedule has not changed. B.K. has had no visitors since being admitted.

16. What is B.K. most likely experiencing, and what actions will you take?

CASE STUDY OUTCOME

You contact the physician with your observations, and he orders scheduled chlordiazepoxide (Librium) and a social services consult to evaluate and treat for possible alcohol abuse. Three days later, B.K. is lucid, tolerating clear liquids, and her pain is controlled with oral pain medications. As she becomes oriented and calmer, B.K. eventually admits to drinking "3 or 4 scotch-on-the-rocks" daily. You also discover that B.K. is estranged from her family because of her drinking. The physician advances her diet to "low-fat/low-cholesterol" and writes orders to discharge that evening if she tolerates the advancement in diet, which she does.

17. What will you include in your discharge teaching with B.K.?

Genitourinary Disorders

5

Case Study 52

Name _____ Class/Group _____ Date _____

Group Members _____

INSTRUCTIONS All questions apply to this case study. Your responses should be brief and to the point. When asked to provide several answers, list them in order of priority or significance. Do not assume information that is not provided. Please print or write clearly. If your response is not legible, it will be marked as ? and you will need to rewrite it.

▶ Scenario

You are working in an extended care facility (ECF) when M.Z.'s daughter brings her mother in for a week's stay while she goes on vacation. M.Z. is an 89-year-old widow with a 4-day history of dysuria, suprapubic pain, incontinence, new onset mental confusion, and loose stools. Her most current vital signs (VS) are 118/60, 88, 18, 99.4° F (37.4° C).

The medical director ordered a postvoid catheterization, which yielded 100 mL of cloudy urine that had a strong odor, and several lab tests on admission. The results were as follows:

■ Chart View

Laboratory Test Results

Complete metabolic panel (CMP): Within normal limits except for the following results:

BUN	25 mg/dL
Sodium	131 mEq/L
Potassium	3.2 mEq/L
White blood cell count	11,000/mm^3

Urinalysis

Appearance	Cloudy
Odor	Foul
pH	6.9
Protein	Negative
Nitrites	Positive
Crystals	Negative
WBC	6 per low-power field
RBC	3

Urine culture and sensitivity results are pending.

1. What condition do the assessment findings and lab reports point toward?

2. The medical director makes rounds and writes orders to start an IV of D5½ NS at 75 mL/hr and insert a Foley catheter to gravity drainage. Because M.Z. is unable to take oral meds, the medical director ordered ciprofloxacin (Cipro) 400 mg q12h IV piggyback (IVPB). Is the type of fluid and rate appropriate for M.Z.'s age and condition? Explain.

3. While administering the IVPB ciprofloxacin, which adverse effects might occur? (Select all that apply.)
   a. Hypotension
   b. Headache
   c. Drowsiness
   d. Restlessness
   e. Nausea
   f. Tendon rupture

4. You enter the room to start the IV and insert the Foley catheter and find that the NAP has taken the patient to the bathroom for a bowel movement. M.Z. asks you to help her, and, as you open the door, you observe the patient wiping herself from back to front. What do you need to do at this time?

5. Because M.Z. has been having diarrhea, what special instructions should you give the NAP assigned to give basic care to M.Z.?

CASE STUDY PROGRESS

The next day, you are the nurse assigned to M.Z.'s care. You notice that the NAP emptying the gravity drain is not wearing personal protection devices. You also observe that the drainage port of the drainage bag was contaminated during the process because the NAP allowed it to touch the floor.

6. What issues need to be considered in protecting M.Z.'s safety? Describe your actions in working with the nursing assistant.

7. As you assess M.Z., you notice that her catheter tubing is not secured. Why does the tubing need to be secured, and where is the correct placement of the catheter tubing?

CASE STUDY PROGRESS

On the third day after M.Z.'s admission, the urinary culture and sensitivity (C&S) results were as follows: *Escherichia coli*, more than 100,000 colonies, sensitive to ciprofloxacin, trimethoprim-sulfamethoxazole, and nitrofurantoin.

8. What changes, if any, will be made to the antibiotic therapy?

9. The NAP reports that M.Z.'s 8-hour intake is 520 mL and the output is 140 mL. Is this significant? Identify two possible reasons that could account for the difference, and explain how you would assess each.

CASE STUDY PROGRESS

M.Z. has completed her antibiotic therapy. Her mental status has cleared, the Foley catheter has been discontinued, and she is ready for discharge.

10. What instructions should you discuss with the daughter?

5 Genitourinary

Case Study **53**

Name _____ Class/Group _____ Date _____

Group Members_____

INSTRUCTIONS All questions apply to this case study. Your responses should be brief and to the point. When asked to provide several answers, list them in order of priority or significance. Do not assume information that is not provided. Please print or write clearly. If your response is not legible, it will be marked as ? and you will need to rewrite it.

▶ Scenario

You are working in the emergency department (ED) when M.B., a 72-year-old man, enters with a chief complaint of the inability to void. His initial vital signs (VS) are 168/92, 88, 20, 98.2° F (36.8° C).

1. Are M.B.'s VS appropriate for a man of his age? If not, offer a rationale for the abnormal readings.

2. Given M.B.'s chief complaint, what would you expect to find during your initial assessment?

CASE STUDY PROGRESS

While you are taking M.B.'s history, he tells you he is generally in good health and leads an active life. His current medications include finasteride (Proscar) 5 mg/day and vitamin supplements. He reports that he has been unable to void for 12 hours and is very uncomfortable. He asks you to help him.

3. What do you need to know about his use of the finasteride (Proscar)?

4. What are your priorities for this patient?

5. After examining M.B., the ED physician asks you to insert an indwelling urethral Foley catheter. What will you include in M.B.'s teaching before placing the Foley?

6. After two unsuccessful attempts to advance the catheter into the bladder, you stop. What is your next intervention? Why? What could be causing this problem?

7. The ED physician successfully inserts the indwelling catheter with the use of a coudé catheter, and urine begins to drain. How is this catheter different?

8. As the physician begins to inflate the catheter balloon, M.B. winces in pain and states, "*Ouch, you are hurting me!*" What happened, and what will the physician do?

9. You watch the urine drain into the bag and note that the amount is approaching 500 mL. What do you do at this time?

10. After the catheter is in place, the ED physician writes orders to discharge M.B. with instructions to see his primary care provider (PCP) on the following day. It is your responsibility to give discharge instructions. Outline your care plan.

5 Genitourinary

11. The next day, M.B. is seen by his PCP, who changes M.B.'s medication to alfuzosin (Uroxatral). The catheter will be discontinued 2 days later. What teaching is essential regarding this new medication?

    a. Alfuzosin needs to be taken in the morning.

    b. This medication might cause fainting when he first starts taking it.

    c. M.B. needs to take each dose on an empty stomach.

    d. M.B. can stop taking the alfuzosin once the urinary symptoms subside.

5 Genitourinary

Case Study **54**

Name _____ Class/Group _____ Date _____

Group Members _____

INSTRUCTIONS All questions apply to this case study. Your responses should be brief and to the point. When asked to provide several answers, list them in order of priority or significance. Do not assume information that is not provided. Please print or write clearly. If your response is not legible, it will be marked as ? and you will need to rewrite it.

▶ Scenario

You are working on a postoperative surgical floor and are assigned to A.T., a 65-year-old woman with a 30-year smoking history who has recently had a radical cystectomy with ileal conduit for invasive bladder cancer.

1. You begin your assessment and look at the transparent urostomy pouch covering the ileal conduit. The stomal opening is red and is draining urine with mucus. Is this normal?

2. A nursing student who is working with you asks you to explain the difference between an ileal conduit and an ileostomy. How do you answer?

3. The student replies, "So, eventually, A.T.'s ileal conduit will become continent, and she won't need to wear a pouch, right?" How do you answer?

4. What is the proper size for an appliance for an ileal conduit?

CASE STUDY PROGRESS

A.T. is quiet and sullen. You ask her if something is wrong, and she confides she is concerned about whether her husband will find her attractive after he sees her "rosebud."

5. What is the underlying problem?

CASE STUDY PROGRESS

You ask A.T. whether she would love her husband or children any less if they had a physical problem that required surgical repair. She quickly tells you, "No, of course not." You suggest that her family will likely respond the same way to her surgery. You suggest that someone from the ostomate program come and talk to her.

6. What is the ostomate program?

7. A.T. is well enough to begin self-care but asks you if you will change her pouch because she doesn't "want to look at it." Is there anyone on the hospital staff who could help teach A.T. ostomy self-care and offer more support?

CASE STUDY PROGRESS

It is now the fourth postop day, and A.T. is now willing to learn how to change her appliance. She tells you the stoma feels wet, and it has no feeling when she touches it.

8. Which statements about the stoma are true? (Select all that apply.)
   a. "The lining of the stoma is the same type of tissue as the inside of your mouth."
   b. "It has touch receptors, just like your skin, and you should have feeling in it."
   c. "The color should be a beefy red, and the stoma should feel wet."
   d. "Normally, the stoma is dry. Feeling moisture is a problem."
   e. "The tissue is tough and rarely bleeds."

9. A.T. asks you, "How will I know when to empty it? What about at night? Do I have to get up at night to empty this little pouch?" How do you answer her?

10. What other topics need to be addressed when doing teaching regarding an ileal conduit?

CASE STUDY PROGRESS

A.T.'s urine looks cloudy, and another nurse suggests that you send a specimen from her pouch to the lab for analysis. Her urine does not smell foul, and she has no fever or flank pain.

11. Should you follow through on this suggestion? Why or why not?

12. What are the signs and symptoms of a urinary tract infection (UTI) in a patient with an ileal conduit?

13. A.T. asks you, "How will they collect a urine specimen when it just dribbles out all the time?" How will you answer her?

14. As you make rounds, you notice that A.T.'s pouch has sprung a urine leak and she has placed a washcloth over the pouch to absorb the urine. She asks you for tape to attach the washcloth to the bag. How will you respond to her request?

CASE STUDY PROGRESS

A.T. eventually masters the pouch application and is discharged to home. She returns to the urology clinic in 6 months for a follow-up visit. She has lost 24 pounds and is seen with a smaller stoma surrounded by a half-inch ring of wartlike skin. The nurse explains to A.T. that her stoma has shrunk, and the bag no longer fits properly; alkaline urine washing over unprotected skin from too large an appliance opening causes a skin reaction that can either appear smooth or wartlike. The wartlike skin buildup is referred to as *hyperkeratotic, hyperplastic, epitheliomatous hyperplasia, metaplasia,* or *acanthosis.*

15. What can be done once a hyperkeratotic lesion forms around a stoma?

CASE STUDY OUTCOME

A.T. mastered her ileal conduit and became a popular ostomate.

Case Study 55

Name _____   Class/Group _____   Date _____

Group Members _____

INSTRUCTIONS All questions apply to this case study. Your responses should be brief and to the point. When asked to provide several answers, list them in order of priority or significance. Do not assume information that is not provided. Please print or write clearly. If your response is not legible, it will be marked as ? and you will need to rewrite it.

▶ Scenario

S.M. is a 68-year-old man who is being seen at your clinic for routine health maintenance and health promotion. He reports that he has been feeling well and has no specific complaints, except for some trouble "emptying my bladder." Vital signs (VS) at this visit are 148/88, 82, 16, 96.9° F (36.1° C). He had a CBC and complete metabolic panel (CMP) completed 1 week before his visit, and the results are listed below.

■ Chart View

Laboratory Test Results	
Sodium	140 mEq/L
Potassium	4.2 mEq/L
Chloride	100 mEq/L
Bicarbonate	26 mEq/L
BUN	19 mg/dL
Creatinine	0.8 mg/dL
Glucose	94 mg/dL
RBC	5.2 million/mm^3
WBC	7400/mm^3
Hgb	15.2 g/dL
Hct	46%
Platelets	348,000/mm^3
Prostate-specific antigen (PSA)	0.23 ng/mL
Urinalysis	WNL

1. What can you tell S.M. about his lab work?

2. What is the significance of the PSA result?

3. What other specific examination will S.M. need to have along with the PSA?

CASE STUDY PROGRESS

While obtaining your nursing history, you record no family history of cancer or other genitourinary (GU) problems. S.M. reports frequency, urgency, and nocturia × 4; he has a weak stream and has to sit to void. These symptoms have been progressive over the past 6 months. He reports he was diagnosed with a large prostate a number of years ago. Last month, he began taking saw palmetto capsules but had to stop taking them because they "made me sick."

4. Why did S.M. try taking the saw palmetto, and why do you think he stopped taking it?

5. S.M. is curious why his enlarged prostate would affect his urination. He is concerned that he has prostate cancer. What would you teach him?

6. The primary care provider (PCP) asked for a postvoiding residual (PVR) urine test. You use a bedside bladder scanner and document that S.M. voided 60 mL and his PVR is 110 mL. You report the PVR to the PCP. What is the significance of his PVR?

7. Commonly used medications for BPH are 5-alpha reductase inhibitors, such as finasteride (Proscar) and alpha-blocking drugs, such as tamsulosin (Flomax). How do these drugs differ?

8. The PCP ordered tamsulosin (Flomax) 0.4 mg/day PO. You enter S.M.'s room to teach him about this medication. What side effects will you tell S.M. about? (Select all that apply.)
   a. Dizziness
   b. Diarrhea
   c. Dry mouth
   d. Insomnia
   e. Heartburn
   f. Orthostatic hypotension

9. S. M. asks, "Will this condition affect my relationship with my wife?" What should you tell him?

10. What would you expect S.M. to report if the medication was successful?

CASE STUDY PROGRESS

S.M. returns in 8 months to report that his symptoms are worse than ever. He has tried several different medications, but medication management failed, and he is told that surgical intervention is necessary.

11. What surgical options are available to S.M.?

CASE STUDY OUTCOME

S.M. elected to undergo a Gyrus transurethral resection of the prostate (TURP). He did well postoperatively and was discharged to home.

Case Study 56

Name _____   Class/Group _____   Date _____

Group Members _____

INSTRUCTIONS All questions apply to this case study. Your responses should be brief and to the point. When asked to provide several answers, list them in order of priority or significance. Do not assume information that is not provided. Please print or write clearly. If your response is not legible, it will be marked as ? and you will need to rewrite it.

▶ Scenario

K.B. is a 32-year-old woman being admitted to the medical floor for complaints of fatigue and dehydration. While taking her history, you discover that she has diabetes mellitus (DM) and has been insulin-dependent since the age of 8. She has undergone hemodialysis (HD) for the past 3 years. Your initial assessment of K.B. reveals a pale, thin, slightly drowsy woman. Her skin is warm and dry to the touch with poor skin turgor, and her mucous membranes are dry. Her vital signs (VS) are 140/88, 116, 18, 99.9° F (37.7° C). She tells you she has been nauseated for 2 days so she has not been eating or drinking. She reports severe diarrhea. Serum calcium, phosphate, magnesium, and a complete blood count (CBC) have been drawn but the results are not yet available. The following blood chemistry results are back:

■ Chart View

Laboratory Test Results

Sodium	145 mEq/L
Potassium	6.0 mEq/L
Chloride	93 mEq/L
Bicarbonate	27 mEq/L
BUN	48 mg/dL
Creatinine	5.0 mg/dL
Glucose	238 mg/dL

1. What aspects of your assessment support her admitting diagnosis of dehydration?

2. Explain any lab results that might be of concern.

3. Identify two possible causes for K.B.'s low-grade fever.

CASE STUDY PROGRESS

The rest of K.B.'s physical assessment is within normal limits. You note that she has an arteriovenous (AV) fistula in her left arm.

4. What is an AV fistula? Why does K.B. have one?

5. What steps do you take to assess K.B.'s AV fistula, and what physical findings are expected? Explain.

6. As you continue the assessment, you notice that a nursing assistive personnel (NAP) comes in to take K.B.'s blood pressure. The NAP places the blood pressure cuff on K.B.'s left arm. What, if anything, do you do?

CASE STUDY PROGRESS

K.B.'s admission CBC yields the following results:

■ Chart View

Laboratory Test Results

WBC	7600/mm³
RBC	3.2 million/mm³
Hgb	8.1 g/dL
Hct	24.3%
Platelets	333,000/mm³

7. Are these values normal? If not, what are the abnormalities?

8. K.B.'s physician notes that she is anemic, which most likely is the cause of her increasing fatigue. Why is K.B. anemic?

CASE STUDY PROGRESS

K.B. is sent for a hemodialysis (HD) treatment. Over the next 24 hours, K.B.'s nausea subsides, and she is able to eat normally. While you are helping her with her morning care, she confides in you that she doesn't understand the renal diet. "I just get blood drawn every week and meet with the dialysis dietitian every month—I just eat what she tells me to eat."

9. Because K.B. is on HD, what are her special nutritional needs?

5 Genitourinary

10. Patients in renal failure have the potential to develop comorbid conditions. Identify five potential problems, determine how you would assess the problem, then delineate nursing interventions and patient education strategies for each.

CASE STUDY PROGRESS

The following day, K.B. is discharged feeling much better and with a good understanding of her dietary restrictions. Her iron stores have been evaluated and found to be low. Her physician has instructed her to resume her preadmission medications, except for the addition of ferrous sulfate elixir 5 mL PO tid with meals and epoetin (Epogen) to be given three times a week IV with dialysis. She is also given a prescription for Nephrocaps vitamin supplements to be taken daily.

11. What information would you give K.B. about her new medications?

12. K.B. asks, "Why do I need a prescription for vitamins? I can just take something on sale at the drug store, right?" How do you respond?

13. When monitoring K.B.'s response to the epoetin, what adverse effect would you expect?
a. Hypertension
b. Tachycardia
c. Drowsiness
d. Diarrhea

14. During the following weeks, which laboratory result is most important to monitor while K.B. is on the epoetin? Explain.

CASE STUDY OUTCOME

K.B. is discharged to home and goes to the local dialysis center three times a week. She also keeps appointments with the registered dietitian and reports that she is feeling much better.

Case Study 57

Name _____ Class/Group _____ Date _____

Group Members _____

INSTRUCTIONS All questions apply to this case study. Your responses should be brief and to the point. When asked to provide several answers, list them in order of priority or significance. Do not assume information that is not provided. Please print or write clearly. If your response is not legible, it will be marked as ? and you will need to rewrite it.

▶ Scenario

A.B. is a 55-year-old man who was referred to the urology clinic by his primary care provider (PCP) for an elevated prostate-specific antigen (PSA). He reports that he has been feeling well and has no specific complaints. He had a CBC, basic metabolic panel (BMP), urinalysis (UA), lipid profile, and screening PSA completed the week before when he was seen by his PCP. His CBC, lipid profile, UA, and blood chemistries are all within normal limits. His PSA is elevated at 11.9 ng/mL, and the prostate is slightly tender on exam.

1. A.B. wonders whether he has prostate cancer. What can you tell A.B. about his PSA?

2. A.B. is scheduled for a transrectal ultrasound (TRUS) of the prostate. What is the purpose of this test?

3. Based on the PSA and TRUS results, A.B. is scheduled for a prostate biopsy. He wonders what he needs to do to prepare for this test. Explain a prostate biopsy procedure and how to prepare for the procedure.

CASE STUDY PROGRESS

A.B.'s prostate biopsy is positive for cancer, with a Gleason grade of 7. He has discussed his diagnosis with the urologist. He is now thinking about his treatment options and asks you to answer some questions. He was told about his Gleason grade but is not sure what this is.

4. What is a Gleason grade?

5. The urologist discusses possible treatment options with A.B. Identify three treatment options for prostate cancer.

CASE STUDY PROGRESS

After consulting with his urologist, A.B. has decided to have his prostate removed with the laparoscopic procedure. He is planning on having surgery in 2 weeks but is concerned about the possible consequences of surgery.

6. Identify the major immediate postoperative concerns for A.B.

7. What are the two main long-term consequences of prostatectomy?

8. The urologist you work for has asked you to give A.B. preoperative instructions. What should you tell him?

CASE STUDY PROGRESS

A.B. returns status post-laparoscopic radical prostatectomy (LRP). Initial postoperative orders are written.

9. Which orders are appropriate for A.B.? (Select all that apply, and correct the inappropriate answers.)
   a. Vital signs per hospital protocol
   b. Notify physician if urinary output is less than 30 mL/hr.
   c. Up ad lib.
   d. Change Foley catheter if clotting occurs.
   e. Oxybutynin (Ditropan XL) 10 mg PO every morning
   f. Docusate (Colace) 100 mg PO qd
   g. Morphine 4 mg IV push q4h prn pain

10. What would be ordered if clotting of the Foley catheter occurs?

11. After giving A.B. a complains of bladder spasms and is given a dose of oxybutynin (Ditropan XL), the nurse will monitor for which adverse effects? (Select all that apply.)
   a. Dry mouth
   b. Watery eyes
   c. Dizziness
   d. Diarrhea
   e. Palpitations

CASE STUDY PROGRESS

A.B. does not require any additional therapy after surgery. At his 6-month follow-up visit, he reports he can get an erection but has difficulty maintaining an erection for sexual relations.

12. You discuss erectile aids with A.B. What options should you address?

Case Study **58**

Name _____ Class/Group _____ Date _____

Group Members _____

INSTRUCTIONS All questions apply to this case study. Your responses should be brief and to the point. When asked to provide several answers, list them in order of priority or significance. Do not assume information that is not provided. Please print or write clearly. If your response is not legible, it will be marked as ? and you will need to rewrite it.

▶ Scenario

It is a hot summer day, and you are a registered nurse in the emergency department (ED). S.R., an 18-year-old woman, comes to the ED with severe left flank and abdominal pain and nausea and vomiting. S.R. looks very tired, her skin is warm to the touch, and she is perspiring. She paces about the room doubled-over and is clutching her abdomen. S.R. tells you that the pain started early this morning and has been pretty steady for the past 6 hours. She gives a history of working outside as a landscaper and takes little time for water breaks. Her past medical history includes three kidney stone attacks, all during late summer. Exam findings are that her abdomen is soft and without tenderness, but her left flank is extremely tender to the touch, palpation, and percussion. You place S.R. in one of the examination rooms and take the following vital signs (VS): 188/98, 90, 20, 99° F (37.2° C). A voided urinalysis (UA) shows RBC of 50 to 100 on voided specimen and WBC of zero.

1. What could be the cause of the blood in her urine? How could you rule out some of these causes?

2. The physician orders an intravenous pyelogram (IVP). What questions do you need to ask S.R. before the test is conducted? What blood tests do you need to check before her having an IVP?

3. S.R. states she had an allergic reaction during her last IVP and was instructed, "Don't let anyone give you dye for any testing." The physician cancels the IVP; what alternative test will be conducted?

5 Genitourinary

The noncontrast CT scan shows a left 2-mm ureteral vesicle junction stone.

4. What are the two most common types of stones?

5. What is the most likely cause of S.R.'s stone?

6. Identify two methods of treating a patient with a ureteral vesicle junction stone.

CASE STUDY PROGRESS

S.R. was discharged with instructions to strain all urine and return if she experienced pain unrelieved by the pain medication or increased N/V.

7. What specific instructions will you give S.R. about her urine, fluid intake, medications, and activity?

S.R. returns to the ED in 6 hours with complaints of pain unrelieved by the pain medication and increased blood in her urine. She is being held in the ED until she can be transported to surgery.

8. What is the immediate plan of care for S.R.?

CASE STUDY PROGRESS

A 2-mm calculus was removed by basket extraction. Pathologic examination reported the stone to be calcium oxalate.

9. If S.R. continues to form stones, what recommendations would the physician make for S.R.?

10. Now that S.R.'s stone has been reported as calcium oxalate, she is referred to a registered dietitian for guidance on a diet that will prevent further development of stones. Which statements are true regarding recommendations for S.R.'s diet? (Select all that apply.)
   a. Decrease animal protein intake.
   b. Avoid eating organ meats, poultry, fish, gravies, red wine, and sardines.
   c. Avoid spinach, black tea, coffee, rhubarb, chocolate, beets, wheat bran, and nuts.
   d. Decrease sodium intake.
   e. Drink at least 3 to 4 liters of water each day.

CASE STUDY OUTCOME

S.R. recovers from this most recent episode and continues to follow the protocol for fluid intake and dietary measures. One year later, she has yet to report a recurrence of stones.

Case Study 59

Name _____ Class/Group _____ Date _____

Group Members _____

INSTRUCTIONS All questions apply to this case study. Your responses should be brief and to the point. When asked to provide several answers, list them in order of priority or significance. Do not assume information that is not provided. Please print or write clearly. If your response is not legible, it will be marked as ? and you will need to rewrite it.

5 Genitourinary

▶ Scenario

F.F., a 58-year-old man with type 2 diabetes mellitus, comes to the emergency department (ED) with severe right flank and abdominal pain and nausea and vomiting (N/V). The abdomen is soft and without tenderness. The right flank is extremely tender to the touch and to palpation. Vital signs (VS) are 142/80, 88, 20, 99° F (37.2° C). Urinalysis shows hematuria. An IV of 0.9% normal saline (NS) is started and set to infuse at 125 mL/hr. An IV pyelogram (IVP) confirms the diagnosis of a staghorn-type stone in the right renal pelvis. The right kidney looks enlarged. F.F. states that he did not sleep well last night and has not eaten much today. He is obviously fatigued. His laboratory results are listed below. F.F. weighs 277 pounds.

■ Chart View

Admission Laboratory Test Results

Sodium	144 mEq/L
Potassium	4.0 mEq/L
Chloride	101 mEq/L
Carbon dioxide	26 mEq/L
BUN	30 mg/dL
Creatinine	3.6 mg/dL
Glucose	260 mg/dL
Uric acid	5.0 mg/dL
Calcium	9.0 mg/L
Phosphorus	3.2 mg/dL
Total protein	7.8 g/dL
Albumin	4.0 g/dL
Total bilirubin	0.3 mg/dL
Direct bilirubin	0.1 mg/dL
Cholesterol	200 mg/dL
Alk phos (ALP)	61 units/L
LDH	Total 100 units/L
ALT (SGPT)	13 units/L
AST (SGOT)	38 units/L
Amylase	98 units/L

1. Review F.F.'s lab work, and note any that might be of concern.

2. Analyze the relationship between creatinine and glomerular filtration rate (GFR) and prediction of kidney function.

3. F.F.'s pain is treated in the ED with IV morphine. It is late afternoon before he is admitted to your unit, and he is scheduled for lithotripsy in the morning. What specific priorities do you identify for F.F.?

4. What problems are possible as a result of the staghorn stone?

5. The physician has ordered gentamicin (Garamycin) 6 mg/kg/day IV piggyback in divided doses q8h. Calculate the dose of gentamicin for F.F. Are there any concerns?

6. How will you bring up your concerns about this dose of gentamicin?

7. The physician reduces the dose of gentamicin to 1 mg/kg q12h and orders daily creatinine and BUN levels, as well as trough gentamicin levels after day 2. As you administer the gentamicin IVPB dose, you will monitor for what signs of toxicity? (Select all that apply.)
   a. Tinnitus
   b. Headache
   c. Dizziness
   d. Hypotension
   e. Restlessness

CASE STUDY PROGRESS

Later, as you walk past F.F.'s bed, you notice him crawling off the end of the bed.

8. What are you going to do?

CASE STUDY PROGRESS

You tell F.F. that radiology called and let him know the time the lithotripsy procedure is scheduled for the next day. He looks at you, panicked, and says, "If that doesn't work, will they do surgery? I can't do that. I don't have any insurance. This is costing me so much already."

9. How will you respond?

Case Study 60

Name _____ Class/Group _____ Date _____

Group Members _____

INSTRUCTIONS All questions apply to this case study. Your responses should be brief and to the point. When asked to provide several answers, list them in order of priority or significance. Do not assume information that is not provided. Please print or write clearly. If your response is not legible, it will be marked as ? and you will need to rewrite it.

▶ **Scenario**

N.H., an 89-year-old widow, recently experienced a left-sided cerebrovascular accident (CVA). She has right-sided weakness and expressive aphasia with minimal swallowing difficulty. N.H. has a past medical history of left-sided CVA $2^{1}/_{2}$ years ago, chronic atrial flutter, and hypertension. She has lived with her daughter's family in a rural town since her previous stroke. Since admission to an acute care facility 5 days ago, N.H. has gained some strength, has become oriented to person and place, and is anxious to begin her rehabilitation program. She is transferred for rehabilitation to your skilled nursing facility with the following orders:

■ **Chart View**

Admission Orders

- Hydrochlorothiazide (HydroDIURIL) 25 mg/day PO
- Digoxin (Lanoxin) 0.125 mg/day PO
- Aspirin (enteric coated) 81 mg/day PO
- Warfarin (Coumadin) 5 mg/day PO
- Acetaminophen (Tylenol) 325 mg q6h PO prn for pain
- Zolpidem (Ambien) 5 mg PO at bedtime prn for sleep
- Diet: mechanical soft, low sodium with ground meat
- Foley catheter to gravity drainage, and then begin bladder training
- Referrals for speech therapy, occupational therapy (OT), and physical therapy (PT) to evaluate and treat swallowing, communication, and functional abilities

1. What lab orders would you anticipate as a result of this specific list of orders? (With each response, describe your rationale.)

CASE STUDY PROGRESS

A week later, at the interdisciplinary care conferences, you report that bladder training is progressing and recommend removing the catheter if N.H.'s mobility and communication abilities have progressed sufficiently. The group and N.H. agree that she is ready for the Foley catheter to be removed.

2. Identify three problems that N.H. is at risk for developing following catheter removal, and describe specific interventions for each problem.

CASE STUDY PROGRESS

Two days after the Foley is removed, you observe that N.H.'s urine is cloudy, is concentrated, and has a strong odor.

3. What are your immediate actions?

CASE STUDY PROGRESS

N.H. is started on sulfamethoxazole 800 mg/trimethoprim 160 mg (Bactrim DS) 1 tab PO bid × 10 days. However, 2 days later, N.H. is in the bathroom, and she is very upset. She has just voided; there is blood on the toilet, and the water is bright red with blood. You help the NAP clean N.H. and help her into bed.

4. Describe your assessment steps.

5. Using SBAR, what information would you provide to the physician when you call?

6. Identify at least two potential causes for N.H.'s hematuria.

CASE STUDY PROGRESS

N.H.'s physician changes her antibiotic to oral ciprofloxacin (Cipro), discontinues the aspirin, and holds the warfarin for 2 days. Two days later, N.H.'s urinary tract infection (UTI) is responding to antibiotics, and she has had no further bleeding in the urine. You want to prepare her and her daughter for eventual discharge.

7. What specific issues must be considered in the teaching and discharge planning to prevent a recurrence of infection?

8. You talk with N.H.'s daughter about her understanding of caregiving responsibilities for her mother. What kind of questions do you ask to assess whether she is capable of taking on this additional burden?

CASE STUDY OUTCOME

N.H.'s daughter takes N.H. home and, with the help of her sister and nieces and a home-health aide, they have adjusted well to living together.

Neurologic Disorders

6

Case Study 61

Name _____ Class/Group _____ Date _____

Group Members _____

INSTRUCTIONS All questions apply to this case study. Your responses should be brief and to the point. When asked to provide several answers, list them in order of priority or significance. Do not assume information that is not provided. Please print or write clearly. If your response is not legible, it will be marked as ? and you will need to rewrite it.

▶ Scenario

M.E. is a 62-year-old woman who has a 5-year history of progressive forgetfulness. She is no longer able to care for herself, has become increasingly depressed and paranoid, and recently started a fire in the kitchen. After extensive neurologic evaluation, M.E. is diagnosed as having Alzheimer's disease. Her husband and children have come to the Alzheimer's unit at your extended care facility for information about this disease and to discuss the possibility of placement for M.E. You reassure the family that you have experience dealing with the questions and concerns of most people in their situation.

1. How would you explain Alzheimer's disease to the family?

2. The husband asks, "How did she get Alzheimer's? We don't know anyone else who has it." How would you respond?

3. After asking the family to describe M.E.'s behavior, you determine that she is in stage 2 of Alzheimer's three stages. Describe common signs and symptoms for each stage of the disease.

4. The daughter expresses frustration at the number of tests M.E. had to undergo and the length of time it took for someone to diagnose M.E.'s problem. What tests are likely to be performed, and how is Alzheimer's disease diagnosed?

CASE STUDY PROGRESS

M.E.'s husband states, "How are you going to take care of her? She wanders around all night long. She can't find her way to the bathroom in a house she's lived in for forty-three years. She can't be trusted to be alone anymore; she almost burnt the house down. We're all exhausted; there are three of us, and we can't keep up with her." You acknowledge how exhausted they must be from trying to keep her safe. You tell the family that there is no known treatment, but Alzheimer's units have been created to provide a structured, safe environment for each person.

5. Describe specific nursing interventions that are part of national patient safety initiatives aimed at minimizing the risk of harm for M.E.

6. Describe the Alzheimer's-related nursing interventions related to each of the following nursing care problems: chronic confusion, inability to perform self-hygiene, disrupted sleep pattern, impaired verbal communication, and agitation.

7. M.E.'s son asks whether there is any medication that might be prescribed to treat Alzheimer's disease. How would you respond?

Copyright © 2013 by Mosby, an affiliate of Elsevier Inc.
Copyright © 2009, 2005, 2001, 1996, by Mosby, Inc. an affiliate of Elsevier Inc. All rights reserved.

8. What other medications might be used with a patient like M.E.?

CASE STUDY PROGRESS

You try to comfort the family by telling them that the problems that they are experiencing are common. You explain that family support is a major focus of your program.

9. List four ways that M.E.'s family might receive the support they need.

Case Study **62**

Name _____ Class/Group _____ Date _____

Group Members _____

INSTRUCTIONS All questions apply to this case study. Your responses should be brief and to the point. When asked to provide several answers, list them in order of priority or significance. Do not assume information that is not provided. Please print or write clearly. If your response is not legible, it will be marked as ? and you will need to rewrite it.

▶ **Scenario**

C.B. is a single, self-supporting 58-year-old man with Guillain-Barré syndrome (GBS). He came to see his family physician in early January with symptoms of fatigue, myalgia, fever, and chills, which were accompanied by a hacking cough. He was diagnosed with viral influenza. Three weeks later, he developed bilateral weakness, numbness, and tingling of his lower extremities, which rapidly progressed into his upper body. He was brought to the emergency department after his brother recognized the seriousness of his condition. Shortly after arrival, he became totally paralyzed and required endotracheal intubation and mechanical ventilation. He was then admitted to the neurology critical care unit, where he spent 1 month. He underwent a tracheotomy before being transferred to a medical floor, where he spent several weeks. He was treated for pneumonia while hospitalized on the medical floor. His pneumonia resolved before a transfer to a skilled care facility 2 days ago for further rehabilitation and continued ventilatory support for continued neuromuscular respiratory paralysis associated with the GBS.

1. What is the etiology of GBS?

2. What type of individual is likely to be diagnosed with GBS?

3. What are the clinical manifestations of GBS?

4. Why does life-threatening respiratory dysfunction occur?

5. How is GBS diagnosed, and what tests would you expect to be performed?

6. Is the history of C.B.'s case typical?

7. What is the medical management for GBS?

8. What are the overall goals of nursing care for C.B. at this time?

9. You are concerned about the possibility of disuse syndrome related to C.B.'s paralysis. Describe an outcome of nursing care for C.B., and describe the independent nursing interventions you would implement to meet that outcome.

10. How would C.B.'s nutritional needs be maintained?

11. What evaluative parameters could you use to determine whether C.B.'s nutritional needs were being met?

12. What interventions can you implement to decrease C.B.'s fear and anxiety?

Case Study **63**

Name _____ Class/Group _____ Date _____

Group Members _____

INSTRUCTIONS All questions apply to this case study. Your responses should be brief and to the point. When asked to provide several answers, list them in order of priority or significance. Do not assume information that is not provided. Please print or write clearly. If your response is not legible, it will be marked as ? and you will need to rewrite it.

▶ **Scenario**

L.C. is a 78-year-old man with a 4-year history of Parkinson's disease (PD). He is a retired engineer, is married, and lives with his wife in a small farming community. He has four adult children who live close by. Since his last visit to the clinic 6 months ago, L.C. reports that his tremors are "about the same" as they were; however, further questioning reveals that he feels his gait is perhaps a little more unsteady, and his fatigue is slightly more noticeable. L.C. is also concerned about increased drooling. Among the medications L.C. takes are carbidopa-levodopa 25/100 mg (Sinemet), one tablet an hour before breakfast and one tablet 2 hours after lunch; carbidopa-levodopa 50/200 mg (Sinemet CR), one tablet at bedtime; and amantadine (Symmetrel) 100 mg at breakfast and bedtime. On the previous visit, he was encouraged to try taking the carbidopa-levodopa (Sinemet) more times throughout the day, but he reports that he became very somnolent with that dosing regimen. He also reports that his dyskinetic movements appear to be worse just after taking his carbidopa-levodopa (Sinemet).

1. What is parkinsonism?

2. What is PD?

3. What are the clinical manifestations of PD? Place a star next to the symptoms L.C. has mentioned.

4. L.C.'s wife asks you, "How do the doctors know L.C. has Parkinson's disease? They never did a lot of tests on him." How is the diagnosis of PD made?

5. L.C.'s wife comments, "I don't even know which one of his medicines he takes for his Parkinson's." What medications are used for PD?

6. L.C. asks, "If I don't have enough dopamine, then why don't they give me a dopamine pill?" Why can't oral dopamine be given as replacement therapy?

7. Levodopa is always given in combination with carbidopa. Why?

8. Why did L.C.'s dyskinetic movements appear to be worse just after taking his carbidopa-levodopa, and what might be done about it?

9. L.C.'s wife asks, "They can do surgery for everything else. Why can't they do surgery to fix Parkinson's?" How would you describe the surgical treatments available for patients with PD?

10. Because L.C. is reporting an increase in drooling, you are concerned about the possibility of his having developed a decreased ability to swallow. What further assessment could you perform to determine whether L.C. is at risk for aspirating?

11. What are three nutrition interventions that should be implemented in caring for L.C?

12. Because L.C. is reporting that his gait is more unsteady, there is an increased risk for falls. Which suggestion could you offer to diminish this risk?
   a. Use a wheelchair to move around.
   b. Stand erect, and use a cane to ambulate.
   c. Keep the feet close together while ambulating, and use a walker.
   d. Consciously think about walking over imaginary lines on the floor.

13. You are giving instructions to L.C. and his wife about maintaining mobility. You determine that they understand the directions if they state that L.C. will:
   a. sit in soft, deep chairs with supportive pillows.
   b. perform his daily exercises in the evening.
   c. rock back and forth to start movement when rising.
   d. buy clothes with many buttons to maintain finger dexterity.

14. As L.C.'s case manager, identify six things that you would need to assess to determine whether L.C. could be cared for in his home.

Case Study **64**

Name _____ Class/Group _____ Date _____

Group Members _____

▶ **Scenario**

N.T., a 79-year-old woman, arrived at the emergency room with expressive aphasia, left facial droop, left-sided hemiparesis, and what is presumed to be symptoms of mild dysphagia. Her husband states that when she awoke that morning at 0600, she complained of a mild headache over the right temple, was fatigued, and felt slightly weak. Thinking that it was unusual for her to have those complaints, he went to check on her and found that she was having trouble saying words and had a slight left-sided facial droop. When he helped her up from the bedside, he noticed weakness in her left hand and convinced her to come to the emergency department. Her past medical history includes paroxysmal atrial fibrillation, hypertension (HTN), hyperlipidemia, and a remote history of deep vein thrombosis. A recent cardiac stress test was normal, and her blood pressure has been well controlled. N.T. is currently taking flecainide (Tambocor), hormone replacement therapy, amlodipine (Norvasc), aspirin, simvastatin (Zocor), and lisinopril (Zestril). After a noncontrast CT scan, she is diagnosed with a thrombolytic stroke. The physician writes the following orders:

■ **Chart View**

Physician's Orders

IV 0.9% NaCl at 75 mL/hr
Activase (tPA) per protocol
STAT CBC, PT/INR, CK isoenzymes
Neurologic assessment every hour
Obtain patient weight
Vital signs every hour
Oxygen at 2 L per nasal cannula (NC)

---

1. Outline a plan of care for implementing these orders.

2. The instructions on the tPA vials read to reconstitute with 50 mL of sterile water to make a total of 50 mg/50 mL (1 mg/mL). The hospital protocol is to infuse 0.9 mg/kg over 60 minutes with 10% of the dose given as a bolus over 1 minute. N.T. weighs 143 pounds. What is the amount of the bolus dose, in both milligrams and milliliters, that you will administer in the first minute? What is the amount of the remaining dose that you will need to administer?

3. What are the three types of cerebrovascular accidents (CVAs)?

4. What role do diagnostic tests play in evaluating N.T. for a suspected CVA?

5. Explain how the type of stroke is an important factor in planning N.T.'s care.

6. Contraindications for beginning fibrinolytic therapy include: (Select all that apply.)
   a. Currently on Coumadin with an INR of 2.4
   b. Major surgery in the last 14 days
   c. Systolic BP of 150
   d. Platelet count of less than 100,000
   e. Blood glucose of less than 50 mg/dL
   f. History of myocardial infarction 1 year ago
   g. Improving neurologic status

7. What is the purpose of monitoring the CPK isoenzyme levels?

CASE STUDY PROGRESS

N.T. is admitted to the neurology unit. A second CT scan (18 hours later) reveals a small CVA in the right hemisphere. She is placed on flecainide (Tambocor), amlodipine (Norvasc), clopidogrel (Plavix), aspirin, simvastatin (Zocor), and lisinopril (Zestril).

8. If N.T.'s deficits are temporary, how long might it take before they are completely reversed?

9. While assessing N.T., you note the following findings. Which one is unrelated to the CVA?
  a. Headache
  b. Lethargy
  c. Lumbar pain
  d. Blurred vision

10. Your co-worker states, "I always heard that atrial fibrillation is a precursor to stroke." Explain whether this statement is true or false.

11. Why was N.T. placed on clopidogrel (Plavix) post-CVA?

12. Because N.T. had a thrombolytic infusion, how many hours should you wait before beginning administration of any anticoagulant or antiplatelet medications?

13. N.T. is not on hormone replacement therapy post-CVA. Why would this medication be discontinued?

14. Is there any benefit from continuing simvastatin (Zocor) after her CVA?

15. As you walk into the nurses' station, the charge nurse is talking to N.T.'s physician, who ordered a modified barium swallow study and referral for a speech-language pathologist (SLP), occupational therapist (OT), and registered dietitian (RD). Give the rationale for these orders.

6 Neurologic

16. N.T.'s BP should be well controlled. What BP level should be considered normal for her, based on the Seventh Report of the Joint National Committee on Prevention, Detection, Evaluation, and Treatment of High Blood Pressure?

Case Study **65**

Name _____ Class/Group _____ Date _____

Group Members _____

INSTRUCTIONS All questions apply to this case study. Your responses should be brief and to the point. When asked to provide several answers, list them in order of priority or significance. Do not assume information that is not provided. Please print or write clearly. If your response is not legible, it will be marked as ? and you will need to rewrite it.

▶ **Scenario**

T.H. is a 55-year-old man with an 8-month history of progressive muscle weakness. Initially, he tripped over things and seemed to drop everything. He lost interest in activities because he was always exhausted. He sought medical assistance when his speech became slurred and he started to drool. During his initial evaluation, the physician noted frequent, severe muscle cramps; muscle twitching; and inappropriate and uncontrollable periods of laughter. After a lengthy period of diagnostic tests, T.H. received the diagnosis of amyotrophic lateral sclerosis (ALS). He is upset and bewildered about this disease that he's "never even heard of." You are a home health nurse who is seeing T.H. for the first time.

1. How would you explain ALS to T.H.?

2. Who gets ALS?

3. How common is ALS?

4. T.H. has many questions. He asks you, "How long can I expect to live?" How should you respond?

5. T.H. asks, "Will I slowly lose my mind?"

6. T.H. then asks, "Are there any treatments for this?"

7. T.H. thinks a moment, then says "How is the doctor even sure this is what I have?"

8. Because ALS affects so many body systems, you will be coordinating efforts with a speech, occupational, respiratory, and physical therapist, as well as a dietitian and psychologist. Define the role that each of the following professionals will play in T.H.'s treatment.

9. You hold a family meeting to recruit adequate help for the caregiver, in this case, T.H.'s spouse. Why is this important?

10. T.H. asks you, "How will the end probably come for me?" What should you tell him?

11. T.H. wants to know whether he has to be put on a "breathing machine." What factors will you take into consideration when deciding what to tell him?

6 Neurologic

Case Study 66

Name _____ Class/Group _____ Date _____

Group Members _____

▶ **Scenario**

J.B. is a 58-year-old retired postal worker who has been on your floor for several days receiving plasmapheresis every other day for myasthenia gravis (MG). About a year ago, J.B. started experiencing difficulty chewing and swallowing, diplopia, and slurring of speech, at which time he was placed on pyridostigmine (Mestinon). Before this admission, he had been relatively stable. His medical history includes hypertension (HTN) controlled with metoprolol (Lopressor) and glaucoma treated with timolol (ophthalmic preparation). Recently, J.B. was diagnosed with a sinus infection and treated with ciprofloxacin (Cipro). On admission, J.B. was unable to bear any weight or take fluids through a straw. There have been periods of exacerbation and remission since admission.

■ **Chart View**

Vital signs	
Blood pressure	170/68 mm Hg
Heart rate	108 beats/min
Respiratory rate	24 breaths/min
Temperature	101.8° F (38.8° C)

1. You note that the nursing assistive personnel has just entered these vital signs into J.B.'s record. What is your priority action at this time?

2. What treatment do you anticipate for J.B.?

3. J.B.'s wife asks you, "What may have caused my husband to get worse, and why does he keep having these episodes?" What explanation should you give her?

4. You are visiting with J.B.'s wife, who tells you she doesn't have a lot of information about MG and she would like to know more about it so that she will feel more comfortable talking to her husband. What should you tell her?

5. J.B.'s wife asks you to explain what to expect in terms of symptoms as her husband's illness progresses. What should you tell her?

6. J.B.'s wife asks, "How do they know that my husband has MG?" What should you tell her about how MG is diagnosed?

7. J.B.'s wife asks, "What are some options for treatment of MG?" How will you explain the different treatments?

8. List four factors that could predispose J.B. to an exacerbation of his illness.

9. J.B.'s wife asks what the physicians and nurses watch for while her husband is in the hospital. How will you explain these activities?

10. J.B.'s wife wants to know when he will be able to go home. How will you respond?

6 Neurologic

11. J.B.'s wife asks you what information she will need before taking her husband home. What will you teach her?

12. J.B.'s wife asks you, "What is the difference between a cholinergic crisis and myasthenic crisis?" What explanation should you give her?

13. You teach J.B. and his wife that the most effective means of preventing myasthenic and cholinergic crises is by:
   a. eating three large, well-balanced meals.
   b. doing muscle-strengthening exercises twice a day.
   c. doing all of their errands early in the day.
   d. taking medications at the same time each day.

14. How will you know that your teaching has been effective?

15. What supportive measures can you suggest to J.B.'s wife that she can undertake or arrange on behalf of her husband?

Case Study 67

Name _____ Class/Group _____ Date _____

Group Members _____

▶ Scenario

You have been asked to see D.V., a 25-year-old man, in the neurology clinic. D.V. has been referred by his internist, who suspects him of having symptoms of multiple sclerosis (MS). D.V. has experienced increasing urinary frequency and urgency over the past 2 months. Because his female partner was treated for a sexually transmitted infection, D.V. also underwent treatment, but the symptoms did not resolve. D.V. has also recently had two brief episodes of eye "fuzziness" associated with diplopia and flashes of brightness. He has noticed ascending numbness and weakness of the right arm with the inability to hold objects over the past few days. Now he reports rapid progression of weakness in his legs.

1. MS is an inflammatory disorder of the nervous system causing scattered, patchy demyelinization of the central nervous system (CNS). What does myelin do? What is demyelinization?

2. MS is characterized by remissions and exacerbations. What happens to the myelin during each of these phases?

3. Isn't D.V. too young to get MS? What is the etiology?

4. Outline the subjective and objective assessment data that you would gather because a diagnosis of MS is suspected. Place a star next to the symptoms that D.V. has.

6 Neurologic

5. What are four common diagnostic tests you can begin to teach D.V. about, and what role will they play in determining whether D.V. has MS?

6. D.V. asks you, "If this turns out to be MS, what is the treatment?"

7. As part of your teaching plan, you want D.V. to be aware of situations or factors that are known to exacerbate symptoms. List four.

CASE STUDY PROGRESS

D.V. is diagnosed with MS. He confides in you that he has been depressed since his parents' divorce and the onset of these symptoms. He tells you that he knows his girlfriend hasn't been faithful, but he's afraid of living alone. He's afraid if he tells her about his MS diagnosis, she'll leave him.

8. What are you going to do with this information?

9. You are concerned with D.V.'s psychological status, particularly the negative feelings he expresses regarding himself and the psychosocial concerns he has voiced. Write a nursing outcome addressing this issue, and identify independent nursing actions that you would implement.

10. In view of his personal history and current diagnosis, what two critical psychosocial issues are you going to monitor in his follow-up visits?

11. List several resources available in the community that D.V. might find helpful.

CASE STUDY OUTCOME

D.V. takes advantage of his time with a psychiatric nurse specialist, joins a local MS support group, and tells his girlfriend to move out. He later marries a woman from the support group.

Case Study 68

Name _____ Class/Group _____ Date _____

Group Members _____

INSTRUCTIONS All questions apply to this case study. Your responses should be brief and to the point. When asked to provide several answers, list them in order of priority or significance. Do not assume information that is not provided. Please print or write clearly. If your response is not legible, it will be marked as ? and you will need to rewrite it.

▶ Scenario

J.G. is a 34-year-old P1G1 (para 1, gravida 1) woman who underwent an emergency cesarean delivery after a prolonged labor, during which she exhibited a sudden change in neurologic functioning and started seizing. Since that time, she has experienced three tonic-clonic (grand mal) seizures. She was diagnosed as having a basal ganglion hematoma with infarct and was started on phenytoin (Dilantin). Post-delivery, J.G. demonstrated dyskinesia, resulting in frequent falls during ambulation. Once the seizure disorder appeared to be under control, she was transferred to a rehabilitation facility for evaluation and 2 weeks of intensive physical therapy (PT). She is now home; she still has occasional falls but has had no seizures. She is receiving PT three times a week in her home. As case manager for J.G.'s health maintenance organization, you make a home visit with her and her family for evaluation of long-term, follow-up care.

1. A seizure is not a disease in itself but a symptom of a disease. What is the term for chronically recurring seizures?

2. Does J.G. have epilepsy?

3. Besides the brain injury, what are some other possible conditions that could be contributing to J.G.'s lowered seizure threshold?

4. What is the pathophysiology of a seizure?

5. J.G. had tonic-clonic, or grand mal, seizures. Describe this type of seizure. List five other types of seizures.

6. The three main phases of a seizure are the preictal, ictal, and postictal. Differentiate among the three phases, and list clinical symptoms you might observe when a patient is having a seizure.

7. Some patients know they are about to have a seizure. What is this preseizure warning called, and what form does it take?

8. List five different classifications of antiepileptic drugs or antiseizure medications, and describe a situation in which each would be expected to be used.

9. What factors are taken into consideration when determining which medication a patient should take?

10. While you are making a home visit, J.G.'s husband asks you what he should do if she has a seizure at home. What should you teach him?

11. Her husband states that he is afraid for J.G. to take care of the baby. What would you say to him?

12. J.G.'s husband tells you that his wife is not good at remembering to take medication. What are some strategies that you should review with J.G. and her husband to increase the likelihood of compliance?

13. J.G. asks, "If I get my blood level under control, will it stay at the same level as long as I take my medicine?" How would you answer her question?

14. You check the chart and note that J.G.'s last phenytoin (Dilantin) level was 14.7 mcg/mL. What action do you expect based on this level?
   a. This level places J.G. at immediate risk for a seizure and she should go to the ER.
   b. Because this level is within normal limits, J.G. would continue therapy as prescribed.
   c. Because this level is on the border of therapeutic, notify the physician.
   d. This level is dangerously high and an immediate reduction in dose is necessary.

15. J.G.'s husband asks whether the drugs could harm his wife in any way. What general information would you give them about antiseizure medications?

16. J.G. states that because she has not had a seizure since she was in the hospital, she questions how long she will have to continue taking the phenytoin (Dilantin). Which is your best response? "This medication:
   a. "will always prevent the occurrence of all seizures."
   b. "might need to be continued for the rest of your life."
   c. "will have to be taken only during periods of emotional stress."
   d. "can usually be stopped after you are seizure free for six months."

17. J.G.'s husband says, "I was watching a TV show set in a hospital last night, and they showed this guy who just kept on having a seizure. That doctor had to give him lots of medicine before he came out of it." How would you explain status epilepticus, and why is it a medical emergency?

Case Study 69

Name _____ Class/Group _____ Date _____

Group Members _____

INSTRUCTIONS All questions apply to this case study. Your responses should be brief and to the point. When asked to provide several answers, list them in order of priority or significance. Do not assume information that is not provided. Please print or write clearly. If your response is not legible, it will be marked as ? and you will need to rewrite it.

▶ Scenario

F.N. is a 57-year-old housewife, happily married with grown children and two new grandchildren. F.N. made an appointment with her optometrist to explore progressive left eye visual loss over a 9-month period. Her eye exam was essentially normal, and the optometrist referred her to a neurologist. After workup, a 2.5-cm brain mass was found, and surgery was scheduled. Her past medical history is hypertension only, for which she takes long-acting metoprolol (Toprol XL) 100 mg/day. Her past surgical history includes tonsillectomy and adenoidectomy as a child, cholecystectomy, and a total abdominal hysterectomy at age 42. She also takes a conjugated estrogen (Premarin) 0.625 mg/day.

1. Name one test that can be done to evaluate for a brain tumor.

2. Using the term *benign* when discussing brain tumors is somewhat misleading. Why?

3. Onset of neurologic symptoms is usually insidious, and patients exhibit symptoms in relation to the area of the brain where the tumor is located. List six general symptoms associated with many brain tumors that F.N. might exhibit.

4. Once the diagnosis is made, F.N. and her family must be involved in the plan for treatment. Treatment depends on the type, grade, and location of the tumor and can include surgery, radiation, chemotherapy, or any combination of these. F.N. also has the right to refuse treatment. Identify four other factors that the medical team, F.N., and her family would consider in devising a treatment plan.

5. Corticosteroids, such as dexamethasone (Decadron) or methylprednisolone (Solu-Medrol), are commonly prescribed when a tumor is diagnosed and the presence of increased intracranial pressure (ICP) is demonstrated. Because F.N. is showing symptoms of ICP, she is immediately placed on dexamethasone (Decadron) 40 mg orally twice daily. What is the expected goal of therapy in using dexamethasone (Decadron), and why should it not be abruptly stopped?

6. Other common supportive medications include antiepileptics, diuretics (including osmotic diuretics), H2 blockers, analgesics, antiemetics, and antidepressants. What is the expected outcome associated with using each of these medications?

7. Describe common psychological responses to a diagnosis of a brain tumor.

8. F.N. draws up a living will and health care power of attorney after she hears the diagnosis. She also sits down with her family and makes her wishes known. Why is this important for F.N., in particular, and for everyone in general?

9. You enter F.N.'s room to take vital signs, and she says, "What if I come out of surgery and I'm different? Or what if I die? My grandbabies will never know me." You hear the concern in her voice and want to provide realistic reassurance about expected outcomes. Suggest several ways that F.N. can communicate with her loved ones in the event that her surgery is unsuccessful.

CASE STUDY PROGRESS

F.N. has a craniotomy and is admitted to ICU postoperatively. She does very well and remains neurologically intact. She has two peripheral IVs, TED hose, oxygen at 4 L by nasal cannula, and a Foley catheter.

■ Chart View

Vital Signs

Heart rate	88 beats/min
Blood pressure	147/68 mm Hg
Respiratory rate	18 breaths/min

Laboratory Testing

Potassium	2.7 mmol/L
Glucose	202 mg/dL

10. As part of conducting a neurologic assessment, the nurse evaluates F.N.'s score on the Glasgow Coma Scale and determines that her score is a 15. What does the nurse evaluate to assess the client's score on the Glasgow Coma Scale? (Select all that apply.)
   a. Ability of the client's pupils to react to light
   b. Degree of purposeful movement by the client
   c. Appropriateness of the client's verbal responses
   d. Stimulus necessary to cause the client's eyes to open
   e. Symmetry of muscle strength of the client's extremities
   f. Appropriateness of thought processes

11. Evaluate the status of F.N.'s potassium and glucose values and identify what, if any, treatment is needed.

12. While caring for F.N., which of these care activities can be safely delegated to a nursing assistive personnel (NAP)? (Select all that apply.)
   a. Performing a capillary blood sugar measurement
   b. Positioning and turning F.N. every 2 hours
   c. Counseling F.N. on pain control measures as needed
   d. Assessing F.N.'s status on the Glasgow Coma Scale
   e. Emptying the Foley catheter collection bag
   f. Monitoring F.N.'s serum potassium levels

CASE STUDY OUTCOME

F.N. did suffer mild neurologic damage as a result of the surgery. She was discharged to a rehabilitation facility and eventually recovered most of her lost function. She continues to enjoy an active life and has become involved in helping others face similar experiences.

Case Study 70

Name _____ Class/Group _____ Date _____

Group Members _____

INSTRUCTIONS All questions apply to this case study. Your responses should be brief and to the point. When asked to provide several answers, list them in order of priority or significance. Do not assume information that is not provided. Please print or write clearly. If your response is not legible, it will be marked as ? and you will need to rewrite it.

▶ **Scenario**

T.W. is a 22-year-old man who fell 50 feet from a chairlift while skiing and landed on hard-packed snow. He is now at the emergency department (ED) with a suspected T5-T6 fracture with paraplegia.

Chart View

Physician's Orders

  Insert Foley catheter
  ECG monitoring
  Immobilize the cervical spine
  Oxygen at 4 L per nasal cannula
  Initiate two large bore IVs
  Neurologic assessment every hour
  Apply warming blankets as needed

---

1. Describe a plan for implementing these physician's orders.

2. What other interventions might be done by the ED nurse?

3. Awareness of the prehospital management of an SCI is critical to each patient's ultimate neurologic outcome. What actions will the nurse take to ensure this goal is met?

4. The physician orders the following for T.W.: IV methylprednisolone (Solu-Medrol), bolus of 30 mg/kg over 15 minutes, followed by a maintenance infusion of 5.4 mg/kg body weight/hr. T.W. weighs 176 pounds. How many milligrams of methylprednisolone (Solu-Medrol) will T.W. receive with the bolus? How many milligrams per hour will T.W. receive with the maintenance infusion? What effect will this medication have on T.W.?

CASE STUDY PROGRESS

The diagnosis of the fracture is confirmed and T.W. is transferred from the ED to the SICU. Although T.W.'s injury is at a level where independent respiratory function is expected, he experiences low oxygen saturation levels and is placed on a mechanical ventilator. The physician states that this is due to spinal shock.

5. How would you explain spinal shock to T.W.'s family and why T.W. requires mechanical ventilation at this time?

6. List three critical potential infections that T.W. will be monitored for throughout his hospitalization.

CASE STUDY PROGRESS

T.W. was taken to surgery 48 hours after the accident for spinal stabilization. He spent 2 additional days in the SICU and 5 days in the neurology unit and now is ready to be transferred to your rehabilitation unit. He continues to have no movement of his lower extremities.

7. Rehabilitation teaching includes teaching T.W. how to manage his urinary drainage system (UDS). What would this teaching include?

8. T.W. is taking vitamin C 2 g orally four times daily. What is the purpose of this and what other nursing actions should accompany vitamin C therapy?

9. What outcome parameters would you use to determine whether your efforts in regards to promoting urinary excretion have been effective?

10. The large bowel musculature has its own neural center that can directly respond to distention caused by fecal material. This is what allows most SCI patients to regain bowel control. What dietary instructions are important for T.W.?

11. T.W. should also be taught bowel training techniques. What would this teaching include?

12. What medications can assist with a bowel program?

13. Describe digital stimulation.

14. T.W. asks you whether he'll ever be able to have sex again. What do you tell him, and what are some possible referrals?

15. You request a consultation with a registered dietitian because you realize that T.W. has special dietary needs. Describe an optimal diet for T.W.

CASE STUDY PROGRESS

T.W. turns on his call light and asks for medication for headache. As you walk into the room, you immediately note that T.W.'s face is flushed. You suspect that T.W. might be experiencing autonomic dysreflexia (AD).

16. What further assessment data do you need to collect?

17. What is AD, and what are its potential causes?

18. What interventions do you need to perform for a patient with AD?

19. AD is a medical emergency. What could happen if it is left untreated?

20. Consider a hierarchy of rehabilitation needs for patients such as T.W. Number the following options from highest (1) to lowest (8) priority as they apply to T.W.
a. Community integration
b. Gainful employment
c. Accomplishment of self-care and ADL
d. Self-actualization
e. Stabilization of the physiologic systems and early psychological support
f. Adjustment to living at home
g. Participation of physical therapy, occupational therapy, and social worker; use of assistive devices; bowel and bladder training
h. Independence

Case Study **71**

Name _____ Class/Group _____ Date _____

Group Members _____

INSTRUCTIONS All questions apply to this case study. Your responses should be brief and to the point. When asked to provide several answers, list them in order of priority or significance. Do not assume information that is not provided. Please print or write clearly. If your response is not legible, it will be marked as ? and you will need to rewrite it.

▶ Scenario

Y.W. is a 23-year-old male student from Thailand studying electrical engineering at the university. He was ejected from a moving vehicle, which was traveling 70 mph. His injuries included a severe closed head injury with an occipital hematoma, bilateral wrist fractures, and a right pneumothorax. During his neurologic intensive care unit (NICU) stay, Y.W. was intubated and placed on mechanical ventilation, had a feeding tube inserted and was placed on tube feedings, had a Foley catheter placed, and a central venous catheter (CVC) inserted. He developed pneumonia 1 week after admission.

1. Define the term *primary head injury.*

2. Define the term *secondary head injury.*

3. What is normal ICP, and why is increased ICP so clinically important?

4. Identify at least five signs and symptoms of increased ICP.

5. List four medication classifications that the NICU nurses could use to decrease or control increased ICP, and describe the primary action of each.

6 Neurologic

6. List eight independent nursing measures and the rationale for the use of each that the NICU nurses could use to decrease or control increased ICP.

7. What outcome criteria would you use to determine whether the independent nursing measures you chose for Y.W. were effective?

8. Y.W.'s medication list includes clindamycin (Cleocin) 150 mg IV q6h, ranitidine (Zantac elixir) 150 mg per PEG tube bid, and phenytoin (Dilantin) 100 mg per PEG tube tid. Indicate the reason Y.W. is receiving each medication.

9. The pharmacy supplies phenytoin (Dilantin) 125 mg per 5 mL. How many milliliters will you administer to correctly fulfill the order of 100 mg per dose?

10. You are preparing to administer Y.W.'s medications through his PEG tube. To safely administer the medications, you will perform which actions? (Select all that apply.)
    a. Position Y.W. in a side-lying position with the HOB flat.
    b. Temporarily stop the feeding while administering the medications.
    c. Flush the PEG tube with water after medication administration.
    d. Hold the tube feeding for 2 hours after administering the medication.
    e. Place the medications into the feeding bag with his tube feed formula.
    f. Aspirate for gastric residual before administering the medications.

11. A STAT portable chest x-ray (CXR) was ordered after Y.W.'s CVC was inserted. According to hospital protocol, no one is permitted to infuse anything through the catheter until the CXR has been read by the physician or radiologist. What is the purpose of the CXR, and why isn't fluid infused through the CVC until after the CXR is read?

CASE STUDY PROGRESS

Y.W. spent 2 months in acute care and is now on your rehabilitation unit. He follows commands but tends to get agitated with too much stimulation. His tracheostomy site is well healed, and the pneumonia is finally resolving. He is receiving a supplemental tube feeding and has some continued incontinence of both bowel and bladder. Y.W. has a supportive group of friends who are students at the university; several of them are also from Thailand. Y.W.'s latest lab results are as follows:

■ Chart View

Laboratory Test Results

Sodium	149 mmol/L
Potassium	4.2 mmol/L
Chloride	119 mmol/L
Total CO_2	21 mmol/L
BUN	12 mg/dL
Creatinine	1.2 mg/dL
Glucose	133 mg/dL
WBC	15,400/mm^3
Hgb	14.9 g/dL
Hct	36.4%
Platelets	140,000/mm^3

12. Are any of these of concern to you, and what actions would you suggest to correct them?

13. Are you surprised by Y.W.'s agitated behavior? Explain.

14. Outline a general rehabilitation plan for Y.W., based on the previous data.

15. Y.W.'s mother has just arrived in the United States and speaks no English. What measures can be taken to facilitate communication between medical personnel and the mother?

16. Y.W.'s mother will need a place to stay while in the United States. What can you do to facilitate the initial contact with the Thai community?

17. What special discharge planning considerations are there, in this case?

Case Study **72**

Name _____ Class/Group _____ Date _____

Group Members _____

INSTRUCTIONS All questions apply to this case study. Your responses should be brief and to the point. When asked to provide several answers, list them in order of priority or significance. Do not assume information that is not provided. Please print or write clearly. If your response is not legible, it will be marked as ? and you will need to rewrite it.

▶ **Scenario**

K.B. is a 21-year-old man with a past medical history (PMH) of seizure disorder controlled with carbamaze-pine (Tegretol). He was accidentally struck in the head by a pitched baseball while batting in a baseball game. He was unconscious momentarily, about 5 seconds, then awakened and was alert and responsive. After a few hours, K.B. returned home with complaints of a "splitting" headache, drowsiness, slight confusion, and some nausea. K.B. was taken to the local hospital emergency department (ED), where a CT scan revealed a left subdural hematoma. He has been transferred to your medical center, which has a neuro-surgeon on call.

1. The ED RN gives you the previous information during a phoned report. What other information do you need to prepare for K.B.?

2. Because you have not taken care of a patient with a head injury recently, you look up subdural hematoma before K.B. arrives. What do you find?

3. Draw a shaded oval in the area where a subdural hematoma occurs.

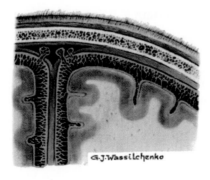

G.J.Wassilchenko

6 Neurologic

4. K.B.'s subdural hematoma is considered acute because symptoms appeared within 24 to 48 hours of injury. What are the other two classifications of subdural hematomas?

5. What are common signs and symptoms (S/S) of an acute subdural hematoma?

6. Why are older patients and alcoholic patients at risk for chronic subdural hematomas?

7. What neurologic changes and indicators would you monitor in K.B. for increased ICP?

8. Why is it important to make certain K.B. is taking his carbamazepine (Tegretol) and has a therapeutic serum level?

9. The decision was made in K.B.'s case not to do a craniotomy. When would a neurosurgeon decide to treat medically versus perform surgery?

10. The resident writes an order for D5W to infuse intravenously at 125 mL/hr. Does this order concern you and, if so, why?

11. How would you instruct the NAP to position K.B. in bed to help control ICP?

12. What other interventions would be appropriate to implement while caring for K.B. that would assist in reducing venous volume?

13. You go in to assess K.B. and find that he is complaining of a headache. His heart rate is 120 and his BP is 90/60. His urine output for the past hour was 685 mL with a specific gravity of 1.002. What do you immediately suspect is occurring?

14. Using SBAR, what information would you provide to the neurosurgeon when you call?

15. What do you anticipate your care of K.B. will include over the next 2-3 hours?

6 Neurologic

16. How would you support the family?

6 Neurologic

Case Study 73

Name _____ Class/Group _____ Date _____

Group Members _____

INSTRUCTIONS All questions apply to this case study. Your responses should be brief and to the point. When asked to provide several answers, list them in order of priority or significance. Do not assume information that is not provided. Please print or write clearly. If your response is not legible, it will be marked as ? and you will need to rewrite it.

▶ **Scenario**

C.J. is a 32-year-old concert pianist. Before her performance this evening, she told a friend that she was experiencing what she called "the worst headache I've ever had" and that she had taken two extra-strength acetaminophen (Tylenol ES), but they "did not touch her headache." During her performance, she stopped playing, reached up, grasped her head, then fell unconscious. When the paramedics arrived, she was intubated and an IV was started with normal saline.

On arrival to the emergency department, she has a Glasgow Coma Scale score of 3. Her husband reports a history of hypertension and states she recently quit taking her medication because it made her feel tired. She is trying to quit smoking; she has cut down to a half pack of cigarettes per day, she drinks alcohol only socially on weekends, and she has a remote history of cocaine use. He says that she has complained of worsening, intermittent headaches for the past few weeks.

1. What is the Glasgow Coma Scale?

2. What is a subarachnoid hemorrhage (SAH)?

3. What are the causes of an SAH?

4. What are C.J.'s risk factors for SAH?

5. How is the diagnosis of SAH made?

6. How are SAHs graded?

7. What kinds of aneurysms cause SAH?

8. What is the recommended treatment for SAH?

9. What are the main complications associated with SAH?

10. Identify the treatment given after SAH to prevent the previously described complications.

11. What considerations should be made for patients with SAH?

CASE STUDY PROGRESS

After a CT scan is done on C.J., the diagnosis of SAH is made and she is transported to the ICU and closely monitored. She is ventilator dependent, unresponsive to verbal or painful stimuli, and has no physical movement. Her husband has remained at her bedside. After C.J. has been in the ICU for 24 hours without a change in her condition, the physician decides to begin testing C.J. to determine whether she is clinically brain dead.

12. What is brain death, and what are the criteria for declaring a patient clinically brain dead?

13. It was determined that C.J.'s condition met the criteria and she was declared legally brain dead. She had previously indicated her willingness to be an organ donor and her husband has agreed to honor her wishes. He asks about the donation process. How will you explain it to him?

Case Study 74

Name _____ Class/Group _____ Date _____

Group Members _____

INSTRUCTIONS All questions apply to this case study. Your responses should be brief and to the point. When asked to provide several answers, list them in order of priority or significance. Do not assume information that is not provided. Please print or write clearly. If your response is not legible, it will be marked as ? and you will need to rewrite it.

▶ Scenario

D.H., a 54-year-old resort owner, has had multiple chronic medical problems, including type 2 diabetes mellitus (DM) for 25 years, which has progressed to insulin-dependent DM for the past 10 years; a kidney transplant 5 years ago with no signs of rejection at last biopsy; hypertension (HTN); and remote peptic ulcer disease (PUD). His medications include insulin, immunosuppressive agents, and two antihypertensive drugs. He visited his local physician with complaints of left ear, mastoid, and sinus pain. He was diagnosed with sinusitis and *Candida albicans* infection (thrush); cephalexin (Keflex) and nystatin were prescribed. Later that evening he developed nausea, hematemesis, and weakness and was taken to the emergency department. He was admitted and started on IV antibiotics, but his condition worsened throughout the night; his dyspnea increased and he developed difficulty speaking. He was flown to your tertiary referral center and was intubated en route. On arrival, D.H. had decreased level of consciousness (LOC) with periods of total unresponsiveness, weakness, and cranial nerve deficits. His diagnosis is meningitis complicated by an aspiration pneumonia and atrial fibrillation. D.H. has continued fever and leukocytosis despite aggressive antibiotic therapy.

1. Why was D.H. at particular risk for infection?

2. Describe bacterial meningitis.

3. What is the probable route of entry of bacteria into D.H.'s brain?

4. When D.H. was admitted, the nurse charted that he could not extend his legs without complaining of extreme pain. This sign of meningitis could have been charted as a positive:
   a. Kernig's sign
   b. Trousseau's sign
   c. Babinski's sign
   d. Brudzinski's sign

5. How do you think D.H. might have developed aspiration pneumonia?

6. What factors influenced the physician's decision to transport D.H. from a smaller hospital to a tertiary referral center?

7. Name four diagnostic tests that are used in patients with suspected meningitis.

8. What type of transmission-based precautions need to be instituted for D.H.? (Select all that apply.)
   a. Placing D.H. in a private room if possible
   b. Wearing a gown for all patient contacts
   c. Wearing a respirator each time upon entering the room
   d. Placing D.H. in a room with negative airflow pressure
   e. Wearing a surgical mask each time upon entering the room
   f. Wearing gloves during contact with oral secretions

6 Neurologic

■ Chart View

Medication Administration Record

NPH 20 units bid
NovoLog per sliding scale ac/hs
Digoxin 0.125 mg IVP daily
Sucralfate (Carafate) 1 g PO q6h
Azathioprine (Imuran) 100 mg daily IVPB in 150 mL D5W
Imipenem–cilastatin sodium (Primaxin) 1 g IVPB q8h in 100 mL 0.9% NaCl
Metronidazole (Flagyl) 500 mg IVPB q6h in 75 mL 0.9% NaCl
Methylprednisolone (Solu-Medrol) 125 mg IVP q8h in 75 mL 0.9% NaCl

9. Indicate the expected outcome for D.H. that is associated with each of the medications he is receiving.

10. The order for the imipenem-cilastatin sodium (Primaxin) reads to infuse 1 g in 100 mL 0.9% NaCl q8h over 30 minutes. You have IV tubing which supplies 15 gtt/mL. At how many gtt/min will you regulate the infusion?

11. When evaluating D.H.'s expected fluid intake over the next 24 hours, you would expect him to receive how many total milliliters from the administration of intravenous piggybacks?

12. The NAP reports to you that D.H. has a glucose result of 450 mg/dL. Identify two factors that could contribute to D.H.'s elevated glucose level.

13. What should you do regarding the elevated glucose level, and why?

14. Outline the nursing management of D.H.'s current problems related to his risks for infection, seizures, increased intracranial pressure, hypovolemia, and acute pain.

15. List six interventions to perform to prevent complications.

16. D.H.'s family is staying at a nearby motel. His adult son brings his mother to the hospital. Mrs. H. says she just wants to stay with her husband around the clock. She states, "I took care of him for 35 years now, and I'm not going to abandon him now when he needs me the most." Recognizing that these are stressful times for all individuals involved, how will you respond?

CASE STUDY PROGRESS

D.H.'s infection destroyed his cadaver kidney. He developed multiple system organ failure and died 7 weeks later.

Case Study 75

Name _____ Class/Group _____ Date _____

Group Members _____

INSTRUCTIONS All questions apply to this case study. Your responses should be brief and to the point. When asked to provide several answers, list them in order of priority or significance. Do not assume information that is not provided. Please print or write clearly. If your response is not legible, it will be marked as ? and you will need to rewrite it.

▶ Scenario

S.B. is a 17-year-old man who lost control of his sport utility vehicle and struck a tree. Witnesses reported he was not restrained, and his face hit the windshield on impact. When paramedics arrived, S.B. was responsive but confused, had significant facial swelling, and complained of pain in his right wrist and left forearm. The paramedics initiated cervical spine precautions, strapped him to a backboard, started oxygen at 15 L/min via a nonrebreather mask, and started a 16-gauge IV with 0.9% normal saline. His vital signs were 120/75, 125, 36, and Sao_2 94%. On arrival to the local emergency department (ED) 5 minutes later, his VS were 110/62, 110 regular, 28 to 32 and shallow, and Sao_2 99%. An additional 16-gauge IV was inserted and the following labs were drawn: CBC, type and crossmatch, complete metabolic panel, PT/PTT INR, and alcohol level. The trauma physician completed a head-to-toe assessment and found the following:

■ Chart View

Physician Note

Obeys commands, responds to voice but not oriented to time or place. Generalized facial edema with full-thickness 2-cm cheek laceration and bilateral mandibular depressed fractures. Blood behind left tympanic membrane, edema with slight discoloration over left mastoid process. Clear drainage coming from the left nare. Mid to upper chest contusions without crepitus, breath sounds clear. Abdomen slightly firm but not tender. Catheterized for 500 mL clear yellow urine; negative for blood, glucose, ketones. Positive deformity of right wrist and diffuse tenderness of left lower forearm.

1. What is the significance of the slight discoloration over the left mastoid process, blood behind the left tympanic membrane, and drainage from the nose?

2. What are the typical signs and symptoms (S/S) of a basilar skull fracture (BSF)? Place a star or asterisk next to those that S.B. has.

3. What physical condition does this picture depict, and why is it a significant finding in a patient with a BSF?

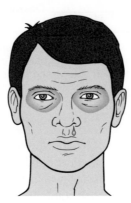

4. S.B.'s skull x-ray study was negative for BSF. How significant is this finding?

5. What is the most reliable diagnostic indicator for BSF?

6. Identify three complications associated with BSF. Which is the most serious?

7. How would you test S.B. for evidence of cerebrospinal fluid (CSF) leakage?

8. What are the symptoms of a posterior fossa fracture (fracture of temporal petrous bone), and how does it compare to a BSF?

9. Because S.B. is suspected of having a BSF, why would you avoid placing a nasogastric tube in S.B.?

10. What is the treatment strategy for a BSF with a limited CSF leak?

11. S.B. remained in the hospital for 48 hours for observation before being discharged. As you are evaluating the discharge teaching for S.B., you would understand that further teaching would be required if he stated:
   a. "I will try to avoid blowing my nose for the next two weeks."
   b. "If I start vomiting, I will return to the hospital immediately."
   c. "Since a headache is expected, I can take aspirin for the pain."
   d. "If I do not move my bowels each day, I will take a Dulcolax."

Endocrine Disorders

Case Study 76

Name_____ Class/Group_____ Date_____

Group Members _____

INSTRUCTIONS All questions apply to this case study. Your responses should be brief and to the point. When asked to provide several answers, list them in order of priority or significance. Do not assume information that is not provided. Please print or write clearly. If your response is not legible, it will be marked as ? and you will need to rewrite it.

▶ Scenario

Y.L., a 34-year-old Asian woman, comes to the clinic with complaints of chronic fatigue, increased thirst, constant hunger, and frequent urination. She denies any pain, burning, or low-back pain on urination. She tells you she has a vaginal yeast infection that she has treated numerous times with over-the-counter medication. She works full time as a clerk in a loan company and states she has difficulty reading numbers and reports, resulting in her making frequent mistakes. She says, "By the time I get home and make supper for my family, then put my child to bed, I am too tired to exercise." She reports her feet hurt; they often "burn or feel like there are pins in them." She has a history of gestational diabetes and reports that, after her delivery, she went back to her traditional eating pattern, which is high in carbohydrates.

In reviewing Y.L.'s chart, you notice she has not been seen since the delivery of her child 6 years ago. She has gained considerable weight; her current weight is 173 pounds. Today, her BP is 152/97 mm Hg, and a random plasma glucose is 291 mg/dL. The primary care provider suspects that Y.L. has developed type 2 diabetes mellitus (DM) and orders the following laboratory studies:

■ Chart View

Laboratory Test Results

Fasting glucose	184 mg/dL
HbA1C	8.8%
Total cholesterol	256 mg/dL
Triglycerides	346 mg/dL
LDL	155 mg/dL
HDL	32 mg/dL
UA	+glucose, −ketones

1. Interpret Y.L.'s laboratory results.

2. Identify the three methods used to diagnose DM.

3. Identify three functions of insulin.

4. Describe the major pathophysiologic difference between type 1 and type 2 DM.

5. What are the risk factors for type 2 DM? Place a star or asterisk next to those that Y.L. exhibits.

CASE STUDY PROGRESS

Y.L. is diagnosed with type 2 DM. The PCP starts her on metformin (Glucophage) 500 mg and glipizide (Glucotrol) 5 mg orally each day at breakfast and atorvastatin (Lipitor) 20 mg orally at bedtime. She is referred to the dietitian for instructions on starting a 1200-calorie diet using an exchange system to facilitate weight loss and lower blood glucose, cholesterol, and triglyceride levels. You are to provide education regarding pharmacotherapy and exercise.

6. What is the rationale for starting Y.L. on metformin (Glucophage) and glipizide (Glucotrol)?

7. What teaching do you need to provide to Y.L. regarding oral hypoglycemic therapy?

8. What potential benefits could Y.L. receive from encouragement to exercise?

CASE STUDY PROGRESS

Y.L. comments, "I've heard many people with diabetes can lose their toes or even their feet." You take this opportunity to teach her about neuropathy and foot care.

9. Which of the symptoms that Y.L. reported today led you to believe she has some form of neuropathy?

10. What findings in Y.L.'s history place her at increased risk for the development of other forms of neuropathy?

11. How would you educate Y.L. about neuropathy?

12. Because Y.L. already has symptoms of neuropathy, placing her at risk for foot complications, you realize you need to instruct her on proper foot care. Outline what you will include when teaching her about proper diabetic foot care.

13. What are some changes that Y.L. can make to reduce the risk or slow the progression of both macrovascular and microvascular disease?

14. Given all of the information in the foregoing scenario, what DM-related complication do you believe Y.L. is most at risk for, and why?

15. What monitoring will be needed for Y.L. in regards to nephropathy and retinopathy?

Case Study 77

Name_____ Class/Group _____ Date _____

Group Members _____

INSTRUCTIONS All questions apply to this case study. Your responses should be brief and to the point. When asked to provide several answers, list them in order of priority or significance. Do not assume information that is not provided. Please print or write clearly. If your response is not legible, it will be marked as ? and you will need to rewrite it.

▶ Scenario

You graduated 3 months ago and are working with a home care agency. Included in your caseload is J.S., a 60-year-old man suffering from chronic obstructive pulmonary disease (COPD) related to cigarette smoking. He has been on home oxygen, 2 L oxygen by nasal cannula (O_2/NC), for several years. Approximately 10 months ago, he was started on chronic oral steroid therapy. His current medications include an ipratropium-albuterol (Combivent) inhaler, beclamethasone (Beclovent) inhaler, dexamethasone (Decadron), digoxin (Lanoxin), and furosemide (Lasix). On the way to J.S.'s home, you make a mental note to check him for signs and symptoms of infection and Cushing's syndrome.

1. Differentiate between Cushing's syndrome and Cushing's disease.

2. Your assessment includes the following findings. Determine whether the findings are attributable to J.S.'s COPD or possible Cushing's syndrome. Place an "L" beside the symptoms consistent with COPD and a "C" next to those consistent with Cushing's syndrome.
   ___1. Barrel chest
   ___2. Full-looking face ("moon face")
   ___3. BP 180/94 mm Hg
   ___4. Pursed-lip breathing, especially when patient is stressed
   ___5. Striae over trunk and thighs
   ___6. Bruising on both arms
   ___7. Acne
   ___8. Diminished breath sounds throughout lungs
   ___9. Truncal obesity with supraclavicular and posterior upper back fat and thin extremities

3. You inform the physician of J.S.'s assessment. The physician believes J.S. has developed Cushing's syndrome and decides to change his prescription from dexamethasone (Decadron) to prednisone (Deltasone) given on alternate days. Explain the rationale for this change.

7 Endocrine

4. Identify possible consequences of suddenly stopping the dexamethasone (Decadron) therapy.

5. Cushing's syndrome can affect memory. Patients can easily forget what medications have been taken, especially when there are several different drugs and some are taken on alternating days. List at least three ways you can help J.S. remember to take his pills as prescribed.

6. J.S. states that his appetite has increased but he is losing weight. He reports trying to eat, but he gets short of breath and cannot eat any more. How would you address this problem?

7. You advise J.S. to take his prednisone (Deltasone) in the morning with food. You ask him a series of questions related to possible gastric discomfort, vision, and joint pain. Discuss the rationale for your line of questioning.

8. Differentiate between the glucocorticoid and mineralocorticoid effects of prednisone (Deltasone).

9. How would your assessment change if J.S. were taking a glucocorticoid that also has significant mineralocorticoid activity?

10. Review J.S.'s list of medications. Based on what you know about the side effects of loop diuretics and steroids, discuss the potential problem of administering these in combination with digoxin.

11. Realizing that patients like J.S. are susceptible to all types of infections, you write guidelines to reduce the risk of infection. Identify four major points that these guidelines will include.

12. Besides measures to reduce the risk of infection, what other information would you want to stress to J.S. at your visit? (Select all that apply.)
   a. Weigh yourself first thing in the morning.
   b. Call the doctor if your weight increases more than 5 lb in 1 day.
   c. Increase intake of foods high in sodium.
   d. Notify the physician if your pulse is lower than 60 beats/min.
   e. Take the furosemide (Lasix) first thing in the morning and again at bedtime.
   f. Drink at least 2500 mL of fluids daily.
   g. Take vitamin and electrolyte supplements as prescribed.

7 Endocrine

Case Study **78**

Name _____ Class/Group _____ Date _____

Group Members _____

INSTRUCTIONS All questions apply to this case study. Your responses should be brief and to the point. When asked to provide several answers, list them in order of priority or significance. Do not assume information that is not provided. Please print or write clearly. If your response is not legible, it will be marked as ? and you will need to rewrite it.

▶ Scenario

You are working in a community outpatient clinic where you perform the intake assessment on R.M., a 38-year-old woman who is attending graduate school and is very sedentary. Her chief complaint is overwhelming fatigue that is not relieved by rest. She is so exhausted that she has difficulty walking to classes and trouble concentrating when studying. She reports a recent weight gain of 15 pounds over 2 months without clear changes in her dietary habits. Her face looks puffy, she has experienced excessive hair loss, and her skin is dry and pale. She complains of generalized body aches and pains with frequent muscle cramps and constipation. You notice she is dressed inappropriately warm for the weather.

■ Chart View

Vital Signs	
Blood pressure	142/84 mm Hg
Heart rate	52 beats/min
Respiratory rate	12 breaths/min
Temperature	96.8° F (36° C)

1. Compare her VS with those of a healthy person at her same age.

2. List eight general questions you might ask R.M. to assist in determining what is going on with her.

3. You know that potential causes for some of R.M.'s symptoms include depression, hypothyroidism, anemia, cardiac disease, fluid and electrolyte imbalance, and allergies. As part of your screening procedures, describe how you would begin to investigate which of these conditions probably do not account for R.M.'s symptoms.

4. Unnecessary diagnostic tests are expensive. What tests do you think would be the most appropriate for R.M., and why?

■ Chart View

Laboratory Test Results	
TSH	20.9 mU/L (2-10 mU/L)
TRH	18.8 ng/dL (2-10 ng/dL)
T_3	24 mU/L (70-205 ng/dL)
Free T_4	0.2 ng/dL (0.8-2.4 ng/dL)

5. Interpret R.M.'s laboratory results.

6. The family practitioner affirms a diagnosis of hypothyroidism. With this diagnosis, what other signs and symptoms would you want to investigate?

7. The family practitioner prescribes levothyroxine (Synthroid) 1.7 mcg/kg body weight/day. At this time, R.M. weighs 130 pounds. What should be her daily dose of levothyroxine in milligrams? How would her prescription read?

8. Why would you want to obtain a complete drug history on R.M.?

9. What general teaching issues will you address with R.M. in regard to hypothyroidism?

10. What teaching needs will you review with R.M. in regards to her medication?

11. R.M. wonders whether she should take iodine supplements if she decreases her salt intake. She recognizes that salt is a significant source of iodine in her part of the country. What would you explain to her?

7 Endocrine

12. What should you teach R.M. regarding prevention of myxedema coma?

13. Before R.M. leaves the clinic, she asks how she will know whether the medication is "doing its job." Outline simple expected outcomes for R.M.

14. Several weeks later, R.M. calls the clinic stating she can't remember whether she took her thyroid medication. What additional data should you obtain, and how would you advise her?

CASE STUDY OUTCOME

R.M. comes in 2 months later for a follow-up visit. You can't believe she is the same person. She looks and walks as if she were 10 years younger. Her skin appears more radiant, and her hair looks much healthier. "You can't believe how different I'm feeling," she says. "I didn't know how bad off I was; I'm starting to live again."

Case Study 79

Name _____ Class/Group _____ Date _____

Group Members _____

▶ Scenario

K.B. is a 65-year-old man admitted to the hospital following a 5-day episode of the "flu" with complaints of dyspnea on exertion, palpitations, chest pain, insomnia, and fatigue. His past medical history includes heart failure and hypertension requiring antihypertensive medications; however, he states that he has not been taking these medications on a regular basis. K.B. was diagnosed with Graves' disease 6 months ago and placed on methimazole (Tapazole) 15 mg/day. Assessment findings are as follows: height 5 feet 8 inches, weight 132 pounds; appears anxious and restless; loud heart sounds; vital signs (VS): 150/90, 124 irregular, 20, 100.2° F (37.9°C); 1+ pitting edema noted in bilateral lower extremities; diminished breath sounds with fine crackles in the posterior bases. K.B. begins to cry when he tells you he recently lost his wife; you notice someone has punched several more holes in his belt so he could tighten it.

■ Chart View

Laboratory Test Results

Hgb	11.8 g/dL
Hct	36%
ESR	48 mm/hr
Sodium	141 mmol/L
Potassium	4.7 mmol/L
Chloride	101 mmol/L
BUN	33 mg/dL
Creatinine	1.9 mg/dL
Free T_4	14.0 ng/dL
T_3	230 ng/dL

1. Which of K.B.'s assessment findings represent manifestations of hypermetabolism?

2. Interpret K.B.'s laboratory results.

3. What additional subjective and objective data would you gather from someone with Graves' disease?

■ Chart View

Physician's Orders

> Propranolol (Inderal) 20 mg PO q6h
> Dexamethasone (Decadron) 10 mg IV q6h
> Verapamil (Calan SR) 120 mg/day PO
> Furosemide (Lasix) 80 mg IV push now, then 40 mg/day IVP
> Diet as tolerated
> STAT ECG and echocardiogram
> Up ad lib
> IV of D5W at 125 mL/hr
> Daily weights with I&O

4. After morning rounds, the physician leaves these orders. Which will you question, and why?

5. Develop four priority problems related to K.B.'s care.

6. Later on your shift, you note that K.B. is extremely restless and is disoriented to person, place, and time. VS are 104/62, 180 and irregular, 32 and labored, 104° F (40° C). His ECG shows atrial fibrillation. What do these findings indicate?

7. What will you do first?

CASE STUDY PROGRESS

K.B. is in thyroid crisis. The physician orders the following:

■ Chart View

Physician's Orders

Oxygen at 2 L per nasal cannula
STAT arterial blood gases, BNP, and cardiac enzymes
Digoxin (Lanoxin) 0.25 mg IV push now, then 0.125 mg IVP q8h × 2 doses
Diltiazem (Cardizem) bolus dose of 0.25 mg/kg IV; after 15 minutes, give a second dose of
    0.35 mg/kg IV for heart rate greater than 140
Increase methimazole (Tapazole) to 15 mg PO q6h
Lugol's solution 10 drops PO tid: start 1 hour after first methimazole dose
Hydrocortisone (HydroCort) 50 mg IVP q6h
Cardiac monitor
Absolute bed rest
Acetaminophen (Tylenol) 650 mg PO q6h prn for temp over 100° F (37.8° C).

8. Describe how you would care for K.B. in the next hour.

9. The label on the vial of diltiazem (Cardizem) states that there are 5 mg/mL. How many total milliliters will you administer for the first dose? How many for the second (if needed)?

10. How would you administer Lugol's solution?

11. Identify four additional measures that would be essential in caring for K.B.

12. Identify two possible factors that might have either precipitated or contributed to K.B.'s thyroid storm.

CASE STUDY PROGRESS

The physician discusses two treatment options with K.B. and his family: radioactive iodine (RAI) therapy using I^{131}, and subtotal thyroidectomy.

13. K.B. is fearful of radiation treatment and asks you for your opinion. How would you respond?

14. K.B. decides to receive I^{131}. During pretreatment instructions, the family asks whether he will be radioactive and what precautions they should take. Outline important guidelines for instructing K.B. and his family on home precautions.

15. Which statement would indicate that K.B. understands the discharge instructions?
   a. "If I get a sore throat, ice chips should help me feel better."
   b. "I should see an improvement in my symptoms by tomorrow."
   c. "I will follow the precautions for two weeks to keep my family safe."
   d. "I will take this medication on a full stomach."

CASE STUDY OUTCOME

Six months later, K.B.'s heart rate, blood pressure, and thyroid hormone levels are within normal limits. He has gained 14 pounds and has started walking in the mornings without any dyspnea. He says he has started to do woodworking and has been doing some volunteer work at the senior center.

Case Study 80

Name _____ Class/Group _____ Date _____

Group Members _____

INSTRUCTIONS All questions apply to this case study. Your responses should be brief and to the point. When asked to provide several answers, list them in order of priority or significance. Do not assume information that is not provided. Please print or write clearly. If your response is not legible, it will be marked as ? and you will need to rewrite it.

▶ Scenario

You are working on the postoperative unit and will be receiving a patient from the recovery room. The post-anesthesia care unit nurse calls and gives the following report: C.P. is a 50-year-old woman with a subtotal thyroidectomy for papillary carcinoma. The estimated blood loss was 25 mL. Vital signs (VS) are 130/82, 80 to 90, 20, and Sao$_2$ 94% on room air. She has a peripheral IV of D5.45NS with 20 mEq KCl infusing at 100 mL/hr. She has received a total of 3 mg morphine sulfate IV push, and she remains awake, but drowsy, and fully oriented. C.P.'s past medical history includes a total abdominal hysterectomy for fibroids and low-level radiation treatments to the neck 30 years ago for eczema. Her medications include lovastatin (Mevacor) and levothyroxine (Synthroid). Both parents are living; her father had a myocardial infarction at 70 years of age; her mother has hypothyroidism but never had thyroid tumors.

1. What preparations will you make before C.P. arrives?

2. You receive C.P. from the recovery room. How will you focus on your initial assessment, and why?

3. During your initial assessment, you document negative Chvostek's and Trousseau's signs. Describe data that would support this conclusion.

4. Identify the major risk factor that might have contributed to the development of thyroid adenoma in C.P.

5. List four complications that C.P. is at risk for postoperatively, and then describe actions you should include in C.P.'s postoperative care related to each complication.

6. Identify measures that reduce the risk for postoperative swelling.

7. After surgery, C.P.'s thyroid hormone levels are elevated, and the physician orders propranolol (Inderal) 80 mg ER orally twice daily for "surgically induced thyrotoxicosis." Is this reaction expected following thyroid surgery, or did something go wrong during surgery? Explain.

8. Eighteen hours after surgery, C.P. calls you into her room complaining of numbness around her mouth and tingling at the tips of her fingers and jitteriness. She appears restless. What is the significance of these findings?

9. Realizing that C.P. might be experiencing hypocalcemia, you notify the physician. What will you do in the interim before the physician returns your call?

10. The physician orders you to give C.P. 1 g calcium gluconate IV over 15 minutes now, and then initiate an infusion of 2 g calcium gluconate in 500 mL D5W over 12 hours. After the bolus is complete, at what rate will you set the IV pump?

11. What precautions do you need to take while administering the calcium gluconate infusion?

CASE STUDY PROGRESS

C.P. is given supplemental calcium gluconate and recovers without further complications. You are preparing her for discharge 2 days postoperatively.

12. As part of your discharge instructions to C.P., you would teach her: (Select all that apply.)
   a. the importance of taking her thyroid replacement therapy as prescribed.
   b. to not return to work until her thyroid hormone is normalized.
   c. to avoid being in extremely warm environments until she is euthyroid.
   d. the importance of keeping follow-up medical appointments.
   e. proper care of the incision and signs of infection to report to the physician.
   f. to avoid foods containing iodine because they increase her risk of recurrent cancer.

Case Study 81

Name _____ Class/Group _____ Date _____

Group Members _____

INSTRUCTIONS All questions apply to this case study. Your responses should be brief and to the point. When asked to provide several answers, list them in order of priority or significance. Do not assume information that is not provided. Please print or write clearly. If your response is not legible, it will be marked as ? and you will need to rewrite it.

▶ Scenario

You work in a diabetes mellitus (DM) treatment center located in a large teaching hospital. The first patient you meet is K.W., a 25-year-old Hispanic female, who was just released from the hospital 2 days ago after being diagnosed with type I DM.

Nine days ago, K.W. went to see the physician after a 1-month history of frequent urination, thirst, severe fatigue, blurred vision, and some burning and tingling in her feet. She attributed those symptoms to working long hours at the computer. Her random glucose level was 410 mg/dL. The next day, her labs were as follows: fasting glucose 335 mg/dL, HbA1C 8.8%, cholesterol 310 mg/dL, triglycerides 300 mg/dL, HDL 25 mg/dL, LDL 160 mg/dL, ratio 12.4, creatinine 0.9 mg/dL, and body mass index 37.6. Her BP is 160/96 mm Hg. She was admitted to the hospital for control of her glucose levels and the initiation of multi-dose injection insulin therapy with carbohydrate (CHO) counting. After discharge, K.W. has been referred to you for comprehensive education. You are to cover four basic areas: pharmacotherapy, glucose monitoring, medical nutrition therapy (MNT), and exercise.

1. K.W. was started on sliding scale lispro (Humalog) four times daily and glargine (Lantus) insulin 30 units at bedtime. What is the most significant difference between these two insulins?

2. What is the peak time and duration for lispro insulin?

3. K.W. states that she knows people who take NPH and regular insulin and wants to know why she can't take them. Explain the advantages of using glargine (Lantus) and lispro (Humalog) insulins.

4. Identify important content to be included under pharmacologic therapy.

5. What specific points would you include in a teaching plan for K.W. regarding managing insulin therapy? (Select all that apply.)
   a. Always administer the injections in the same, easy-to-reach location.
   b. Two injections will be needed to administer lispro (Humalog) and glargine (Lantus).
   c. The current vial of lispro (Humalog) can be kept at room temperature for 1 month.
   d. Ideally, the glargine (Lantus) should be administered at bedtime.
   e. The insulin can still be used if it is yellowed but not expired.
   f. Unused insulin needs to be kept in the freezer.
   g. Administer the lispro (Humalog) within 15 minutes of eating.

6. Identify important content to be included under glucose monitoring.

7. K.W. states that her diet is mostly fast foods, and the foods cooked at home are high in starch and fat. She also states that because of her work schedule, mealtimes often vary from day to day. What is CHO counting, and why would this method work well for K.W.?

8. Identify important points to be covered under MNT.

9. K.W. states that she currently does not exercise at all. What benefits will K.W. receive from participating in an exercise program?

10. What do you need to teach K.W. regarding exercise precautions?

11. K.W. states that she and her husband were planning to have another child in a year to two. She wants to know how her DM will affect a pregnancy. Pregnancy in persons with DM is a complex issue. What basic information can you share with K.W. today without overwhelming her?

12. What evaluative parameters could you use to determine whether your teaching with K.W. was effective?

CASE STUDY PROGRESS

K.W. calls the clinic several days later complaining of having the "flu." She says that she has been nauseated and vomited once during the night. She says she has had two loose stools. Upon questioning, she states that she does have a few chills and might have a low-grade fever but does not have a thermometer to check her temperature. She states she did not check her glucose level this morning or take her insulin because she has "not eaten."

13. Describe the instructions that you need to give K.W. regarding the management of her illness and DM.

Immunologic Disorders

8

Case Study 82

Name _____ Class/Group _____ Date _____

Group Members_____

INSTRUCTIONS All questions apply to this case study. Your responses should be brief and to the point. When asked to provide several answers, list them in order of priority or significance. Do not assume information that is not provided. Please print or write clearly. If your response is not legible, it will be marked as ? and you will need to rewrite it.

▶ Scenario

You are a nurse at a university student health clinic. T.Q. comes in to your clinic and informs you of his immunodeficiency problem. He has just moved here to go to school. He gives you a letter from his attending physician, hands you a vial of gamma globulin, and asks you to give him his "shot." The letter from T.Q.'s physician states that he was diagnosed with primary immunodeficiency disease 18 years ago. He has an adequate number of B cells, but they fail to mature properly and become plasma cells or immunoglobulin. T.Q. states he has a history of chronic respiratory and gastrointestinal infections. He is maintained on 0.66 mL/kg gamma globulin IM every 3 weeks and has tolerated this well. He has no known drug allergies. His vital signs are stable.

1. Can you honor this patient's prescription? Why or why not? How could you provide him with his injection?

2. What should you do while the physician is verifying information?

3. You note on T.Q.'s health record that he has not received his polio, measles, mumps, or rubella vaccines. What explanation can be given for the lack of these vaccinations?

4. The clinic physician receives confirmation from T.Q.'s physician and orders the gamma globulin. What questions would you ask T.Q. that would reassure you that the medication he brought was safe to administer?

5. Briefly describe the maturation cycle of the B cell.

6. Compare how primary immunodeficiencies differ from secondary immunodeficiencies.

7. What is the most common primary immunodeficiency?

8. How do you know what type of immunoglobulin deficiency T.Q. has?

9. Explain why T.Q. is at greater risk for developing infections than his classmates.

10. Before T.Q. leaves, you assess his knowledge and give specific precautions. What will you assess, and what precautions will you give?

CASE STUDY PROGRESS

T.Q. returns in 3 weeks with complaints of a stuffy nose. He is also due for his next injection of gamma globulin.

11. What will you assess to further evaluate his stuffy nose?

12. If T.Q. is developing a sinus infection, what signs are you likely to encounter on examining him?

13. T.Q.'s nares do not appear swollen or red, although he does have some clear mucus drainage. His temperature is normal at 98.4° F (36.9° C). Should you give the medication or ask him to return when he is no longer having nasal stuffiness? Why or why not?

14. What do you need to teach T.Q. before leaving the clinic?

Case Study 83

Name _____ Class/Group _____ Date _____

Group Members _____

INSTRUCTIONS All questions apply to this case study. Your responses should be brief and to the point. When asked to provide several answers, list them in order of priority or significance. Do not assume information that is not provided. Please print or write clearly. If your response is not legible, it will be marked as ? and you will need to rewrite it.

▶ **Scenario**

You are working at a physician's office, and you have just taken C.Q., a 38-year-old woman, into the consultation room. C.Q. has been divorced for 5 years, has two daughters (ages 14 and 16), and works full time as a legal secretary. She is here for a routine physical examination and requested that a human immunodeficiency virus (HIV) test be performed. C.Q. stated that she is in a serious relationship, is contemplating marriage, and just wants to make certain she is "okay." No abnormalities were noted during C.Q.'s physical examination, and blood was drawn for routine blood chemistries and hematology studies. The physician requests you perform a rapid HIV test, which is an antibody test. Within 20 minutes, the results are available and are positive.

1. Does a positive rapid HIV test mean that C.Q. definitely has HIV? If it is negative, does it mean she definitely doesn't have HIV?

2. What counseling do you need to provide to C.Q.?

CASE STUDY PROGRESS

The physician informs you that C.Q.'s Western blot test results confirm that she is HIV positive; he requests that you be present when he talks to her. Before leaving C.Q.'s room, the physician requests that you give C.Q. verbal and written information about local HIV support groups and help C.Q. call a friend to accompany her home this evening. She looks at you through her tears and states, "I can't believe it. J. is the only man I've had sex with since my divorce. He told me I had nothing to worry about. I can't believe he would do this to me."

8 Immunologic

3. C.Q.'s statement is based on three assumptions: (1) J. is HIV positive; (2) he intentionally withheld the information from her; and (3) he intentionally transmitted the HIV to her through unprotected sex. Based on your knowledge of HIV infection, how would you counsel C.Q.?

4. In addition to offering alternative explanations and exploring options, what is your most important role at this time?

5. C.Q. asks you whether she has AIDS. What do you tell her?

6. Why is it a good idea for C.Q. to have someone she trusts transport her home this evening?

7. C.Q. gives you the name and phone number of a relative she wants you to call. You remain with her until she leaves with her relative. Has C.Q.'s right to privacy been violated? Explain why or why not.

CASE STUDY PROGRESS

C.Q. returns to the office 4 days later to discuss her diagnosis.

8. What are your goals for C.Q. at this time?

9. What additional laboratory tests would you anticipate for C.Q.?

10. C.Q. asks whether there is any treatment available. How would you respond?

11. C.Q. asks why she has to take so many drugs instead of a "big dose" of one drug. What would you tell her?

12. The physician starts C.Q. on a regimen of Truvada (tenofovir and emtricitabine), Reyataz (atazanavir), and Norvir (ritonavir). What general information will you give C.Q. about ART therapy?

13. What other issues will you discuss with C.Q. at this visit?

14. Does C.Q. have a legal responsibility to inform J. of her HIV status?

CASE STUDY PROGRESS

Two weeks later, C.Q. visits the office and asks to speak to you in private. She thanks you for talking to her the day she received the news of her diagnosis. She tells you that J. confessed to her that he was afraid to tell her about his hemophilia because she might leave him. J. tested positive in the 1980s after being infected through contaminated recombinant factor VIII products. C.Q. tells you that they are going to get married and invites you to the wedding.

Case Study 84

Name _____ Class/Group _____ Date _____

Group Members _____

▶ Scenario

J.P., a 56-year-old man, developed a severe viral infection and suffered fatigue, fever, and myalgia. Although he recovered from the acute episode, J.P. never quite regained his normal activity level. Six months later, J.P. continues to find it difficult to work a 10-hour day as a brick mason, so he returns to his physician. Diagnostic studies reveal heart failure (HF) related to postviral cardiomyopathy.

Following medical management with metoprolol (Toprol XL) and furosemide (Lasix), his condition stabilizes and he returns to work, but his attendance is erratic. J.P.'s condition gradually deteriorates. Sixteen months later he is readmitted to the hospital complaining of dyspnea with minimal exertion, fatigue, orthopnea, chest pain, anorexia, and feelings of abdominal fullness. He has 1+ peripheral edema and is diaphoretic. Further studies reveal that J.P. has cardiac dilation, moderate to gross ventricular hypertrophy, and a systolic ejection fraction of 17%, consistent with severe congestive cardiomyopathy. Because J.P.'s only other health problem is mild hypertension, a heart transplant evaluation is recommended. J.P. and his wife discuss his prognosis, and he agrees to an evaluation for possible heart transplantation.

1. If J.P. is accepted for cardiac transplantation, what data will be collected in addition to his past medical history, current diagnostic findings, and cardiac evaluation?

2. What criteria does J.P. meet that will make him eligible for cardiac transplantation?

3. Identify five contraindications for cardiac transplant.

4. J.P. is accepted for cardiac transplant and placed on the waiting list. What fears or concerns might J.P. experience during this waiting period?

CASE STUDY PROGRESS

Three weeks later, J.P. receives a phone call to report to the hospital immediately because a donor heart has become available.

5. What compatibility tests are performed to determine eligibility for transplantation and to ensure as close a match as possible?

6. As the nurse on the transplant unit, how can you best help J.P. prepare for his heart transplant?

CASE STUDY PROGRESS

J.P.'s surgery and recovery are uncomplicated, and he is sent home and referred to cardiac rehabilitation after adjustment of his immunosuppression therapy and appropriate teaching. J.P. is readmitted for low-grade fever and dyspnea 6 weeks after surgery. Cardiac biopsy demonstrates moderate acute rejection.

7. What is the etiology of acute rejection, and how does it differ from chronic rejection?

8. The nurse can anticipate that prompt immunosuppressive therapy will be instituted using what drugs? How do these alter the rejection process?

9. The tacrolimus (Prograf) dosage is 0.03 mg/kg/day IV as a continuous infusion. J.P. currently weighs 187 pounds. The pharmacy sends 5 mg of tacrolimus (Prograf) in 100 mL of 0.9% sodium chloride injection. How many total milligrams per day will J.P. receive? At how many milliliters per hour will you set the infusion pump?

10. What is the most important intervention for J.P. at this time, and why?

CASE STUDY PROGRESS

J.P. responds positively to steroid therapy and is released to home after 5 days. J.P. is admitted to the hospital 7 months later with complaints of dyspnea, low-grade fever, and ankle swelling. Both J.P. and his wife are anxious and fearful.

11. Explain what might be happening to J.P. physiologically.

12. Compare the treatment for this episode of graft rejection to the treatment from his earlier episode of rejection.

13. J.P.'s prognosis for the future will depend on what factors?

Case Study 85

Name _____ Class/Group _____ Date _____

Group Members _____

INSTRUCTIONS All questions apply to this case study. Your responses should be brief and to the point. When asked to provide several answers, list them in order of priority or significance. Do not assume information that is not provided. Please print or write clearly. If your response is not legible, it will be marked as ? and you will need to rewrite it.

▶ Scenario

W.V. is a 57-year-old man who lives with his wife and two teenage sons. W.V. developed chronic kidney disease 20 years ago after he developed acute kidney disease from using a drug for migraine headaches that was later shown to cause severe nephrotoxicity. W.V. underwent hemodialysis for 5 years before receiving a cadaveric transplant, or cadaver kidney. He recovered without complications, and his serum laboratory values returned to normal. He was placed on triple immunosuppression therapy, including prednisone (Deltasone), cyclosporine (Imuran), and tacrolimus (Prograf), and was discharged to home.

Today, W.V. reports to his physician for a 12-week follow-up. He returned to work 3 weeks ago. W.V. has gained 5 pounds since his last appointment 2 weeks ago.

■ Chart View

Vital Signs	
Blood pressure	148/82 mm Hg
Pulse rate	88 beats/min
Respiratory rate	24 breaths/min
Temperature	99.2° F (37.3° C)
Laboratory Test Results	
Creatinine	1.2 mg/dL
BUN	22 mg/dL

1. What histocompatibility studies are generally performed before renal transplant, and why are they important?

2. By what criteria was W.V. considered a good candidate for renal transplantation?

3. If W.V.'s kidney is producing sufficient urine and he is feeling well, why is it necessary to monitor his laboratory data?

4. What is the possible significance of W.V.'s blood pressure?

5. How would the physician determine whether W.V. was experiencing organ rejection?

6. If W.V. begins to reject his kidney, how would the rejection be classified?

7. What interventions would be implemented to save the transplant if rejection is present?

8. The physician decides to add mycophenolate (CellCept) 1 g twice daily to W.V.'s immunosuppressive regimen. How does mycophenolate (CellCept) protect W.V.'s kidney from rejection, and what points should you include in a teaching plan for W.V.?

9. Identify at least four ways that W.V. might experience difficulty adjusting to his organ transplant.

10. How can you best support W.V. and his family?

11. Why is it necessary for W.V. to be concerned about infection?

12. Which of these statements would indicate that W.V. might need more teaching regarding immunosuppressant therapy?
   a. "I should wash my hands frequently."
   b. "Now I can watch all of my son's basketball games."
   c. "I will need to have regular laboratory testing."
   d. "I will call the doctor if I urinate less frequently."

8 Immunologic

Case Study 86

Name _____ Class/Group _____ Date _____

Group Members _____

INSTRUCTIONS All questions apply to this case study. Your responses should be brief and to the point. When asked to provide several answers, list them in order of priority or significance. Do not assume information that is not provided. Please print or write clearly. If your response is not legible, it will be marked as ? and you will need to rewrite it.

▶ Scenario

K.D. is a 36-year-old gay professional man who has been human immunodeficiency virus (HIV) infected for 6 years. He had been on antiretroviral therapy (ART) with Combivir (zidovudine and lamivudine) and nelfinavir (Viracept). He self-discontinued his medications 6 months ago because of depression. The appearance of purplish spots on his neck and arms persuaded him to make an appointment with his physician. When he arrived at the physician's office, the nurse performed a brief assessment. His vital signs (VS) were 138/86, 100, 30, 100.8° F (38.2° C). K.D. stated that he had been feeling fatigued for several months and was experiencing occasional night sweats, but he also had been working long hours, skipped meals, and had been particularly stressed over a project at work. The remainder of K.D.'s physical examination was within normal limits. The doctor ordered a chest x-ray, CBC, lymphocyte studies, including CD4 T-cell count, ultra sensitive viral load, cytomegalovirus assay, and a tuberculin test.

Over the next week, K.D. developed a nonproductive cough and increasing shortness of breath (SOB). Last night, he developed a fever of 102° F and was acutely short of breath, so his roommate, J.F., brought him to the emergency department. He was admitted with probable *Pneumocystis jiroveci* pneumonia (PJP), which was confirmed with bronchoalveolar lavage examination under light microscopy. K.D.'s admission WBC and lymphocyte studies demonstrate an increased pattern of immunodeficiency compared with earlier studies. K.D. is admitted to your medical unit and placed on nasal oxygen, IV fluids, and IV trimethoprim-sulfamethoxazole (Bactrim).

1. What is PJP?

2. What is the significance of the purplish spots over K.D.'s neck and arms?

3. Differentiate between HIV-positive status and AIDS.

4. Why is K.D.'s development of KS and PJP of particular importance in light of his HIV status?

5. K.D. has been seropositive for several years, yet he has been asymptomatic for AIDS. What factors might have influenced K.D.'s development of PJP and KS?

6. Identify four problems you must manage regarding K.D.

7. What precautions will you need to use when caring for K.D.?

8. What is the focus of your ongoing assessment?

9. What major side effects of his antibiotic should you monitor K.D. for?

10. What aspects of K.D.'s care can you delegate to the LPN? (Select all that apply.)
   a. Administering first dose of IV trimethoprim-sulfamethoxazole (Bactrim)
   b. Monitoring K.D.'s pulse oximeter readings, reporting values under 95%
   c. Developing a plan of care to improve K.D.'s oxygenation status
   d. Providing instructions about a high-calorie, high-protein diet
   e. Reinforcing teaching with K.D. regarding good handwashing techniques
   f. Repositioning K.D. and having him deep breathe every 2 hours

CASE STUDY PROGRESS

K.D. is responding well to treatment for PJP, and plans are being made for discharge. His ART regimen will be restarted, and he will be starting radiation treatments for Kaposi's sarcoma. He will receive follow-up care at the outpatient clinic.

11. K.D. is kept on trimethoprim/sulfamethoxazole (Bactrim) two tablets once daily. He asks why he has to keep taking the drug "since the pneumonia is gone." How would you respond?

12. K.D. was taught about disease transmission and safer sex and encouraged to maintain moderate exercise, rest, and dietary habits when he was first diagnosed as HIV positive. Give at least four additional topics that should be discussed with K.D. before he goes home.

13. What laboratory data will most likely be monitored in K.D. in the future?

14. List at least five other opportunistic infections that K.D. is at risk for developing.

8 Immunologic

Case Study 87

Name _____ Class/Group _____ Date _____

Group Members _____

INSTRUCTIONS All questions apply to this case study. Your responses should be brief and to the point. When asked to provide several answers, list them in order of priority or significance. Do not assume information that is not provided. Please print or write clearly. If your response is not legible, it will be marked as ? and you will need to rewrite it.

▶ Scenario

D.W. is a 25-year-old married woman with three children under 5 years old. She came to her physician 7 months ago with vague complaints of intermittent fatigue, joint pain, low-grade fever, and unintentional weight loss.

Her physician noted small, patchy areas of vitiligo and a scaly rash across her nose, cheeks, back, and chest at that time. Laboratory studies revealed that D.W. had a positive antinuclear antibody (ANA) titer, positive dsDNA (positive lupus erythematosus), positive anti-Sm (anti-smooth muscle antibody), elevated C-reactive protein (CRP) and erythrocyte sedimentation rate (ESR), and decreased C3 and C4 serum complement. Joint x-ray films demonstrated joint swelling without joint erosion. D.W. was subsequently diagnosed with systemic lupus erythematosus (SLE). She was initially treated with hydroxychloroquine (Plaquenil) 400 mg and Deltasone (Prednisone) 20 mg orally per day, bed rest, and ice packs. D.W. responded well to treatment, the steroid was tapered and discontinued, and she was told she could report for follow-up every 6 months unless her symptoms became acute. D.W. resumed her job in environmental services at a large geriatric facility.

1. What is the significance of each of D.W.'s laboratory findings?

2. Given that most tests are nonspecific, how is SLE diagnosed?

3. What priority problems were addressed in D.W.'s care plan at that time of diagnosis?

CASE STUDY PROGRESS

Eighteen months after diagnosis, D.W. seeks out her physician because of puffy hands and feet and increased fatigue. D.W. reports that she has been working longer hours because of the absence of two of her fellow workers.

■ Chart view

Laboratory Test Results

Sodium	129 mmol/L
Potassium	4.2 mmol/L
Chloride	119 mmol/L
Total CO_2	21 mmol/L
BUN	34 mg/dL
Creatinine	2.6 mg/dL
Glucose	123 mg/dL
Urinalysis	2+ protein
	1+ RBCs

4. Which laboratory findings concern you, and why?

5. How will D.W.'s treatment and care plan likely change?

6. The physician orders cyclophosphamide (Cytoxan) 100 mg/m²/day orally in two divided doses. D.W. weighs 140 pounds and is 5 feet, 4 inches tall. How much will she receive with each dose?

CASE STUDY PROGRESS

D.W. is seen in the immunology clinic twice monthly during the next 3 months. Although her condition does not worsen, her BUN and creatinine remain elevated. While at work one afternoon, D.W. begins to feel dizzy and develops a severe headache. She reports to her supervisor, who has her lie down. When D.W. starts to become disoriented, her supervisor calls 911, and D.W. is taken to the hospital. D.W. is admitted for probable lupus cerebritis related to acute exacerbation of her disease.

7. What other findings indicative of central nervous system (CNS) involvement from SLE should D.W. be assessed for?

8. What preventive measures need to be instituted to protect D.W. at this time?

9. While caring for D.W., which of these care activities can be safely delegated to the NAP? (Select all that apply.)
   a. Measuring D.W.'s blood pressure every 2 hours
   b. Assisting D.W. with personal hygiene measures
   c. Counseling D.W. on seizure safety precautions
   d. Assessing D.W.'s neurologic status every 2 hours
   e. Emptying the urine collection device and measuring the output
   f. Monitoring D.W.'s BUN and creatinine levels

CASE STUDY PROGRESS

The physician orders pulse therapy with methylprednisolone (Solu-Medrol) 125 mg IV every 6 hours and plasmapheresis once daily.

10. What major complicationsns associated with immunosuppression therapy will D.W. have to be monitored for?

11. D.W. asks about what plasmapheresis does and why might it help her feel better. Describe how you would respond.

■ Chart View

Vital Signs

Blood pressure	86/43 mm Hg
Pulse rate	108 beats/min
Respiratory rate	18 breaths/min
Temperature	97.2° F (36.2° C)

12. D.W. returns to the floor following the plasmapheresis. The NAP reports to you D.W.'s vital signs. You go in to assess D.W. and find that she is complaining of a headache and some dizziness. What do you immediately suspect is occurring?

13. What do you anticipate your care of D.W. will include over the next 2-3 hours?

14. What outcome criteria would support that D.W.'s condition is stabilizing?

15. Identify at least five topics that D.W. must be taught before she is discharged that might help her lead as normal a life as possible.

16. You note that D.W.'s husband is visiting her this afternoon. You enter the room to ask whether they have any questions. D.W.'s husband states, "I have tried to tell her that she cannot go back to work. Sure, we need the money, but the kids and I need her more. I'm afraid that this lupus has weakened her whole body and it will kill her if she goes back to work. Is that right?" How should you respond to his concerns?

Oncologic and Hematologic Disorders

Case Study 88

Name _____ Class/Group _____ Date _____

Group Members _____

INSTRUCTIONS All questions apply to this case study. Your responses should be brief and to the point. When asked to provide several answers, list them in order of priority or significance. Do not assume information that is not provided. Please print or write clearly. If your response is not legible, it will be marked as? and you will need to rewrite it.

▶ Scenario

You are a home health nurse who has been seeing P.C., who was diagnosed with small-cell lung cancer approximately 1 year ago. She has been treated with radiation and chemotherapy; however, her provider recently informed her that her cancer is no longer treatable because it has spread to her bones and liver and that the focus of her treatment will change from curative measures to symptom relief. She is confused and somewhat bewildered. She vaguely remembers the term *palliative treatment* when discussing her situation with her provider but doesn't know what it means.

1. How would you describe palliative treatment?

CASE STUDY PROGRESS

P.C. confides that she has never formally written down her wishes concerning what types of treatments she would or would not want. You advise her to complete an advance directive and/or living will or to complete a medical durable power of attorney and/or a surrogate decision maker form. In current practice, it is very likely that a part of the home health intake process will be completion of a Physician Orders for Life-Sustaining Treatment (POLST) Paradigm form.

2. What is the purpose of these documents?

3. What health care decisions are considered in these documents?

4. How are advance directives and living wills formalized?

5. P.C. states that she is confused and has mixed feelings about her health care wishes right now. She asks, "If I fill out this form, can I change my mind down the road?" How should you answer this question?

6. You inform P.C. that you will help with symptomatic control of her illness. Outline four areas of care you will focus on.

7. As P.C. becomes frailer and incoherent, how will her treatment be given?

CASE STUDY OUTCOME

P.C. discusses her wishes with her family and completes the documents describing what she would like her plan of care to be over the remainder of her life span. She passes away peacefully 7 weeks later in her home, supported by her family and friends, under her terms.

Case Study 89

Name _____ Class/Group _____ Date _____

Group Members _____

▶ Scenario

G.C. is a 78-year-old widow who relies on her late husband's Social Security income for all of her expenses. Over the past few years, G.C. has eaten less and less meat because of her financial situation and the trouble of preparing a meal "just for me." She struggles financially to buy medicines for the treatment of hypertension and arthritis. Over the past 2 to 3 months, she has felt increasingly tired, despite sleeping well at night. When she goes to the senior clinic, the nurse practitioner orders blood work. G.C.'s chemistry panel is all within normal limits and a stool guaiac test is negative. Her other results include the following:

■ Chart View

Laboratory Test Results

WBC	$7600/mm^3$
Hct	27.3%
Hgb	8.3 mg/dL
Platelets	$151,000/mm^3$
RBC indices	
Mean corpuscular volume (MCV)	$65 mm^3$
Mean corpuscular hemoglobin (MCH)	31.6 pg
MCH concentration (MCHC)	35.1%
Red cell distribution width (RDW)	15.6%
Iron (Fe)	30 mcg/dL
Total iron-binding capacity (TIBC)	422 mcg/dL
Ferritin	8 mg/dL
Vitamin B_{12}	414 pg/mL
Folate	188 ng/mL

1. Which lab values are normal, and which are abnormal?

2. Explain the significance of each abnormal result.

3. What type of anemia does G.C. have?

4. What are some causative factors for the type of anemia G.C. has?

5. Which individuals are at risk?

6. Describe the signs and symptoms of this type of anemia.

7. Discuss some of the treatment options for her disease.

8. The physician starts G.C. on ferrous sulfate (Feosol) 325 mg orally per day. What teaching needs to be done regarding this medication?

9. Discuss some ideas that might help her with her meal planning.

10. You teach G.C. about foods she should include in her diet. You determine that she understands your teaching if she states she will increase her intake of which of the following foods?
    a. Whole wheat pastas and skim milk
    b. Lean cuts of poultry, pork, and fish
    c. Cooked cereals, such as oats, and bananas
    d. Beans and dark green, leafy vegetables

11. What evaluative parameters could you use to determine whether G.C.'s nutritional needs are being met?

Case Study **90**

Name _____ Class/Group _____ Date _____

Group Members _____

INSTRUCTIONS All questions apply to this case study. Your responses should be brief and to the point. When asked to provide several answers, list them in order of priority or significance. Do not assume information that is not provided. Please print or write clearly. If your response is not legible, it will be marked as? and you will need to rewrite it.

▶ Scenario

You are a nurse working as a preoperative evaluation nurse. J.B., a well-known 62-year-old homeless alcoholic, is sent to you before a total laryngectomy with left radical neck dissection with placement of a permanent tracheostomy for squamous cell carcinoma. He has a long history of tobacco use, poor diet, and no dental care. Over the past several months, he has experienced increasing shortness of breath, hoarseness, and odynophagia. A piriform sinus mass was found on bronchoscopy. The large mass extends to and is fixed to the left true vocal cord. His chest x-ray is normal with the exception of changes related to chronic tobacco use. Past medical history includes reactive airway disease and hypertension. On examination, you find two palpable left-sided cervical nodes, which are firm and fixed.

1. Identify risk factors for head and neck cancer present in this case.

2. Name the warning signals listed on the American Cancer Society's list of warning signs of cancer. Place a star or asterisk next to those J.B. has.

3. Describe the surgical intervention J.B. will undergo.

4. J.B. has several important postoperative needs. Identify two serious complications for which he is most at risk.

5. What type of follow-up therapy is J.B. likely to undergo after his initial wound heals?

6. J.B. will require placement of a percutaneous endoscopic gastrostomy (PEG) feeding tube postoperatively to maintain adequate nutritional intake. Discuss one immediate postoperative problem related to each of the following: nutrition, airway maintenance, and communication.

7. J.B. has several factors that make discharge planning especially problematic. Describe three specific discharge problems, and list possible solutions.

CASE STUDY PROGRESS

J.B. undergoes surgery, which ends up being complicated by pneumonia and poor wound healing. After being hospitalized for 6 weeks, he is discharged to a long-term care facility for care while recuperating and external radiation therapy. He is scheduled to receive 2000 cGy to the head and neck three times weekly for the next 8 weeks. As J.B.'s nurse, you are concerned about the effects of radiation therapy, particularly the development of mucositis and xerostomia, which are common in those receiving radiation to the head and neck.

8. Outline independent nursing actions that will assist in managing J.B.'s risks for mucositis and xerostomia.

9. What instructions will you provide the nursing assistive personnel (NAP) caring for J.B. regarding skin care? (Select all that apply.)
 a. "Assist J.B. with selecting loose-fitting shirts."
 b. "Remove the ink marked on his neck with a washcloth."
 c. "Make sure you thoroughly rinse away all of the soap."
 d. "Dry the area with patting motions using a soft cloth."
 e. "After his shower, apply lotion to the radiated area."
 f. "He can have the heat lamp placed for 15 minutes each evening."

10. What other interventions would you anticipate in your plan of care while J.B. receives radiation therapy?

9 Oncologic/Hematologic

9 Oncologic/Hematologic

CASE STUDY OUTCOME

Despite receiving radiation therapy, J.B.'s disease progresses and he develops metastases to his lung and brain. He chooses to remain in the long-term care facility until he passes away from pneumonia 5 months later.

Case Study 91

Name _____ Class/Group _____ Date _____

Group Members _____

INSTRUCTIONS All questions apply to this case study. Your responses should be brief and to the point. When asked to provide several answers, list them in order of priority or significance. Do not assume information that is not provided. Please print or write clearly. If your response is not legible, it will be marked as ? and you will need to rewrite it.

▶ Scenario

R.T. is a 64-year-old man who went to his primary care provider's office for a yearly examination. He initially reported having no new health problems; however, on further questioning, he admitted to having developed some fatigue, abdominal bloating, and intermittent constipation. His physical examination was normal except for a stool positive for guaiac. A CBC with differential, BMP, and carcinoembryonic antigen (CEA) were ordered. R.T. was referred to a gastroenterologist for a colonoscopy. A 5-cm mass found in the sigmoid colon was diagnosed as an adenocarcinoma of the colon. The pathology report described the tumor as a Dukes' stage B, meaning the cancer extends into the muscle or connective tissue and invades adjacent organs and lymph nodes. A distant metastatic workup is negative, and R.T. is being referred for surgery.

1. What is a risk factor?

2. Identify six risk factors for colon cancer.

3. Describe the American Cancer Society's current recommended screening procedures related to colon cancer.

405

4. What are the warning signs of colon cancer? Place a star or asterisk next to those that R.T. has.

5. Compare the common early versus late signs and symptoms found in individuals with colorectal cancer.

6. What is a CEA? How does it relate to the diagnosis of colon cancer?

7. After bowel prep, R.T. is admitted to the hospital for an exploratory laparotomy, small bowel resection, and sigmoid colectomy. List at least five major potential complications for R.T.

CASE STUDY PROGRESS

After surgery, R.T. is admitted to the surgical intensive care unit (SICU) with a large abdominal dressing. The nurse rolls R.T. side to side to remove the soiled surgical linen, and the dressing becomes saturated with a large amount of serosanguineous drainage.

8. Would the drainage be expected after abdominal surgery? Explain.

9. What are the goals of nursing care after surgery?

Four weeks after surgery, R.T. is scheduled to begin chemotherapy.

10. Describe three chemotherapy regimens used to treat adenocarcinoma of the colon.

11. Discuss the major toxicities and side effects associated with these drugs.

12. Given the profiles of the drugs used to treat colon cancer, develop a teaching plan for R.T. focusing on common side effects.

9 Oncologic/Hematologic

Case Study 92

Name _____ Class/Group _____ Date _____

Group Members _____

INSTRUCTIONS All questions apply to this case study. Your responses should be brief and to the point. When asked to provide several answers, list them in order of priority or significance. Do not assume information that is not provided. Please print or write clearly. If your response is not legible, it will be marked as? and you will need to rewrite it.

▶ Scenario

M.D. is a 50-year-old woman whose routine mammogram showed a 2.3 × 4.5 cm lobulated mass at the 3:00 position in her left breast. M.D. underwent a stereotactic needle biopsy and was diagnosed with infiltrating ductal carcinoma that was both estrogen and progesterone receptor positive. The staging workup was negative for distant metastasis. Her final staging was stage IIB. She had a modified radical mastectomy with lymph node dissection. The sentinel lymph node and 11 of 16 lymph nodes were positive for tumor cells. An implanted port was placed during surgery. She is prescribed a chemotherapy regimen of six cycles of CAF (cyclophosphamide [Cytoxan], fluorouracil [5-FU], and doxorubicin [Adriamycin]).

1. Describe the biopsy technique used to diagnosis M.D.'s cancer.

2. Discuss the implications of a positive sentinel node.

3. Using the TNM staging system, what would her classification be?

4. What is the significance of her hormone receptor status?

5. Surgical intervention is the primary treatment for breast cancer. Describe the surgical procedure that M.D. had.

6. M.D. asks you why she has to have chemotherapy with so many drugs if the surgeon removed all of the cancer. How would you respond?

7. Compare the drug actions of cyclophosphamide (Cytoxan), fluorouracil (5-FU), and doxorubicin (Adriamycin).

8. List any side effects and special considerations associated with the use of CAF.

9. M.D. is ordered doxorubicin at $75\,mg/m^2$. Her height is 5 feet, 7 inches, and her weight is 155 pounds. Calculate the dose she will receive.

10. You have finished teaching M.D. regarding the effects of CAF. You know that she understands instructions regarding cyclophosphamide (Cytoxan) when she states:
a. "This medication should be taken with food."
b. "I will drink 2000 to 3000 mL of fluids each day."
c. "Taking this drug at nighttime will reduce nausea."
d. "I will increase my intake of foods with potassium."

CASE STUDY PROGRESS

M.D. has now completed three cycles of CAF. Her last treatment with doxorubicin, cyclophosphamide, and 5-fluorouracil was approximately 12 days ago. She comes to the emergency department with a 2-day history of fever, chills, and shortness of breath. On arrival, she is disoriented and agitated. Vital signs are 86/43, 119, 28, 103.6° F (39.8° C), Sao_2 85% on room air. Chest x-ray demonstrates diffuse infiltrates in the left lower lung. Her chem 14 is within normal limits, with the exception of BUN 28 mg/dL, creatinine 1.6 mg/dL, and lactic acid 2.4 mg/dL.

■ Chart View

Complete Blood Count

WBC	1200/mm^3
Neutrophils	34%
Segmented (Polys)	30%
Bands	4%
Lymphocytes	60%
Monocytes	3%
Eosinophils and basophils	2%
Hct	24.9%
Hgb	8.7 g/dL
Platelets	85,000/mm^3

11. Interpret M.D.'s CBC results.

12. Calculate M.D.'s absolute neutrophil count (ANC) and describe its significance.

13. What is the single most important nursing intervention for a patient with an ANC less than 500/mm^3?

14. What are the probable causes of the abnormal laboratory findings listed previously?

15. What is the significance of the lactic acid level?

16. What treatment do you anticipate for M.D.?

17. The physician orders a 500-mL normal saline bolus now, with orders to infuse over 2 hours. You decide to use M.D.'s implanted port for IV access. After accessing the port and connecting the fluid, the infusion pump alarms that the line is occluded. What will you do?

CASE STUDY OUTCOME

M.D. requires endotracheal intubation and spends 3 days in the ICU receiving antibiotics and respiratory support. She is able to be extubated and returns to the oncology unit, where she remains for a few more days before being discharged to home.

Case Study 93

Name _____ Class/Group _____ Date _____

Group Members _____

INSTRUCTIONS All questions apply to this case study. Your responses should be brief and to the point. When asked to provide several answers, list them in order of priority or significance. Do not assume information that is not provided. Please print or write clearly. If your response is not legible, it will be marked as? and you will need to rewrite it.

▶ **Scenario**

C.P. is a 71-year-old married farmer, with a past medical history of hernia surgery in 1986 and prostate surgery in 2005 for benign prostatic hyperplasia. C.P. does not drink, but he has smoked for 40 years; the past 3 years he has smoked two to three packs per day. Two weeks ago, C.P. visited the local rural health clinic with complaints of a progressive cough and chest congestion. Despite a week of antibiotic therapy, C.P. continued to worsen; he experienced progressive dyspnea and productive cough, and he began to have night sweats. C.P. refused to be admitted to the hospital because "there's no one to look after the cows," but he agreed to go for a chest x-ray (CXR). The radiologist reads C.P.'s CXR as "left hilar lung mass, probable lung cancer." C.P. is scheduled for a diagnostic fiberoptic bronchoscopy with endobronchial lung biopsy as an outpatient this morning to confirm the diagnosis.

1. What is fiberoptic bronchoscopy, and what information will fiberoptic bronchoscopy with endobronchial lung biopsy provide?

2. As the nurse who works with the pulmonologist, it is your responsibility to prepare C.P. for the fiberoptic bronchoscopy procedure. What will you include in your teaching plan?

3. What is your responsibility during and immediately after the bronchoscopy?

4. C.P. tolerates the procedure well. He returns to the office in 4 days to learn the results of his test. The pulmonologist tells C.P. and his wife that he has poorly differentiated oat cell lung cancer and explains that it is a very fast-growing cancer with a poor prognosis. This kind of lung cancer is directly related to C.P.'s history of smoking. What is your role at this time?

5. What does poorly differentiated mean?

CASE STUDY PROGRESS

C.P. undergoes a metastatic workup and is found to have disease in a number of lymph nodes. The physician tells C.P. and his wife that surgery is not an option and schedules C.P. to begin combination chemotherapy.

6. How would you explain combination chemotherapy and how it works to C.P. and his wife?

7. C.P. says he doesn't know if he should take chemotherapy if he "isn't going to live anyway." What are the goals of administering chemotherapy in patients such as C.P.?

8. C.P.'s wife tells you she's heard that chemotherapy makes you really sick. How would you explain chemotherapy side effects?

9. C.P. agrees to chemotherapy and is scheduled to receive cisplatin (Platinol) 60 mg in 100 mL normal saline (NS) IV over 1 to 2 hours daily, and etoposide (VePesid) 200 mg in 250 mL NS IV over 1 to 2 hours daily, both during the first 3 days of each month. What is the nadir for each drug, and what implications does the nadir have for C.P.?

10. Based on your knowledge of the most common side effects of cisplatin (Platinol) and etoposide (VePesid), list at least seven interventions that should be incorporated into C.P.'s care plan.

11. C.P. plans to continue to work the farm as long as possible and says his brother-in-law has promised to help him. C.P. needs to have a working understanding of how to balance his treatment with his work. You sit down with C.P. to plan a daily work, activity, rest schedule to accommodate his treatments and side effects. List at least four concepts you would emphasize.

9 Oncologic/Hematologic

CASE STUDY PROGRESS

A month later, when C.P. returns for his second round of chemotherapy, he complains of shortness of breath, chest tightness, and palpitations. He looks exhausted. An ECG reveals new onset atrial fibrillation, and a CXR suggests a large left lower lobe pleural effusion. C.P. is admitted to the hospital for supportive care. The pulmonologist performs a thoracentesis and drains 985 mL of fluid, immediately relieving some of C.P.'s dypsnea and chest discomfort.

■ Chart View

Laboratory Test Values

WBC	2500/mm³
RBC	4.9 millions/mm³
Hgb	12.7 g/dL
Hct	37.6%
Platelets	152,000/mm³
Sodium	131 mmol/L
Potassium	4.2 mmol/L
Chloride	90 mmol/L

12. What do these lab values indicate?

13. You assess C.P. 2 hours after the thoracentesis. Which information is important to report to the physician? C.P.:
  a. has a small amount of serosanguineous drainage on the dressing.
  b. complains of occasional chest pain when taking deep breaths.
  c. has a blood pressure of 90/50 mm Hg and some increase in dyspnea.
  d. states that he has some burning and stinging at the thoracentesis site.

14. C.P. tells you he doesn't want to live like this and that he would like to stop chemotherapy, but his physician wants him to continue with aggressive therapy. Discuss the pros and cons of continuing therapy and what role you can play in helping him.

CASE STUDY OUTCOME

C.P. refuses the second round of chemotherapy and is discharged to home. He receives no further treatment and dies 3 weeks later with his wife at his side.

Case Study **94**

Name _____   Class/Group _____   Date _____

Group Members _____

INSTRUCTIONS All questions apply to this case study. Your responses should be brief and to the point. When asked to provide several answers, list them in order of priority or significance. Do not assume information that is not provided. Please print or write clearly. If your response is not legible, it will be marked as? and you will need to rewrite it.

▶ **Scenario**

H.J. is a 46-year-old man diagnosed with Burkitt's lymphoma 4 months ago. He has received three of six chemotherapy courses and is seen today at his physician's office with a complaint of malaise and fever. He is found to have splenomegaly on examination. Chest x-ray (CXR) demonstrates patchy infiltrates in bilateral lower lobes, right greater than left. He is sent for a CT of the abdomen, which showed metastatic disease in the liver, spleen, and pancreas. He is admitted to the hospital with progressive disease.

■ **Chart View**

BMP

Na	136 mmol/L
K	5.2 mmol/L
Cl	97 mmol/L
CO_2	28 mmol/L
Glucose	98 mg/dL
BUN	24 mg/dL
Creatinine	1.7 mg/dL
Ca	7.9 units/L
Total protein	5.4 g/dL
Albumin	2.8 g/dL
Phosphorus	4.5 mg/dL
Uric acid	23.7 mg/dL
Total bilirubin	0.8 mg/dL
Alkaline phosphatase	172 units/L
AST	254 units/L
ALT	74 units/L
LDH	214 IU/L

CBC

WBC	51,900/mm³
Neutrophils	66%
Lymphocytes	16%
Monocytes	15%
Eosinophils	5%
Hgb	8.3 g/dL
Hct	23.6%
Platelets	21,000/mm³

1. H.J. is diagnosed with acute tumor lysis syndrome (TLS). Briefly describe this syndrome.

2. Which of the above labs confirm the diagnosis of TLS?

3. What assessment findings would you anticipate in H.J.?

9 Oncologic/Hematologic

■ Chart View

Medication Record

IV 0.9% saline at 150 mL per hour
Add 100 mEq sodium bicarbonate to the first liter of IV fluid
Allopurinol (Aloprim) 500 mg orally twice daily
Furosemide (Lasix) 40 mg IV now then every 6 hours
Sodium polystyrene (Kayexalate) 15 g orally every 6 hours
Aluminum hydroxide (Amphojel) two caps orally with meals

4. What is the expected outcome for H.J. associated with each medication he is receiving?

5. Identify two additional complications or emergencies for which H.J. is at risk.

6. List four things you would do for H.J.

7. As soon as H.J. is stabilized, the physician orders a round of chemotherapy. Because the TLS is just resolving, what interventions would you include in your plan of care?

8. What precautions should you take when preparing H.J.'s chemotherapy to reduce your risk of injury? (Select all that apply.)
   a. Prepare the infusion in the medication room by yourself.
   b. Wear surgical gloves and a disposable long-sleeved gown.
   c. Place an absorbent plastic-backed pad on the work area.
   d. Wear goggles when preparing an intravenous infusion.
   e. Dispose of all waste in special biohazard containers.

9. The NAP you are working with states she is unfamiliar with caring for patients who just received chemotherapy. What instructions do you give to the NAP to reduce her risk of injury?

■ Chart View

BMP

Na	138 mmol/L
K	4.8 mmol/L
Cl	109 mmol/L
CO_2	26 mmol/L
Glucose	148 mg/dL
BUN	34 mg/dL
Creatinine	1.0 mg/dL
Ca	7.3 units/L
Total protein	5.4 g/dL
Albumin	2.8 g/dL
Phosphorus	3.8 mg/dL
Uric acid less than	0.5 mg/dL
Total bilirubin	1.0 mg/dL
Alkaline phosphatase	96 units/L
AST	49 units/L
ALT	48 units/L
LDH	224 IU/L

CBC

WBC	1400/ mm³
Hgb	8.3 g/dL
Hct	23.8%
Platelets	10,000/mm³

10. On hospital day 5, his labs are repeated after the ordered chemotherapy has been completed. Comparing current laboratory data to those on admission, how has his condition changed?

11. H.J. requires blood product support, including leukocyte-poor pheresed platelets and leukocyte-reduced packed RBCs (PRBCs). Acetaminophen (Tylenol) and diphenhydramine (Benadryl) are ordered as premedication for transfusion. H.J. will be closely monitored for intravascular and extravascular hemolytic reactions; febrile, allergic, and hypervolemic reactions; transfusion-related acute lung injury; and bacterial sepsis. Identify the signs and symptoms, usual cause, and treatment for each.

Reaction Type	Signs/Symptoms	Usual Cause	Treatment
Intravascular hemolytic (immune)			
Extravascular hemolytic (immune)			
Febrile			
Allergic (mild to severe)			
Hypervolemic			
Transfusion-related acute lung injury			
Bacterial sepsis			

9 Oncologic/Hematologic

Case Study 95

Name _____ Class/Group _____ Date _____

Group Members _____

INSTRUCTIONS All questions apply to this case study. Your responses should be brief and to the point. When asked to provide several answers, list them in order of priority or significance. Do not assume information that is not provided. Please print or write clearly. If your response is not legible, it will be marked as? and you will need to rewrite it.

▶ Scenario

R.M. is a 49-year-old woman with a history of stage III ovarian carcinoma. She was initially treated with an exploratory laparotomy that included a total abdominal hysterectomy, an ileocecal resection and anastomosis, omentectomy, and peritoneal biopsies. The postoperative CA-125 level was 69 units/mL; currently, it is 328 units/mL. She has received four courses of chemotherapy consisting of paclitaxel (Taxol) and cisplatin (Platinol). She is being admitted with shortness of breath, complaints of nausea, and early satiety with recent weight loss of 10 pounds. Her abdomen is distended, and her Sao_2 is 86% on room air.

1. What is the most common reason ovarian cancer is usually stage III or stage IV when initially diagnosed?

2. List three common presenting signs and symptoms of ovarian cancer.

3. Explain the significance of R.M.'s CA-125 levels.

4. Knowing the chemotherapeutic agents R.M. has received, what laboratory data will the nurse monitor?

5. Identify five side effects of R.M's chemotherapeutic agents.

6. You perform R.M.'s admission assessment. Which finding needs to be reported to the physician immediately?
   a. A temperature greater than 101° F (38.3° C)
   b. Bleeding gums and mouth ulcerations
   c. Numbness in her lower legs bilaterally
   d. Dark amber colored urine

7. R.M.'s chest x-ray reveals bilateral pleural effusions. How do these relate to her underlying disease? How might they be treated?

CASE STUDY PROGRESS

The physician orders an MRI of the abdomen and pelvis, which reveals a mass in the left lower quadrant and a malignant bowel obstruction. He immediately schedules R.M. for a tumor debulking and possible placement of an ostomy.

8. Delineate four appropriate topics to be included in preoperative teaching.

9. R.M. is undergoing a palliative surgical intervention. How will you explain this to the patient and family?

10. How can you support R.M. and her family at this time?

CASE STUDY PROGRESS

Family history analysis reveals a strong positive occurrence of breast and ovarian cancer in R.M.'s family. Her mother died of breast cancer at the age of 56, and a maternal aunt died of ovarian cancer at the age of 59. The physician suggests testing for the presence of the *BRCA1* and *BRCA2* genes and, if positive, testing R.M.'s two daughters and son.

11. Describe the meaning of this test.

12. Discuss pros and cons of genetic testing for cancer.

13. R.M. tests positive for the *BRCA2* gene. What implications does this have for her children?

Case study 96

Name _____ Class/Group _____ Date _____

Group Members _____

INSTRUCTIONS All questions apply to this case study. Your responses should be brief and to the point. When asked to provide several answers, list them in order of priority or significance. Do not assume information that is not provided. Please print or write clearly. If your response is not legible, it will be marked as? and you will need to rewrite it.

▶ Scenario

V.M. is a 39-year-old African-American man who has sickle cell disease (SCD), sometimes called *sickle cell anemia,* marked by frequent episodes of severe pain. His anemia has been managed with multiple transfusions, and he started showing signs of chronic renal failure 6 months ago. His regular medications are pentoxifylline (Trental), oxycodone-acetaminophen (Percocet), hydroxyurea (Droxia), and folic acid. In the hematology clinic this morning, V.M.'s hemoglobin measured 6.7 g/dL. He received 2 units packed RBCs over 3 hours and then went home. He developed dyspnea and shortness of breath approximately 1 to 1½ hours later, and his wife called 911. The emergency medical system crew initiated oxygen and transported V.M. to the emergency department (ED).

1. What is SCD, and how is it related to race?

2. The stiff, sickled RBCs tend to cause vascular occlusions with subsequent local infarction. As a rule, the spleen suffers so many vasoocclusive/infarction episodes that it is greatly increased in size and is rendered nonfunctional by the time the individual is 6 years of age. What are the implications of having a nonfunctioning spleen?

3. Identify two mechanisms that contribute to anemia in patients with SCD.

4. When V.M. arrives at the ED, the physician asks him whether he is in pain and whether he needs pain medication. V.M. answers no to both questions. Why did the physician ask these two questions?

5. V.M.'s arterial blood gases on 8 L O_2 by simple face mask show Pao_2 (partial pressure of oxygen in arterial blood) 74 mm Hg. Is V.M. being adequately oxygenated?

6. V.M. complains of being short of breath. Do you believe the low hemoglobin level is responsible for his complaints?

CASE STUDY PROGRESS

You perform a quick assessment and note a systolic murmur and crackles in V.M.'s bases bilaterally. Vital signs (VS) are 176/102, 94, 28, 97.8° F (36.6° C). Acting according to the standing orders for your institution, you start an IV and draw blood for CBC with differential, basic metabolic panel, calcium, and phosphorus and send it for analysis.

7. Your assessment findings are consistent with fluid overload. What four findings led you to that conclusion?

8. What action will you expect the physician to take next, and why?

■ Chart View

Laboratory Test Values

Sodium	137 mmol/L
Potassium	4.9 mmol/L
Chloride	110 mmol/L
CO_2	16 mmol/L
BUN	27 mg/dL
Creatinine	2.7 mg/dL
WBC	4300/mm³
Hgb	7.8 g/dL
Hct	20.9%
Platelets	208,000/mm³

9. What is the significance of the lab results, and why?

CASE STUDY PROGRESS

The physician prescribes furosemide (Lasix) 40 mg IV push now, methylprednisolone (Solu-Medrol) 75 mg IVP now, and ceftriaxone (Rocephin) 1 g IV piggyback after the furosemide (Lasix).

10. Indicate the expected outcome for V.M. that is associated with each of the medications he is receiving.

11. The methylprednisolone (Solu-Medrol) 75 mg IV is supplied as a 125 mg/2 mL solution. Shade in the dose to be administered on the syringe.

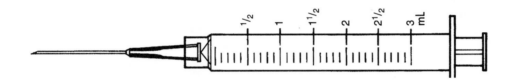

12. Why is it difficult to crossmatch blood to transfuse V.M.? What precautions should be taken with each unit of blood?

13. Identify three outcomes that you expect for V.M. as a result of your interventions.

CASE STUDY PROGRESS

V.M. voids 1900 mL within 2 hours of the furosemide (Lasix) administration. As V.M.'s dyspnea is relieved, he shakes the physician's hand and thanks him for asking about the presence of pain and the need for pain medication. V.M. states, "One of my biggest fears is that I'll come in here in crisis and the doctor won't treat my pain aggressively enough. I don't want to be labeled as a drug seeker or an emergency room abuser."

14. Why would V.M. be concerned about obtaining adequate pain control in the ED?

15. What issues will you address with V.M. before discharge?

Case Study 97

Name _____ Class/Group _____ Date _____

Group Members _____

INSTRUCTIONS All questions apply to this case study. Your responses should be brief and to the point. When asked to provide several answers, list them in order of priority or significance. Do not assume information that is not provided. Please print or write clearly. If your response is not legible, it will be marked as? and you will need to rewrite it.

▶ Scenario

C.O. is a 43-year-old woman who noted a nonpruritic nodular rash on her neck and chest approximately 6 weeks ago. The rash became generalized, spreading to her head, abdomen, and arms and was accompanied by polyarticular joint pain and back pain. She experienced three episodes of epistaxis in 1 day about 2 weeks ago. Over the past week, her gums have become swollen and tender. Because of the progression of symptoms and increasing fatigue, she sought medical attention. Lab work was performed, and C.O. was directly admitted to the referred hematology/oncology unit of a teaching hospital under the care of a hematologist for diagnostic evaluation. Her chest x-ray (CXR) showed normal lung expansion, heart size normal, and no lymphadenopathy. Skin biopsy showed cutaneous leukemic infiltrates, and a bone marrow biopsy showed moderately hypercellular marrow and collections of monoblasts. Her lumbar puncture was free of blast cells. The final diagnosis was acute myeloblastic leukemia.

C.O. is to begin remission induction therapy with cytarabine (Ara-C) 100 mg/m^2/day as continuous infusion for 7 days and idarubicin (Idamycin) 12 mg/m^2/day IV push for 3 days. She is scheduled in angiography for placement of a triple-lumen subclavian Hickman catheter before beginning her therapy.

■ Chart View

Laboratory Test Results	
CBC	
WBC	39,000/mm^3
Monocytes	64%
Lymphocytes	15%
Neutrophils	4%
Blasts	17%
Hgb	10.4 g/dL
Hct	28.7%
Platelets	49,000/mm^3

1. Interpret C.O.'s CBC results. What does the presence of blasts in the differential mean?

2. What is the purpose of a bone marrow biopsy?

3. Considering all the admission data listed previously, what potential problem will the nurse be alert for after the patient returns to the unit following insertion of the catheter?

4. What assessments are essential for the nurse to make regarding the central catheter throughout the hospitalization?

5. What are the side effects of cytarabine (Ara-C) and idarubicin? Identify five nursing interventions related to the side effects of each chemotherapeutic agent.

CASE STUDY PROGRESS

On the fifth day of continuous infusion of cytarabine (Ara-C), the NAP reports to you C.O.'s vital signs:

■ Chart View

Vital Signs

Blood pressure	110/54 mm Hg
Heart rate	115 beats/min
Respiratory rate	26 breaths/min
Temperature	101.6° F (38.7° C)

6. What additional assessments should you make at this time?

CASE STUDY PROGRESS

You notify the intern on duty of your findings, who evaluates C.O. and writes the following orders:

■ Chart View

Physician's Orders

Blood cultures now × 2 sites
Acetaminophen (Tylenol) suppository 650 mg q4-6 h prn
Primaxin (Imipenem) 500 mg IVPB q8h
Notify physician for temp over 100.0° F (37.8° C)

7. Do these orders seem appropriate for this patient? Explain.

8. What will your next step be?

■ Chart View

Laboratory Test Values

WBC	$1200/mm^3$
Monocytes	25%
Lymphocytes	65%
Neutrophils	5%
Blasts	5%
Bands	0%
Hgb	6.8 g/dL
Hct	21.3%
Platelets	$17,000/mm^3$

9. These are C.O.'s labs on the last day of the continuous chemotherapy. What does this count indicate about her immune system?

10. Calculate C.O.'s absolute neutrophil count (ANC) and describe its significance.

11. Considering the previous data, what blood products will most likely be ordered for C.O.?

CASE STUDY PROGRESS

On day 14 after completion of her therapy, a bone marrow biopsy shows the patient is in complete remission. With continued blood product support and antibiotic coverage, her marrow recovers and she is discharged from the hospital. HLA (human lymphocyte antigen) typing has been performed on all siblings. Her oldest brother is a perfect HLA match and has agreed to donate bone marrow or stem cells. C.O. is to be readmitted to the bone marrow transplant unit within the next few weeks.

12. What does "complete remission" mean for C.O., and what impact did it have on the decision to perform a bone marrow transplant?

13. What type of bone marrow transplant will she have? Briefly describe the transplant process.

14. On day 17 after the transplant, she develops severe nausea and vomiting in addition to diarrhea of more than 1200 mL in 24 hours. Graft-versus-host disease of the gut is suspected. Describe graft-versus-host disease.

15. Is there a potentially positive result of this complication? Explain your answer.

16. Identify four priority problems for a patient undergoing a bone marrow transplant, then develop interventions and expected outcomes for each problem

Problem List	Interventions	Expected Outcomes

Continued

9 Oncologic/Hematologic

Problem List	Interventions	Expected Outcomes

Pediatric Disorders

Case Study 98

Name _____ Class/Group _____ Date _____

Group Members _____

INSTRUCTIONS All questions apply to this case study. Your responses should be brief and to the point. When asked to provide several answers, list them in order of priority or significance. Do not assume information that is not provided. Please print or write clearly. If your response is not legible, it will be marked as? and you will need to rewrite it.

▶ Scenario

A.P. is an 8-year-old who is sent to the nurse's office because she has had a several-day history of scratching her head so badly that she complains that her "head hurts." You complete a general examination of A.P.'s head and notice that she has red, irritated areas with several scratch marks; a few open sores; and sesame seed–sized, silvery white and yellow nodules (bugs) that are adhered to many of her hair shafts. You determine that A.P. has pediculosis capitis.

1. What is pediculosis capitis?

2. What will be your next steps in A.P.'s care?

3. What should be included in the educational plans for A.P. and her parents?

4. The parents take A.P. home to treat her. Which statement by A.P.'s mother would help make A.P. the most comfortable during this treatment period? Explain.
   a. "Here is the shampoo. Be sure to scrub your head for several minutes."
   b. "We can pretend you are at the beauty parlor! Lean back while I wash your hair."
   c. "I sure hope this works. I never thought this would happen!"
   d. "It might be best to go ahead and cut your hair. It will grow back quickly."

5. Why would head lice occur in school-aged children?

6. What possible complications can occur as a result of failing to treat head lice?

7. What should your nursing actions include regarding A.P.'s classmates?

10 Pediatric

Case Study **99**

Name _____ Class/Group _____ Date _____

Group Members _____

INSTRUCTIONS All questions apply to this case study. Your responses should be brief and to the point. When asked to provide several answers, list them in order of priority or significance. Do not assume information that is not provided. Please print or write clearly. If your response is not legible, it will be marked as? and you will need to rewrite it.

▶ Scenario

Z.O. is a 3-year-old boy with no significant medical history. He is brought into the emergency department (ED) by the emergency medical technicians after experiencing a seizure lasting 3 minutes. His parents report no previous history that might contribute to the seizure. Upon questioning, they state that they have noticed that he has been irritable, has had a poor appetite, and has been clumsier than usual over the past 2 to 3 weeks. Z.O. and his family are admitted for diagnosis and treatment for a suspected brain tumor. A CT scan of the brain shows a 1-cm mass in the posterior fossa region of the brain, and Z.O. is diagnosed with a cerebellar astrocytoma. The tumor is contained, and the treatment plan will consist of a surgical resection followed by chemotherapy.

1. What are the most common presenting symptoms of a brain tumor?

2. Outline a plan of care for Z.O., describing at least two nursing interventions that would be appropriate for managing fluid status, providing preoperative teaching, facilitating family coping, and preparing Z.O. and his family for surgery.

CASE STUDY PROGRESS

Z.O. returns to the unit after surgery. He is arousable and answers questions appropriately. His pupils are equal and reactive to light. He has a dressing to his head with small amount of serosanguineous drainage. His IV is intact and infusing to a new central venous line as ordered. His breath sounds are equal and clear, and O_2 saturations are 98% on room air. You get him settled in his bed and leave the room.

3. You check the postop orders, which are listed below. Which orders are appropriate, and which would you question? State your rationale.

■ **Chart View**

Postoperative Orders

1. Vital signs every 15 minutes × 4, then every hour × 4, then every 4 hours.
2. Contact MD for temperature less than 36° C or over 38.5° C (96.8° F to 101.3° F).
3. Maintain NPO until fully awake. May offer clear liquids as tolerated.
4. Maintain Trendelenburg's position.
5. Reinforce bandage as needed.
6. Neuro checks every 8 hours.

---

4. You return to the room later in the shift to check on Z.O. Which of these assessment findings would cause concern? (Select all that apply.)
   a. BP 90/55 mm Hg
   b. Increased clear drainage to dressing
   c. Increased choking while sipping water
   d. Photophobia
   e. HR 130 beats/min

10 Pediatric

CASE STUDY PROGRESS

Z.O.'s wound and neurologic status are monitored, and he continues to improve. Z.O. is transferred to the Oncology Service on postoperative day 7 for initiation of chemotherapy.

5. Outline a plan of care that addresses common risks secondary to chemotherapy, describing at least two nursing interventions that would be appropriate for managing risks for infection, bleeding, dehydration, altered growth and nutrition, altered skin integrity, and body image.

6. The nursing assistive personnel (NAP) is in the room caring for Z.O. Which of these safety observations would you need to address? Explain your answer.
   a. NAP encourages Z.O. to use a soft toothbrush for oral care.
   b. NAP applies the disposable probe cover to the rectal thermometer.

  c. NAP applies hand gel before and after assisting Z.O. to the restroom.

  d. NAP assists Z.O. out of bed to prevent a fall.

On Day 10 after initiation of chemotherapy, you receive the following laboratory results:

■ Chart View

Laboratory Test Results

Hemoglobin (Hgb)	12.5 g/dL
Hematocrit (Hct)	36%
White blood cells (WBCs)	7.5/mm^3
Red blood cells (RBCs)	4.0 million/mm^3
Platelets	80,000/mm^3
Albumin	2.8 mg/dL
Absolute neutrophil count (ANC)	75

7. Which of the lab results would you be concerned about, and why?

8. Discuss some of the emotional issues Z.O.'s parents will experience during the immediate postoperative period.

9. Z.O. has a 5-year-old sister. She has been afraid of visiting at the hospital because her "brother might die." Discuss a preschooler's concept of death and strategies to help cope with the illness of a sibling.

10. Postoperatively, Z.O. completed his initial course of chemotherapy. Now, 4 months later, he is experiencing new symptoms, including behavior changes and regression in speech and mobility. His tumor has recurred. The physician suggests hospice care to Z.O.'s parents. List some of the goals of hospice care for this patient and family.

CASE STUDY OUTCOME

Z.O. dies at home just before his fourth birthday. The hospice nurse helps the family by assessing their coping strategies and offers them family bereavement resources.

10 Pediatric

Case Study **100**

Name _____ Class/Group _____ Date _____

Group Members _____

INSTRUCTIONS   All questions apply to this case study. Your responses should be brief and to the point. When asked to provide several answers, list them in order of priority or significance. Do not assume information that is not provided. Please print or write clearly. If your response is not legible, it will be marked as? and you will need to rewrite it.

▶ Scenario

S.G. is a 6-month-old girl who is scheduled for sequential repair of her cleft lip (cheiloplasty) and palate (palatoplasty). She has recently been adopted from China and her past medical history is unknown. S.G. is scheduled for her cleft lip repair, and Mrs. G. brings her to the same-day surgery unit the week before for her preoperative workup. As you do her workup, you recognize that care of the child with clefting uses a multidisciplinary approach.

1. Discuss additional health problems for which these patients are at risk and who on the craniofacial team would address each issue:

2. S.G. weighs 6.5 kg. Plot this finding on the Centers for Disease Control and Prevention (CDC) growth chart (see http://www.cdc.gov/growthcharts/data/set1clinical/cj41l018.pdf). Which of these statements best summarizes your findings?
   a. S.G. falls below the 5th percentile.
   b. S.G.'s weight is at or near the 25th percentile.
   c. S.G.'s weight is at or near the 75th percentile.
   d. S.G.'s weight is greater than the 95th percentile.

3. What information regarding her health history will you obtain from her mother? (Select all that apply and explain your rationale.)
   a. Current known health status
   b. Current source of feeding
   c. Parent's employment status
   d. Immunization status
   e. Adoption status
   f. Gross motor milestones

4. Choose the labs/tests that you expect to be obtained preoperatively, and discuss the rationale for your choices.
   a. Chem 7
   b. Urinalysis
   c. Stool sample for fat content
   d. ABGs (arterial blood gases)
   e. Complete blood count (CBC) with differential

CASE STUDY PROGRESS

The laboratory test results and findings of S.G.'s preoperative workup are normal, and she is scheduled for her cheiloplasty.

5. What will you include in your preoperative teaching to S.G.'s parents?

6. Determine S.G.'s daily fluid maintenance requirements. How can her parents ensure this intake and determine adequate hydration status?

10 Pediatric

7. Mr. and Mrs. G. are advised that S.G. will return 6 months later for the palatoplasty. They are concerned about the delay between surgeries. What will your response be?

CASE STUDY PROGRESS

S.G. returns to your unit 6 months later for her cleft palate repair (palatoplasty).

8. Which of these nursing interventions are appropriate as you plan her care? (Select all that apply, and explain why or why not.)
   a. Position patient side-lying or on abdomen postoperatively.
   b. Use elbow restraints as needed.
   c. Clear fluids; advance as tolerated. Patient may use a straw.
   d. Administer pain medications as ordered.
   e. Oral suction as needed.
   f. Maintain strict intake and output.

9. S.G. has a normal recovery and is being discharged. When giving her parents discharge instructions, what will you advise them concerning diet and signs and symptoms to report?

CASE STUDY OUTCOME

S. G. is discharged to home with instructions for follow-up with a speech pathologist and surgeon.

Case Study **101**

Name _____ Class/Group _____ Date _____

Group Members _____

INSTRUCTIONS All questions apply to this case study. Your responses should be brief and to the point. When asked to provide several answers, list them in order of priority or significance. Do not assume information that is not provided. Please print or write clearly. If your response is not legible, it will be marked as? and you will need to rewrite it.

▶ Scenario

Mr. and Mrs. B. present to the emergency department (ED) with their 6-week-old infant, S.B. As the triage nurse, you ask the couple why they have brought S.B. to the ED. Mrs. B. states, "My baby breastfed well for the first couple of weeks but has recently been throwing up all the time, sometimes a lot and really forcefully. He looks skinny and is hungry and fussy all the time." You determine that the couple is homeless and has been living out of their car for the past month. S. B. has had no primary care since discharge after delivery.

1. What additional information will you need to obtain from Mr. and Mrs. B.?

2. What would you include in your physical assessment of S.B.?

3. The emergency physician orders a complete blood count (CBC), complete metabolic profile (CMP), urinalysis (UA), blood pH, and x-rays. The physician suspects dehydration and metabolic alkalosis secondary to hypertrophic pyloric stenosis. Which of these lab findings would you expect with metabolic alkalosis?
    a. Na: 128 mEq/L, K: 2.6 mEq/L, Cl: 90 mEq/L, HCO_3: 28 mEq/L
    b. Na: 130 mEq/L, K: 5.7 mEq/L, Cl: 94 mEq/L, HCO_3: 22 mEq/L
    c. Na: 130 mEq/L, K: 3.9 mEq/L, Cl: 98 mEq/L, HCO_3: 17 mEq/L
    d. Na: 148 mEq/L K: 4.1 mEq/L, Cl: 108 mEq/L, HCO_3: 13 mEq/L

4. What is the underlying cause of S.B.'s diagnosis of metabolic alkalosis?

10 Pediatric

5. Which of these clinical manifestations might you find with metabolic alkalosis? (Select all that apply.)
   a. Increased respiratory rate
   b. Tetany
   c. Increased risk for seizures
   d. Hyperthermia
   e. Neuromuscular irritability

6. What additional assessment findings might reflect the consequences of frequent prolonged vomiting in the infant?

CASE STUDY PROGRESS

S.B. is diagnosed with hypertrophic pyloric stenosis, admitted to the pediatric unit, and scheduled for surgery.

7. S.B.'s parents are concerned that their living situation contributed to S.B.'s diagnosis. How would you respond to their concerns?

8. Mr. and Mrs. B. have questions about the necessity of surgery and question what is going to be done next. What are your responsibilities as you respond to Mr. and Mrs. B.'s concerns?

9. Which of these preoperative orders would you question?

■ Chart View

Preoperative Orders

1. Vital signs q4h
2. Strict I&O
3. 30 mL Pedialyte q3h PO
4. Place IV and begin D5 1/3 NS at maintenance
5. NG tube placed to low continuous wall suction
6. Daily weights

10. Which of these interventions can be delegated to nursing assistive personnel (NAP)? (Select all that apply.)
    a. Teaching parents rationale for NG tube insertion
    b. Reminding parents to save diapers to be weighed
    c. Obtaining vital signs every 4 hours and reporting any abnormal findings to the RN
    d. Assisting parents in holding infant without removing NG tube
    e. Assessing for NG tube placement every shift

CASE STUDY PROGRESS

S.B. returns to your unit following a pyloromyotomy. Mrs. B. is concerned when she will be able to resume breastfeeding and what they need to do for their baby.

11. What postoperative teaching would you provide to them?

CASE STUDY OUTCOME

S.B. progresses well and is tolerating normal breastfeeding within 48 hours with minimal vomiting. He is discharged with follow-up in 2 weeks with their new primary care provider. A social worker has helped Mr. and Mrs. B. obtain temporary housing and file for temporary insurance for the patient.

Case Study **102**

Name _____ Class/Group _____ Date _____

Group Members _____

INSTRUCTIONS All questions apply to this case study. Your responses should be brief and to the point. When asked to provide several answers, list them in order of priority or significance. Do not assume information that is not provided. Please print or write clearly. If your response is not legible, it will be marked as? and you will need to rewrite it.

▶ **Scenario**

K.B. is a 16-year-old who fell while skiing. She was transported down the hill by the ski patrol after being stabilized and then was flown to the hospital. She has a fractured right femur and humerus. She is admitted to your unit after an open reduction and internal fixation (ORIF) of the femur fracture and casting of her leg and arm.

1. What information should you receive from the post-anesthesia care unit (PACU) nurse?

2. How will you use this information in planning your immediate assessment and care of K.B.?

3. Prioritize the following orders from the most important (1) to the least important (9), and be prepared to explain the priorities you assigned.
   a. VS per routine
   b. Neurologic checks every 2 hours
   c. Turn, cough, and deep breathe and incentive spirometer (IS) every 2 hours while awake
   d. Ice pack and elevate right lower extremity and right upper extremity
   e. Neurovascular checks every 1 hour
   f. NPO
   g. IV fluids D5½NS at 100 mL/hr
   h. Morphine sulfate 5 mg IV every 4-6 hours prn
   i. Cefazolin (Ancef) 880 mg IV every 6 hours

CASE STUDY PROGRESS

K.B. has been settled into her room and begins to complain of pain (7/10) in her leg and arm. She weighs 65 kg. You note the previously mentioned dose, and your drug reference states that the appropriate dose is 0.05-0.1 mg/kg every 4-6 hours.

4. Is this dose safe for your patient?

5. The morphine for injection comes in a concentration of 2 mg/mL. How much will you draw up and double check with an RN? Indicate the amount on the syringe.

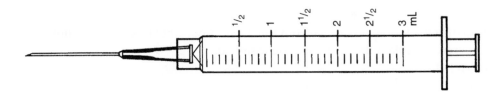

CASE STUDY PROGRESS

K.B. has been on the unit for approximately 6 hours. You identify the following changes in your assessment data: K.B. is difficult to arouse, but when awake she is able to identify who and where she is; PERRLA (Pupils Equal, Round, Reactive to Light and Accommodation) is 1+ with slower reaction time than earlier; color is pale, pink; skin is cool and clammy; heart rate is 126 beats/min, respiratory rate is 28 breaths/min, temperature (oral) is 102° F (39° C); Sao_2 is 90%. You find that neurovascular checks of the affected extremities are unchanged.

6. What will your immediate nursing interventions include?

7. K.B.'s Glasgow Coma Scale begins to decline. What are possible reasons for changes in her neurologic status?

CASE STUDY PROGRESS

K.B. is transferred to the pediatric ICU and treated for changes in her neurologic status. The following day, her primary care provider (PCP) determines she is stable and has her transferred back to the pediatric unit. It is now 36 hours postop. K.B. suddenly begins to complain of extreme pain in her lower right leg. She rates her pain as a 10/10.

8. Which of these findings are early signs of compartment syndrome? (Select all that apply.)
   a. Diminished pedal pulse
   b. Macular rash
   c. Edema
   d. Paresthesia
   e. Cap refill less than 2 seconds
   f. Increased pain

9. You page the orthopedic surgeon. Use SBAR (situation, background, assessment, recommendation) to address patient status.

10. K.B.'s cast is split and her foot pulses are restored. K.B. and her parents are extremely anxious. What education and support will be provided to K.B. and her parents?

10 Pediatric

K.B.'s status continues to improve. Physical and occupational therapists work with her on transfers and performing activities of daily living (ADL). She has many questions about how she will be able to go to school and resume her normal routine.

11. Recognizing her developmental and cognitive stage, which of these statements are appropriate as you explain her care on discharge?
    a. Adolescents are capable of thinking in concrete terms only.
    b. Adolescents are preoccupied with the immediate situation rather than future events.
    c. Adolescents can anticipate future implications of current decisions.
    d. Family acceptance is more important than peer acceptance.

12. The multidisciplinary team is made aware of K.B.'s progress in discharge rounds. How will you use the following disciplines?
    • Discharge planning
    • Education
    • Physical/Occupational therapy
    • Nutrition

CASE STUDY OUTCOME

K.B. is discharged to home on postop day 5 with homebound schooling ordered and follow-up with orthopedics in 2 weeks.

Case Study **103**

Name _____ Class/Group _____ Date _____

Group Members _____

INSTRUCTIONS All questions apply to this case study. Your responses should be brief and to the point. When asked to provide several answers, list them in order of priority or significance. Do not assume information that is not provided. Please print or write clearly. If your response is not legible, it will be marked as? and you will need to rewrite it.

▶ **Scenario**

J.R., a 13-year-old with cystic fibrosis, is being seen in the outpatient clinic for a biannual evaluation. J.R. lives at home with his parents and 7-year-old sister, C.R., who also has cystic fibrosis. J.R. reports that he "doesn't feel good," explaining that he has missed the last week of school, doesn't have any energy, is coughing more, and is having "a hard time breathing."

1. What additional data should be obtained from J.R. and his parents?

2. Describe the pathophysiology of cystic fibrosis (CF). Be sure to address the multisystem component of this disorder.

CASE STUDY PROGRESS

J.R. is admitted to the hospital for a suspected respiratory infection. Your assessment includes the following: color, pale pink with bluish tinged nail beds; respiratory rate, 28 breaths/min and somewhat labored; oral temperature, 38.8° C (101.8° F); Sao$_2$, 88%; rhonchi noted throughout; thorax has a barrel-chest appearance; appears thin, weighs 30 kg.

3. Why is J.R. at risk for developing pulmonary infections?

4. What are the common microorganisms that cause respiratory infections in children with cystic fibrosis?

■ Chart View

Medication Orders

Ceftazidime (Fortaz) 2 g IV q8h
Gentamicin (Gentak) 100 mg IV q8h
Vancomycin (Vancocin) 450 mg IV q8h

5. You review the drugs that have been ordered to treat J.R.'s suspected infection. What will you do before administering these drugs?

6. Use a nursing drug reference book to find the safe dosage ranges for the previously mentioned antibiotics, and calculate the dosage of each antibiotic J.R. will receive with the previous orders. Are the prescribed doses within the safe ranges? (Show all work.) J.R. weighs 30 kg.

7. What factor will affect the selection of antibiotics and dosages?

8. You are reviewing the physician orders for respiratory care. Which of these nursing interventions would you expect to perform, and why?
   a. Administer aerosolized albuterol (a bronchodilator).

   b. Administer chest physiotherapy (CPT) before administering the bronchodilator.

   c. Monitor continuous pulse oximetry.

   d. Administer aerosolized Pulmozyme (dornase alfa) after administration of bronchodilator.

   e. Administer nebulized NS (normal saline).

   f. Administer antibiotic via JET nebulizer.

   g. Limit fluid intake.

9. J.R.'s weight is below the 5th percentile. He has been on a high-calorie, high-protein diet at home; however, he reports that he hasn't been hungry and really hasn't been eating much. Describe the link between malnutrition and cystic fibrosis.

10. Which of these actions can be delegated to the nursing assistive personnel (NAP)?
   a. Charting daily weights and intake and output
   b. Instructing the parents on correct administration of normal saline nebulizers.
   c. Administering pancreatic enzymes from home supply with each snack.
   d. Increasing O_2 during an episode of desaturation.

10 Pediatric

11. Which of these strategies are appropriate to manage the GI dysfunction that patients with CF often experience? (Select all that apply.)
    a. Administer fat-soluble vitamins daily.
    b. Administer pancreatic enzymes with meals and snacks.
    c. Restrict fat intake.
    d. Encourage a high-protein diet.
    e. Breastfeeding is contraindicated in infants with CF.
    f. Encourage snacks between meals.

12. What clinical sign assists in determining the effective dosage of pancreatic enzymes?

13. Discuss the common GI disorders that children with CF might be prone to.

CASE STUDY PROGRESS

J.R. will be spending 14 to 21 days in the hospital for treatment of his pulmonary infection. How will this hospitalization affect J.R.'s normal development?

14. How can you foster his development while he is hospitalized?

15. J.R. is an adolescent and asks you, "Will I be able to have children when I grow up?" Your best response would be:
    a. "You should discuss this with your parents. I will let them know you asked."
    b. "Most males have a significant chance of being sterile and you won't need to consider use of contraception."

c. "Although nearly 95% of males are sterile, you can discuss this with your physician and family."

d. "CF does not affect the male reproductive system; however, it does affect the female reproductive tract."

CASE STUDY OUTCOME

J.R. improves with antibiotic therapy and is being discharged to home.

16. Discuss health promotion behaviors that need to be reinforced with J.R. and his parents.

10 Pediatric

Case Study **104**

Name _____ Class/Group _____ Date _____

Group Members _____

INSTRUCTIONS All questions apply to this case study. Your responses should be brief and to the point. When asked to provide several answers, list them in order of priority or significance. Do not assume information that is not provided. Please print or write clearly. If your response is not legible, it will be marked as? and you will need to rewrite it.

▶ Scenario

J.H. is a 2-week-old infant brought to the emergency department (ED) by his mother, who speaks little English. Her husband is at work. She is young and appears frightened and anxious. Through a translator, Mrs. H. reports that J.H. has not been eating, sleeps all of the time, and is "not normal."

1. What are some of the obstacles you need to consider, recognizing that Mrs. H. does not speak or understand English well?

2. You perform your primary assessment and question Mrs. H. with a translator. Which of these findings are abnormal and need to be reported? (Select all that apply and state rationale.)
   a. Anterior fontanel palpable and tense
   b. Pupils equal and +3
   c. Temperature 36° C rectally
   d. Heart rate: 85 beats/min
   e. Positive Babinski's reflex
   f. High-pitched cry
   g. Refusal of PO intake per mom

CASE STUDY PROGRESS

J.H. is admitted to the medical unit with the diagnoses of meningitis and rule out sepsis.
The ED physician orders the following:

■ Chart View

Emergency Department Orders

    CBC with differential

    Blood culture

    Complete metabolic panel (CMP)

    Urinalysis (UA)

    Cerebrospinal fluid (CSF) for culture, glucose, protein, cell count (following lumbar puncture)

    Ceftriaxone (Rocephin) 260 mg IV now (loading dose)

    Acetaminophen (Tylenol) 50 mg suppository per rectum for irritability

---

3. Prioritize the order of your interventions, with 1 being your first action and 7 being your last action.

    ___Administer ceftriaxone (Rocephin)

    ___Place IV

    ___Straight catheterization for urine specimen

    ___Place on contact isolation and droplet precautions

    ___Assist with lumbar puncture

    ___Administer Tylenol

    ___Obtain blood culture, CMP

4. Before administering the ceftriaxone (Rocephin), you must verify the dose with another RN. The therapeutic range is 100 mg/kg/day divided in two doses. J.H. weighs 3.5 kg. Is the dose ordered safe? (Show your work.)

10 Pediatric

5. Interpret J.H.'s lab findings, and explain the rationale for abnormal results.

■ Chart View

Laboratory Test Results

Urine

pH	7.2
Color	Clear
Leukocytes	Negative

Complete blood count

Hct	32%
HgB	10.5 g/dL
WBC	22,000/mm^3
Sodium	125 mEq/L

6. Interpret the CSF findings. Would you suspect bacterial or viral meningitis? Why?

■ Chart View

Cerebrospinal Fluid Analysis

CSF	Clear
Gram stain	Pending
Protein	300 mg/dL (elevated)
Leukocytes	1030 cells/microliter (elevated)
Glucose	40 mg/dL (decreased)

7. What are the most common pathogens in this age group?

10 Pediatric

CASE STUDY PROGRESS

J.H. is diagnosed with *Escherichia coli* meningitis. His medical care plan will include 14 to 21 days of antibiotic therapy. You are developing his nursing plan of care.

8. Outline a plan of care for J.H., describing nursing interventions that would be appropriate for managing pain and infection, maintaining hydration, assisting with increased intracranial pressure (ICP), and teaching to review with his parents.

CASE STUDY PROGRESS

Mrs. H., through her translator, asks you what could have caused her baby to be sick since he had an immunization when he was born. She asks whether he should get "more shots" so this won't happen again. You reinforce to Mrs. H. that infants have immature immune systems, and they are vulnerable to infections until they have been immunized. Mrs. H. asks when J.H. will get more shots and what will they be?

9. According to the CDC immunization schedule, which of the following immunizations will J.H. receive at 2 months? You can refer to the current immunization schedules posted at http://www.cdc.gov/vaccines/recs/schedules/child-schedule.htm.
   a. Hib
   b. MMR
   c. OPV
   d. IPV
   e. Rotavirus
   f. DTaP

    g. Varicella

    h. Hep B

    i. Pneumococcal

10. What is the impact of hospitalization on J.H.'s growth and development?

11. J.H. is being discharged after 3 weeks of IV antibiotic therapy. What educational topics will be important to discuss with J.H.'s parents when he is discharged?

CASE STUDY OUTCOME

J.H. is discharged to home with his parents. He will continue PO antibiotics for 1 week and receive a home health visit for infant care follow-up. He is to return to his PCP in 1 week or call for any concerns.

10 Pediatric

Case Study 105

Name _____ Class/Group _____ Date _____

Group Members _____

INSTRUCTIONS All questions apply to this case study. Your responses should be brief and to the point. When asked to provide several answers, list them in order of priority or significance. Do not assume information that is not provided. Please print or write clearly. If your response is not legible, it will be marked as? and you will need to rewrite it.

▶ Scenario

L.S. is a 7-year-old who has been brought to the emergency department (ED) by his mother. She immediately tells you he has a history of ED visits for his asthma. He uses an inhaler when he wheezes, but it ran out a month ago. She is a single parent and has two other children at home with a babysitter. Your assessment finds L.S. alert, oriented, and extremely anxious. His color is pale, and his nail beds are dusky and cool to the touch; other findings are heart rate 136 beats/min, respiratory rate 36 breaths/min regular and even, oral temperature 37.3° C (99.1° F), Sao_2 89%, breath sounds decreased in lower lobes bilaterally and congested with inspiratory and expiratory wheezes, prolonged expirations, and a productive cough.

1. As you ask Ms. S. questions, you note that L.S.'s respiratory rate is increasing; he is sitting on the side of the bed, leaning slightly forward, and is having difficulty breathing. You are concerned that he is experiencing status asthmaticus. Which interventions are appropriate at this time? (Select all that apply and explain rationale.)
   a. Monitor HR and RR every 2 hours.
   b. Administer oxygen via nasal cannula to keep Sao_2 greater than 90%.
   c. Have L.S. lie flat.
   d. Administer albuterol (Proventil) and ipratropium bromide (Atrovent) via hand-held nebulizer (HHN).
   e. Reassess in 20 minutes and if no improvement, administer salmeterol (Serevent) via multidose inhaler (MDI).
   f. Administer methylprednisolone IV stat.
   g. Have L.S. perform incentive spirometry.
   h. Encourage PO fluids.

2. Identify the nursing responsibilities associated with giving albuterol.

CASE STUDY PROGRESS

L.S. is admitted to the PICU (pediatric intensive care unit) for close monitoring. He improves and 24 hours later is transferred to the floor. Asthma teaching is ordered. You assess Ms. S.'s understanding of asthma and her understanding of the disorder.

10 Pediatric

3. Which of these statements by Ms. S. would indicate a need for further teaching?
   a. "He should go to the doctor regularly to make sure his asthma is being treated correctly."
   b. "If he takes medications for a while, he will outgrow his asthma."
   c. "Part of L.'s treatment should be avoiding things that irritate his lungs."
   d. "If I recognize early warning signs, he might be able to take medicine and not go to the ER."

4. You are educating L.S. and his mother on possible triggers in their environment. They live in public housing in an apartment without air conditioning. Which of these statements indicate possible triggers? (Select all that apply, and discuss strategies to avoid these triggers.)
   a. "The building has copper pipes."
   b. "He coughs when we have cold nights after a warm day."
   c. "We have a pet fish."
   d. "There are hardwood floors."
   e. "L. collects stuffed animals."
   f. "Our visitors smoke outside."
   g. "There are dark stains in our bathroom."
   h. "The housing authority puts a foam down for bugs."

CASE STUDY PROGRESS

The following day, L.S. gets the following discharge orders.

■ Chart View

Discharge Orders

Discharge to home
Follow up with primary care provider in 3 days for evaluation
Albuterol (Proventil HFA) MDI: 2 puffs with spacer every 4 hours prn
Prednisolone (Prelone) 1 mg/kg PO every day for 5 days (L.S. weighs 23 kg.)
Fluticasone (Flovent HFA) MDI: 1 puff twice a day
Montelukast sodium (Singulair) 5 mg every evening PO
Regular diet

10 Pediatric

5. Ms. S. asks why she will use the spacer with the medicine L.S. breathes in. Explain the purpose of a multi-dose inhaler (MDI) and spacer, and how they are used together.

6. During your medication teaching session with Ms. S. and L.S., Ms. S. makes this statement: "So, if he has to take both inhalers at the same time, he should take the Flovent first, then the albuterol. Right?" Is this statement true or false? If false, explain your answer.

7. As you continue your medication teaching, you explain the difference between controller and reliever medications. Place a C beside the controller medication(s) and R beside the reliever medication(s).
_____a. Albuterol
_____b. Prelone
_____c. Flovent
_____d. Singulair

8. After L.S. takes a dose of the inhaled corticosteroid Flovent, what is the most important action he should do next?
a. Hold his breath for 45 seconds.
b. Rinse out his mouth with water.
c. Repeat the dose in 5 minutes if he feels short of breath.
d. Check his peak flow meter reading for an improvement of function.

10 Pediatric

9. Ms. S. comes back from the pharmacy with the Prelone and asks you to show her how much to give. Prelone is dispensed 15 mg/5 mL. You give her a 10-mL oral dosing syringe. How much will she draw up for this dose?

10. L.S. tells you that he loves to play basketball and football and asks you whether he can still do these activities. How will you respond?

11. What additional information should be included in your discharge teaching regarding how to prevent acute asthmatic episodes and how to manage symptoms of exacerbation of asthma?

CASE STUDY OUTCOME

L.S. is discharged to home and has a follow-up appointment scheduled in 2 weeks. He plans to try out for his school's swim team.

10 Pediatric

Case Study **106**

Name _____ Class/Group _____ Date _____

Group Members _____

INSTRUCTIONS All questions apply to this case study. Your responses should be brief and to the point. When asked to provide several answers, list them in order of priority or significance. Do not assume information that is not provided. Please print or write clearly. If your response is not legible, it will be marked as? and you will need to rewrite it.

▶ ## Scenario

E.M., a 5-month-old female, presents to the emergency department (ED) with respiratory distress, hypoxia, and fever. Her parents state that she has had mild cold symptoms for a few days. She has fed poorly over the last few days with a decreased number of wet diapers. You take her vital signs and complete an initial assessment.

■ Chart View

Vital Signs

Blood pressure	130/72 mm Hg
Respiratory rate	83 breaths/min
Heart rate	188 beats/min
Temperature	38.4° C (101.1° F)
Sao_2	88% on room air
Weight	8 kg

Initial Assessment

Neurologic	Alert, fussy, consoles briefly, anterior fontanel soft and slightly depressed
Cardiovascular	Tachycardia; capillary refill less than 3 seconds
Respiratory	Upper airway congestion; coarse cough; tachypnea, transient bilateral wheezing; breath sounds coarse and decreased slightly at bases; mild intercostal retractions
GI	Positive bowel sounds; last bowel movement yesterday
GU	Decreased urine output (per history); no urine output in last 4 hours
Skin	No rashes; slightly flushed
Other	Mucous membranes "sticky"; decreased tearing

Emergency Department Orders

a. Acetaminophen (Tylenol) 60 mg PO for fever
b. Normal saline (NS) bolus 20 mL/kg IV bolus
c. Oxygen to keep saturations greater than 93%
d. Nebulizer trial of albuterol (Proventil) 2.5 mg

10 Pediatric

1. Review the standing ED orders. Prioritize your interventions with rationales.

2. Based on E.M.'s vital signs and assessment, what diagnostic tests would you anticipate?

3. Calculate how much normal saline E.M. will receive as a bolus.

CASE STUDY PROGRESS

E.M. begins coughing and has copious nasal secretions. You provide nasopharyngeal suctioning and obtain a large amount of thick secretions. She is allowed to recover and is reassessed. The respiratory rate and retractions have not changed significantly. Her breath sounds are less coarse but are diminished in the bases. The Sao_2 is now 92% to 93% on 1.5 L oxygen. After E.M. settles, her mother asks whether she can feed her because she has not eaten much for the past few days. You tell her that with a current respiratory rate of greater than 65 breaths/min, she should not be fed.

4. What is the rationale for holding feeds?

5. When E.M.'s respiratory rate decreases, what teaching would you provide the parents concerning feeding?

6. You are reviewing the medication administration record. Which order(s) would you question? Explain.

■ Chart View

Medication Administration Record

Normal saline drops to nares q3hr with suctioning
Acetaminophen (Tylenol) 60 mg PO q4-6 h prn for fever
Amoxicillin (Amoxil) 45 mg/kg/day PO tid × 7 days

CASE STUDY PROGRESS

E.M.'s mother calls you to the room because her baby is "not right." You note E.M.'s respiratory rate is 23 breaths/min, and the retractions have increased. The Sao_2 is 89% on 1.5 L of oxygen. She is pale and listless and does not cry with stimulation.

7. Why is the respiratory rate significantly lower even though other signs of respiratory distress have increased?

CASE STUDY PROGRESS

You are concerned and call the Rapid Response Team. The Senior Resident orders a portable chest x-ray (CXR) and capillary blood gas (CBG). The CXR is consistent with bronchiolitis with atelectasis.

■ Chart View

Capillary Blood Gas

pH	7.31
$Paco_2$	72 mm Hg
HCO_2	29 mEq/L

8. Interpret E.M.'s CBG results.

CASE STUDY PROGRESS

E.M. is transferred to the pediatric ICU and is placed on a continuous positive airway pressure (CPAP) machine. You know from experience that patients are usually on CPAP for a couple of days before they are ready to be taken off and continue to improve until they are ready for discharge. You explain this to the parents who are very distressed.

10 Pediatric

9. What resources might you seek for E.M.'s parents during this unanticipated change in status?

Following 2 days in the PICU, E.M. is transferred back to your unit. You note that she is taking increased oral fluids and requiring less suctioning. Her Spo$_2$ is 96% to 98% on room air. As you are preparing the parents for discharge, they want to know how they can prevent this in the future. They ask whether there is a "shot" E.M. can get to avoid getting this again.

10. How would you address their concerns?

11. Mr. and Mrs. M. ask you for instructions about the treatment of cold symptoms if E.M. develops them again. Which answer is your best reply?
   a. "Over-the-counter cough suppressants may be safely administered at night."
   b. "If a fever is present, you can treat the fever with baby aspirin."
   c. "Saline nose drops and bulb suctioning can be done before feedings."
   d. "You do not need to worry if she is not drinking; intake should improve in a day or so."

Case Study **107**

Name _____ Class/Group _____ Date _____

Group Members _____

INSTRUCTIONS All questions apply to this case study. Your responses should be brief and to the point. When asked to provide several answers, list them in order of priority or significance. Do not assume information that is not provided. Please print or write clearly. If your response is not legible, it will be marked as? and you will need to rewrite it.

▶ Scenario

You admit L.M., a 2-month-old girl with a history of hydrocephalus and ventriculoperitoneal (VP) shunt placement 1 month earlier. Her parents report that she has been more irritable than usual and, for the past 3 days, has fed poorly and had emesis five or six times every day.

1. Explain the pathophysiology of hydrocephalus and cerebral spinal fluid (CSF) imbalance.

2. Explain how the placement of a VP shunt helps the patient.

CASE STUDY PROGRESS

You get L.M. settled on the unit and promptly perform her admission assessment.

3. Your assessment includes the following findings. Select the abnormal findings and state a possible rationale for each.

System	Assessment and Vital Signs	If Abnormal, State Rationale
Weight	4.5 kg	
Neurologic	Irritable, awake, and fussy; difficult to console FOC: 44 cm, "increased 2 cm from measurement yesterday" per mother	
	Anterior fontanel slightly bulging Unable to palpate posterior fontanel Pupils equal and reactive	
Respiratory	Bilateral breath sounds equal and clear Sao$_2$ 95% on room air Respiratory rate: 55 breaths/min	
Cardiovascular	Rectal temp: 38.8° C	
	HR: 182 BP: 111/70 Pulses 2+ and equal bilaterally	
GI	Postive bowel sounds Emesis during exam Last feeding 6 hours ago	

4. The doctors order a CT scan and lumbar puncture with a cell count, culture, Gram stain, glucose, and protein run on the cerebrospinal fluid (CSF). What is the rationale for each procedure?

CASE STUDY PROGRESS

It is determined that the VP shunt is infected. L.M. is taken to surgery to have a temporary left extraventricular drain (EVD) placed. She returns to your unit in stable condition. You get her settled back into her room and perform her assessment. You note that her EVD is correctly leveled and draining CSF. The dressing is clean/dry and intact under a sterile dressing.

5. Which of these medications would you expect to see on L.M.'s Medication Administration Record (MAR)? Select all that apply and state the rationale for the ones you choose.

■ Chart View

Medication Administration Record

Acetaminophen (Tylenol) 15 mg/kg PO q4h
Morphine sulfate 0.05-0.1 mg/kg IV q4h
Enalapril (Vasotec) 5 mcg/kg q24h
Cefotaxime sodium (Claforan) 150 mg/kg/day IV in divided doses q8h
Baclofen (Lioresal) 10 mg/kg/day PO q8h
Ondansetron (Zofran) 0.1 mg/kg IV now

6. You are preparing to give the first dose of the antibiotic that is ordered. Referring to L.M.'s MAR, calculate the dose of the antibiotic that you will administer.

7. Which of these tasks can be appropriately delegated to the nursing assistive personnel (NAP)?
   a. Performing the every-2-hour neurologic check
   b. Obtaining a complete set of vital signs and charting
   c. Instructing the parents on changes in neurologic status
   d. Changing the dressing on the surgical site

8. Which of the following positions should L.M. be placed immediately postop?

    a. Flat, left side-lying

    b. Flat, right side-lying

    c. Supine HOB 45 degrees

    d. Supine, Trendelenburg's

9. What will you teach the parents about the EVD system?

CASE STUDY PROGRESS

Several days later, Mrs. M. is changing L.M.'s diaper, and she tells you that she is worried because L.M. has started having diarrhea recently, and it is getting worse.

10. Based on the medications that L.M. is receiving, what is the most likely cause of the diarrhea? What is a possible concern you should consider, and what should your care plan include?

CASE STUDY PROGRESS

L.M. responds well to the antibiotics, and her shunt is internalized 2 weeks later. She is released from the hospital after observation for 2 days.

11. During your discharge instructions, Mrs. M. states that she normally gives L.M. 1 mL of Tylenol Elixir (acetaminophen) (160 mg/5 mL) and asks whether this is the correct dose. L.M.'s current weight is 4.5 kg and the therapeutic range of acetaminophen dosage is 10-15 mg/kg q 4-6 hours. Which of these statements would be your best response?

    a. "This is a safe amount; you should continue to give that dose every four hours."

    b. "You can continue to give her that amount; you can give her a dose every two hours."

    c. "You should give 1.4 to 2.1 milliliters every four to six hours based on her current weight."

    d. "Tylenol should not be given to a child her age."

10 Pediatric

CASE STUDY OUTCOME

L.M. returns for her postop check 2 weeks later and is playful and alert. The neurologist will continue to monitor her closely with follow-up visits.

Case Study **108**

Name _____ Class/Group _____ Date _____

Group Members _____

INSTRUCTIONS All questions apply to this case study. Your responses should be brief and to the point. When asked to provide several answers, list them in order of priority or significance. Do not assume information that is not provided. Please print or write clearly. If your response is not legible, it will be marked as? and you will need to rewrite it.

▶ **Scenario**

The charge nurse tells you that you will be admitting a 1-hour-old girl, Baby Girl R., with a myelomeningocele that was discovered in utero. You know that the mother will still be at the local medical center recovering from her cesarean delivery.

1. What is the rationale for doing a cesarean delivery for babies with myelomeningocele?

CASE STUDY PROGRESS

The infant arrives accompanied by her aunt and father. While you are getting vital signs (VS), the father tells you that he has been trying to research myelomeningocele on the Internet, but he is still confused, especially about the difference between myelomeningocele and meningocele.

2. Using lay terms, what would you tell the father about the pathophysiology of myelomeningocele? What is the difference between myelomeningocele and meningocele?

3. Following your discussion with the family, which of these statements by the father would indicate a need for more teaching? (Select all that apply.)
   a. "My baby's malformation can also be referred to as spina bifida (SB) cystica."
   b. "My baby will probably not require surgery until she is a year old."
   c. "My baby will need to lie on her stomach in her incubator."
   d. "I need to wash my hands carefully to prevent spread of germs."

10 Pediatric

CASE STUDY PROGRESS

Baby Girl R. is in an open warmer. You document the following information:

■ Chart

Admission Data

Blood pressure	67/33 mm Hg
Pulse	173 beats/min
Respirations	52 breaths/min
Rectal temperature	37.1° C (98.8° F)
Sao_2	95%
Weight	3.5 kg
FOC	37 cm

Fontanel soft and flat

Pupils 2 cm, brisk reaction

Sleepy, squirms and fusses during pupil check

Breath sounds clear; bowel sounds present

Pulses 2+ and capillary refill time less than 3 seconds

Bilateral clubfeet, and no reaction when pulse oximeter is placed on right foot

Sac in sacral region covered with sterile gauze that is moistened with saline

4. Which of the previous assessment and monitoring data are abnormal for a 1-hour-old infant?

5. Explain the rationale for the following orders:

Orders	Rationale
Place in prone position.	
Place PIV with D5 1/3 NS at 15 mL/hr.	
Administer IV antibiotics as ordered.	
PT (physical therapy) consult	
Open warmer.	
Orthopedic consult	
Place Foley catheter.	
NPO	
Maintain sterile gauze with NS to sac/monitor q1h.	
Measure FOC (frontal occipital circumference) every shift.	

6. The surgeon orders cefazolin sodium (Ancef) 140 mg on call to the OR. You add 10 mL of sterile water to the 1 g vial for concentration of 100 mg/1 mL. Calculate how many milliliters you will draw up for this dose. Note on the syringe how much you will draw up to send with the patient.

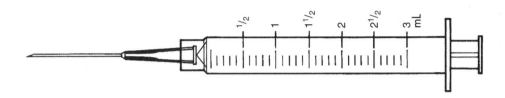

The next day in report, you hear that Baby Girl R. did well overnight. She goes to surgery at 0815. Later, the post-anesthesia care unit (PACU) nurse tells you that Baby Girl R. is ready to return to your unit. When she arrives, you and the NAP start putting on the monitors. Mr. R. is present, and he asks you to give the baby some pain medication. The open warmer starts alarming because the patient's skin temperature is reading 35° C. You look down at her to see whether the temperature probe has fallen off. You see that it is still on, but you also notice that the suture from surgery is no longer intact. Then the oxygen (O_2) monitor reads 71% saturated with an accurate waveform, and the pulse oximeter probe is correctly placed on the patient. The patient's respiratory rate is 25 breaths/min and the heart rate is 102 beats/min.

7. Which of the issues should you address first? Give rationale.

Baby Girl R. stabilizes. Her temperature is 36.7° C (98.1° F) per skin probe. Respiratory rate and heart rate improve and her Sao_2 is 98% on ¼ LPM oxygen per nasal cannula. The surgeon is at the bedside and patient returns to the OR for revision of incision.

Two days later, you are caring for Baby Girl R. at night. In report, you hear that the parents really want to hold their baby, but they have not yet because they are afraid of causing the suture to open again. They are currently at the bedside, and the infant is due for a feeding.

8. How can you help the parents become comfortable with holding their baby?

10 Pediatric

9. When you take the bottle in to the patient's room, you notice a growth chart next to the bed tracking the patient's frontal occipital circumference (FOC) that is measured at least once per shift. Baby Girl R.'s FOC has increased to 38.5 cm. Using the appropriate CDC growth chart (http://www.cdc.gov/growthcharts/data/set2/chart%2010.pdf), is the following statement true or false?
The FOC is close to the 95% and can be monitored less frequently because this is a normal finding.

CASE STUDY OUTCOME

Baby Girl R. is followed closely in the Level 2 nursery. She stabilizes and is able to be discharged to home in 2 weeks with close multidisciplinary follow-up.

Case Study **109**

Name _____ Class/Group _____ Date _____

Group Members _____

INSTRUCTIONS All questions apply to this case study. Your responses should be brief and to the point. When asked to provide several answers, list them in order of priority or significance. Do not assume information that is not provided. Please print or write clearly. If your response is not legible, it will be marked as? and you will need to rewrite it.

▶ Scenario

R.O. is a 12-year-old girl who lives with her family on a farm in a rural community. R.O. has four siblings who have recently been ill with stomach pains, vomiting, diarrhea, and fever. They were seen by their primary care provider (PCP) and diagnosed with viral gastroenteritis. A week later, R.O. woke up at 0200 crying and telling her mother that her stomach "hurts really bad!" She had an elevated temperature of 37.9° C (100.2° F). R.O. began to vomit over the next few hours, so her parents took her to the local emergency department (ED). R.O.'s vital signs (VS), complete blood count (CBC), and complete metabolic panel were normal, so she was hydrated with IV fluids and discharged to home with instructions to call their PCP or to return to the ED if she did not improve or worsened. Over the next 2 days, R.O.'s abdominal pain localized to the right lower quadrant (RLQ), she refused to eat, and she had slight diarrhea. On the third day, she began to have more severe abdominal pain, increased vomiting, and fever that did not respond to acetaminophen. R.O. returns to the ED. Her VS are 128/78, 130, 28, 39.5° C (103.1° F). R.O. is guarding her lower abdomen, prefers to lie on her side with her legs flexed, and is crying. IV access is established, and morphine sulfate 2 mg IV is administered for pain. An abdominal CT (computed tomography) confirms a diagnosis of appendicitis. R.O.'s white blood count (WBC) is 12,000 mm³.

1. Identify the clinical manifestations exhibited by R.O. that most clearly reflect the classic presentation of appendicitis.

2. Discuss why R.O.'s presenting clinical manifestations make diagnosis more difficult; identify two other possible diagnoses.

3. The abdominal CT confirms that R.O. has appendicitis. Which of these orders are appropriate? Explain rationale. If the order is inappropriate, explain why.

■ Chart View

Emergency Department Orders

1. Make patient NPO.
2. Place a peripheral IV and begin D5½NS at 80 mL/hr.
3. Administer Fleet Enema to rule out impaction.
4. Administer morphine sulfate 2 mg IV q2h for pain.
5. Obtain surgical consent from patient.
6. Administer cefotaxime (Claforan), a broad spectrum antibiotic, at 150 mg/kg/day q6h.

4. R.O.'s weight is 42 kg, and height is 155 cm. Calculate her maintenance fluid needs and discuss how this will be met.

5. Mr. and Mrs. O. give informed consent, and R.O. assents to the surgery after the procedure is explained to her. Why is it important for R.O. to provide her assent for the procedure?

6. What should be included in the preoperative teaching for R.O. and her parents?

CASE STUDY PROGRESS

R.O. undergoes an appendectomy; the appendix has ruptured. The peritoneum is inflamed, and abscesses are seen near the colon and small intestine. R.O. is admitted to the surgical unit; she is NPO, has a nasogastric tube (NGT), Foley catheter, IV, abdominal dressing, and a Penrose drain.

7. Identify five priority nursing considerations.

CASE STUDY PROGRESS

Postop Day 2: R.O. continues to improve and is tolerating ice chips. Breath sounds are clear, and she is performing her pulmonary hygiene. NGT has minimal drainage. Foley catheter has been removed, and the patient has adequate urine output. The Penrose drain has been removed. The incision is well approximated with no drainage or redness. Her pain is 4-6 out of 10 with pain medication every 4 hours.

Postop Day 3: Assessment shows that R.O. is pale and listless; bowel sounds are absent; abdomen is distended and tender to the touch; the NGT is draining an increased amount of dark, greenish black fluid. Her lung sounds are moist bilaterally, and her temperature has spiked to 40.2° C (104.4° F). She rates her pain at 10 out of 10 and is having difficulty taking deep breaths because of the pain, which she says "hurts over my whole stomach."

8. What should your priority nursing care include?

9. Using SBAR (**s**ituation, **b**ackground, **a**ssessment, **r**ecommendation), what would you communicate to the surgeon?

10 Pediatric

10. What will you consider as part of your nursing management of R.O.'s pain?

CASE STUDY PROGRESS

The surgeon assesses R.O. and orders a return to the operating room. R.O. returns to surgery, where she has lysis of adhesions, removal of necrotic bowel, and drainage of an abscess. The surgeon has left her abdominal wound open and has ordered wound packing changes twice daily and abdominal irrigation with normal saline (NS). R.O. cries and becomes agitated when you go to perform the procedure.

11. What should you consider in your approach to help R.O. cope with the procedure?

12. In anticipation of R.O.'s discharge, identify expected outcomes that must be achieved before her leaving the hospital.

13. You provide discharge teaching to R.O. and her parents. Which of these statements would indicate that more teaching is required?
   a. "We need to return if R.O. begins vomiting again or develops a fever."
   b. "R.O. should wait 2 weeks before returning to her gymnastics program."
   c. "We will keep the incision clean and call if we see redness or drainage."
   d. "R.O. can advance her diet to the regular foods that she likes to eat."

CASE STUDY OUTCOME

R.O. is discharged to her home with her parents and has an uneventful recovery. She is scheduled for a follow-up visit with the surgeon in 2 weeks.

Case Study 110

Name _____ Class/Group _____ Date _____

Group Members _____

▶ Scenario

T.M. is a 3-year-old boy with cerebral palsy (CP) who has been admitted to your unit preoperatively. He will have surgery for a femoral osteotomy and tendon lengthening to stabilize hip joints and to help reduce spasticity. You are orienting the parents to the unit and have a nursing student assisting you.

1. After getting the family settled, you return to the nursing station, and the nursing student asks you to explain what CP is and what might have caused cerebral palsy. How would you answer the student's question?

2. The nursing student asks what the family might have noticed that would indicate CP in T.M. when he was a baby. Which of these findings will you include in your discussion with the student? (Select all that apply and state rationale.)
   a. Head lag at 5 months
   b. Able to sit unassisted at 7 months
   c. Positive Moro (startle) reflex at 2 months
   d. Leg scissoring
   e. Right hand preference at 12 months
   f. Use of pincer grasp at 9 months
   g. Increased irritability

CASE STUDY PROGRESS

You and the nursing student finish a health history with the family and determine that T.M. has impaired vision (wears glasses), speech impairment, seizure disorder, and has had poor weight gain and feeding issues since birth. He has a skin-level feeding device (Mic-Key button). He is not able to ambulate without braces and wears AFOs (ankle-foot orthotics). He receives physical therapy and occupational therapy and speech therapy on an outpatient basis. T.M. is verbal and able to communicate age appropriately. T.M. weighs 12 kg.

3. The admitting physician orders the following. Explain the rationale for each order.

■ Chart View

Admission Orders

Baclofen (Lioresal) 5 mg every 8 hours PO
Diazepam(Valium) 2 mg twice a day PO
Lamotrigine (Lamictal) 60 mg twice a day PO
Diet as tolerated; NPO after midnight
Place IV and begin D5 ½ NS at 45 mL/hr.
Vital signs every 4 hours

4. Calculate maintenance fluid requirements for this patient. Do the IV fluids ordered meet this requirement? Show your work.

CASE STUDY PROGRESS

T.M. returns to your unit the following afternoon from PACU. He is in a bilateral spica cast, Foley catheter, and has a family-controlled PCA (patient-controlled analgesia) for pain control. You assess your patient and chart the following findings.

10 Pediatric

■ Chart View

Postoperative Assessment

Neuro	Awake and alert, verbalizes and responds to commands
Resp	RR 25 breaths per minute, bilateral breath sounds, equal, clear, good air exchange, O_2 saturations 98% on room air
CV	Peripheral IV to right forearm infusing D5$^1/_2$ NS at 45 mL/hr, HR 85 beats/min, Temperature 36.8° C (98.2° F) (axillary)
GI	Positive bowel sounds; taking sips of juice PO; Mic-Key button to abdomen clamped; skin clean, dry, and intact
GU	8 French Foley catheter intact and secured, draining yellow clear urine to collection bag. Diaper to spica cast opening
NM	Bilateral spica cast to legs with hip abductor bar intact. Toes warm to touch; able to move, unable to palpate pedal pulses. Cap refill less than 2 seconds
Pain	T.M. occasionally shines and frowns but is comforted by parents; his PCA is Y- connected to his IV and infusing morphine at 0.01 mg/kg continuous and 0.015 mg/kg PCA with 15-minute lockout.
Psychosocial	Parents at bedside active in care

5. What are your top five priorities while providing nursing care to T.M. postoperatively? How will you address these areas?

6. Using the FLACC pain scale, what pain score would you assign T.M.? Why is the FLACC scale an appropriate tool?

10 Pediatric

7. Which of these nonpharmacologic interventions would be age appropriate for this patient? (Select all that apply.)
   a. Encourage "positive self-talk" such as statements like, "I will feel better when the cast comes off."
   b. Offer a favorite DVD or video.
   c. Use bubbles to "blow the hurt away."
   d. Educate T.M. on pain and relationship to the procedure.
   e. Read a favorite book.
   f. Use guided imagery.

CASE STUDY PROGRESS

T.M. is stable throughout the day, and the physician writes the following orders:
   Patient can PO ad lib. Resume home schedule of 520 mL PediaSure via G-tube from 10 PM to 6 AM. Remove Foley catheter.

8. Describe instructions for setting up with a Mic-Key button. What is the hourly rate you will set your pump?

9. When you remove the Foley catheter, what will your education and nursing plan include for T.M. and his mother?

CASE STUDY PROGRESS

T.M. continues to improve and you provide discharge education. Mrs. M. asks how she will care for his cast when he gets home. You discuss with her the care of a synthetic spica cast.

10. Which of these statements by T.M.'s mother would indicate that further education is needed? (Select all that apply.)
   a. "I need to check the toes on T.'s feet several times a day for the first week or so to see if they are warm and he is able to wiggle them."
   b. "I need to keep his feet elevated when I get him home."
   c. "It is okay if I give him a tub bath. Because it is a synthetic cast, I can dry it with a blow dryer."
   d. "Because T. uses pull-up diapers, I will need to use plastic tape to protect the cast opening."
   e. "If he has an itch, it is okay to use a knitting needle to scratch under the cast."

11. What additional information should be included in your discharge teaching?

Mrs. M. verbalizes understanding of the discharge instructions, and T.M. is discharged to home with a wheelchair and a home-health follow-up. He will return to the orthopedic surgeon in 2 weeks.

10 Pediatric

Case Study **111**

Name _____ Class/Group _____ Date _____

Group Members _____

INSTRUCTIONS All questions apply to this case study. Your responses should be brief and to the point. When asked to provide several answers, list them in order of priority or significance. Do not assume information that is not provided. Please print or write clearly. If your response is not legible, it will be marked as? and you will need to rewrite it.

▶ Scenario

Three-week-old J.T. arrives at the cardiac catheterization lab for her cardiac catheterization with her parents. She was born at term with Down syndrome, and her pediatrician is concerned because of lack of weight gain and poor feeding. You are getting the patient and her parents prepared for the procedure.

1. As you obtain her history and take vital signs, which statements/findings would be concerning and suggestive of heart failure (HF)? (Select all that apply.)
   a. "J. takes thirty to forty minutes to take two to three ounces of formula."
   b. Rectal temperature: 36.6° C
   c. "J. gets damp and sweaty when she feeds."
   d. HR: 195 at rest
   e. Peripheral pulses = +3
   f. "J. seems to have fewer wet diapers than when we brought her home from the hospital."

2. What teaching would you include as you prepare J.T.'s parents?

10 Pediatric

After the catheterization, J.T. returns to the unit in a crib. These orders were written:

Chart View

Physician's Orders

Daily weights: current weight of 4 kg
Strict intake and output
O_2 per NC as needed to maintain O_2 saturations greater than 93%
VS every 15 minutes × 4, then every 1 hour × 4, then every 4 hours
Digoxin (Lanoxin) 60 mcg PO now, then 20 mcg PO every 12 hours
Furosemide (Lasix) PO 4 mg now, then every 12 hours

3. What would you include in your post-procedure assessment? (Include rationale.)

4. You are reviewing her medications. What is the purpose of starting J.T. on digoxin (Lanoxin)?

5. You have a student nurse working with you and she asks why the first ordered dose is high. What would be a possible explanation for this?

6. The student nurse asks whether there are any precautions to observe when giving digoxin to an infant. What medication safety precautions should be observed when giving this medication?

CASE STUDY PROGRESS

You administer the ordered medication and proceed with your assessment.

7. Which of these are possible complications to monitor for after a cardiac catheterization? (Select all that apply.)
   a. Hemorrhage
   b. Hematoma
   c. Hyperglycemia
   d. Dysrhythmia
   e. Decreased pulse in unaffected leg
   f. Vasospasm

8. You are preparing to administer J.T.'s furosemide. Your drug reference gives the following therapeutic range: 0.5-1 mg/kg/dose every 8-24 hours. Is the ordered dose of 4 mg a safe dose for J.T?

CASE STUDY PROGRESS

You note the following serum metabolic panel on J.T.

▨ Chart View

Lab Results

Glucose	85 mg/dL
Calcium	9.1 mg/dL
Sodium	142 mEq/L
Potassium	3.3 mEq/L
Chloride	101 mEq/L

9. Which lab finding would concern you, and why?

10. The cardiologist is present and tells J.T.'s parents that J.T. has a ventricular septal defect (VSD). On the diagram, circle the area affected by this defect.

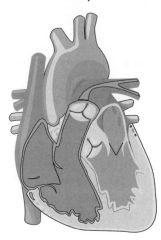

11. This defect would create decreased pulmonary flow. True or False? Explain your answer.

CASE STUDY PROGRESS

The cardiologist consults with the family, and it is decided that J.T. will be discharged to home the following day with medications and close monitoring and will return in several months for surgical repair.

12. You begin your discharge teaching. What will you include?

Case Study **112**

Name _____ Class/Group _____ Date _____

Group Members _____

INSTRUCTIONS All questions apply to this case study. Your responses should be brief and to the point. When asked to provide several answers, list them in order of priority or significance. Do not assume information that is not provided. Please print or write clearly. If your response is not legible, it will be marked as? and you will need to rewrite it.

▶ Scenario

Three-year-old C.E. is admitted to the Emergency Department (ED) fast track clinic. Her mother tells the nurse that C.E. has had a low-grade fever for 2 days and is complaining of ear pain and a sore throat. Mrs. E. states that C.E.'s appetite has been "off," but she has been drinking and using the bathroom as usual.

1. As you get C.E. settled in the exam room, what routine information regarding risk factors for otitis media (OM) would you want to obtain from Mrs. E.?

2. Mrs. E. asks, "Why does C. keep getting ear infections? Is there something I should do?" Explain the etiology of ear infections.

3. What will you include in your physical examination, and why?

CASE STUDY PROGRESS

As you continue to get a history from Mrs. E., you learn that C.E. has had "ear problems" and throat infections since she was a baby. She is in daycare each weekday, Dad smokes outside of the house, and there is a family history of seasonal allergies. C.E. is allergic to penicillin. Her weight is 14 kg. The PCP diagnoses C.E.

with bilateral otitis media and strep pharyngitis. C.E. is given a prescription for Augmentin 600 mg bid PO ×
7 days. She is to be discharged to home with instructions to follow-up with the ENT (ear, nose, and throat)
specialist.

4. You review the order before completing discharge teaching. What is your first action?

CASE STUDY PROGRESS

Mrs. E. is given a new prescription for azithromycin (Zithromax) PO 160 mg qd × 5 days.

5. Azithromycin is dispensed 200 mg/5 mL. Calculate the dosage for Mrs. E. to administer to C.E.

6. You are providing Mrs. E. with information on medication administration. Which of these
statements by Mrs. E. indicates need for further teaching? (Select all that apply.)
   a. "I will place the correct amount of antibiotic in the ear canal once a day."
   b. " I will monitor for vomiting, diarrhea, or stomachaches because this might be a side
   effect of the medication."
   c. "If C. refuses to take her medication, I will tell her it tastes like the candy we get at the
   movies."
   d. "This medicine can be given with or without food."
   e. "I don't have to finish the medication if she feels better after a few days."

7. Mrs. E. asks when C.E. can return to daycare. Which of these statements is your best
response?
   a. "She should be able to return in about a week."
   b. "She can return twenty-four hours after her last documented normal temperature."
   c. "She can return twenty-four hours after she starts her antibiotics."
   d. "She can return forty-eight hours after her last documented normal temperature."

CASE STUDY PROGRESS

Mrs. E. takes C.E. to an ENT specialist. It is determined that her enlarged tonsils might be contributing to
the frequent throat and ear infections, and a tonsil and adenoidectomy (T&A) is scheduled. She will be
admitted postoperatively for 24-hour observation.

After the surgery, the postoperative nurse receives C.E. to the short-stay unit from the
post-anesthesia care unit (PACU). C.E. is awake and alert, bilateral breath sounds are clear, and her
oxygen saturation is 98% on room air. She has tolerated sips of clear fluids, and her parents are with her.

8. Which of these orders would you expect to see in her postoperative orders? (Select all that apply, and discuss the rationales for your choices.)
   a. Vital signs q4h
   b. Clear liquids. Advance to regular toddler diet.
   c. Methylprednisolone (Solu-Medrol) 2.3 mg IV q8h × 3 doses
   d. Acetaminophen (Tylenol) (120 mg) with codeine (12.5 mg) 5 mL PO q6h prn for pain
   e. Home prescription for amoxicillin (Amoxil) 120 mg PO q8h
   f. Maintain peripheral IV with D5½ NS at 50 mL/hr until taking PO well and then saline lock
   g. Aggressively gargle and swish with water after eating or drinking.

9. State at least two nursing interventions for each of these commonly encountered nursing problems during the postoperative phase of care.
   a. Airway
   b. Pain
   c. Fluid and electrolyte balance
   d. Bleeding risk

10. How would the nurse monitor C.E. for pain?

11. You are reviewing discharge instructions with Mrs. E. She asks, "How would I know if we need to come back?" Discuss common findings and when Mrs. E. would need to seek immediate medical attention for C.E.

CASE STUDY OUTCOME

Mrs. E. indicates an understanding of discharge instructions and follow-up care. C.E. continues to take oral fluids well and meets discharge criteria and is discharged to home to follow up with the ENT physician in 2 weeks.

Maternal and Obstetric Disorders 11

Case Study 113

Name _____ Class/Group _____ Date _____

Group Members _____

INSTRUCTIONS All questions apply to this case study. Your responses should be brief and to the point. When asked to provide several answers, list them in order of priority or significance. Do not assume information that is not provided. Please print or write clearly. If your response is not legible, it will be marked as? and you will need to rewrite it.

▶ Scenario

T.N. delivered a healthy male infant 2 hours ago. She had a midline episiotomy. This is her sixth pregnancy. Before this delivery, she was para 4014. She had an epidural block for her labor and delivery. She is now admitted to the postpartum unit.

1. What is important to note in the initial assessment?

2. You find a boggy fundus during your assessment. What corrective measures can be instituted?

3. The patient complains of pain and discomfort in her perineal area. How will you respond?

4. The nurse reviews the hospital security guidelines with T.N. The nurse points out that her baby has a special identification bracelet that matches a bracelet worn by T.N. and reviews other security procedures. Which statement by T.N. indicates a need for more teaching?
   a. "If I have a question about someone's identity, I can ask about it."
   b. "If someone comes to take my baby for an exam, that person will usually carry my baby to the exam room."
   c. "Nurses on this unit all wear the same purple uniforms."
   d. "Each staff member who takes my baby somewhere should have a picture identification badge."

5. An hour after admission, you recheck T.N.'s perineal pad and find that there is a very small amount of drainage on the pad. What will you do next?
   a. Ask T.N. to change her perineal pad.
   b. Check her perineal pad again in 1 hour.
   c. Check the pad underneath T.N.'s buttocks.
   d. Document the findings in T.N.'s medical record.

6. That evening, the NAP assesses T.N.'s vital signs. Which vital signs would be of concern at this time?

■ Chart View

Vital Signs	
Temperature	99.9° F (37.7° C) oral
Pulse rate	120 beats/min
Blood pressure	100/50 mm Hg
Respiratory rate	16 breaths/min

11 Maternal/Obstetric

7. What will you do next?

8. T.N.'s condition is stable and you prepare to provide patient teaching. What patient teaching is vital after delivery?

9. T.N. tells you she must go back to work in 6 weeks and is not sure she can continue breastfeeding. What options are available to her?

CASE STUDY OUTCOME

T.N. is discharged to home and plans to consult a lactation specialist before returning to work.

11 Maternal/Obstetric

Case Study 114

Name _____ Class/Group _____ Date _____

Group Members _____

INSTRUCTIONS All questions apply to this case study. Your responses should be brief and to the point. When asked to provide several answers, list them in order of priority or significance. Do not assume information that is not provided. Please print or write clearly. If your response is not legible, it will be marked as? and you will need to rewrite it.

▶ Scenario

P.M. comes to the obstetric (OB) clinic because she has missed two menstrual periods and thinks she might be pregnant. She states she is nauseated, especially in the morning, so she completed a home pregnancy test and it was positive. As the intake nurse in the clinic, you are responsible for gathering information before she sees the physician.

1. What are the two most important questions to ask to determine possible pregnancy?

2. You ask whether she has ever been pregnant, and she tells you she has never been pregnant. How would you record this information?

3. What additional information would be needed to complete the TPAL record?

4. It is important to complete the intake interview. What categories will you address with P.M.?

CASE STUDY PROGRESS

According to the clinic protocol, you obtain the following for her prenatal record: CBC, blood type, urine for urinalysis (UA) (protein, glucose, blood), vital signs (VS), height, and weight. Next, the nurse-midwife does a physical examination, including a pelvic exam and confirms that P.M. is pregnant. P.M. has a gynecoid pelvis by measurement, and the fetus is at approximately 6 weeks' gestation.

■ Chart/Exhibit

Vital Signs

Blood pressure	116/74 mm Hg
Heart rate	88 beats/min
Respiratory rate	16 breaths/min
Temperature	98.9° F (37.2° C)

5. Do any of these vital signs cause concern? What should you do?

6. P.M. tells you that the date of her last menstrual period (LMP) was February 2. How would you calculate her due date? What is her due date?

7. What is the significance of a gynecoid pelvis?

8. What specimens are important to obtain when the pelvic examination is done?

CASE STUDY PROGRESS

Nursing interventions focus on monitoring the woman and fetus for growth and development; detecting potential complications; and teaching P.M. about nutrition, how to deal with common discomforts of pregnancy, and activities of self-care.

9. A psychological assessment is done to determine P.M.'s feelings and attitudes regarding her pregnancy. How do attitudes, beliefs, and feelings affect pregnancy?

10. P.M. asks you whether there are any foods that she should avoid while pregnant. She lists some of her favorite foods. Which foods, if any, should she avoid eating while she is pregnant? (Select all that apply.)
   a. Hot dogs
   b. Sushi
   c. Yogurt
   d. Deli meat
   e. Cheddar cheese

11. As the nurse, you know that assessment and teaching are vital in the prenatal period to ensure a positive outcome. What information is important to include at every visit and at specific times during the pregnancy?

11 Maternal/Obstetric

12. After her examination, P.M. states that she is worried because her sister had an ectopic pregnancy and had to have surgery. She asks you, "What are the signs of an ectopic pregnancy?" Which of these are correct? (Select all that apply.)
   a. Fullness and tenderness in her abdomen, near the ovaries
   b. Pain, either unilateral, bilateral, or diffuse over the abdomen
   c. Nausea
   d. Dark red or brown vaginal bleeding
   e. Increased fatigue

13. P.M. asks the nurse about what should be reported to her doctor. List at least six of the "danger signs of pregnancy."

14. Changes in the body caused by pregnancy include relaxation of joints, alteration to center of gravity, faintness, and discomforts. These changes can lead to problems with coordination and balance. In teaching P.M. about safety during pregnancy, what will you include in your teaching?

15. P.M. asks, "Is a vaginal exam done at every visit?" What is your response? Explain your answer.

CASE STUDY OUTCOME

P.M. makes an appointment for her next checkup. You tell her that an ultrasound may be done at about 8 to 12 weeks' gestation to check fetal growth.

Case Study 115

Name _____ Class/Group _____ Date _____

Group Members _____

INSTRUCTIONS All questions apply to this case study. Your responses should be brief and to the point. When asked to provide several answers, list them in order of priority or significance. Do not assume information that is not provided. Please print or write clearly. If your response is not legible, it will be marked as? and you will need to rewrite it.

▶ Scenario

You are the charge nurse working in labor and delivery at a local hospital. D.H. comes to the unit having contractions and feeling somewhat uncomfortable. You take her to the intake room to provide privacy, have her change into a gown, and ask her three initial questions to determine your next course of action, that is, whether to do a vaginal exam or to continue asking her more questions.

1. What three initial questions will you ask, and why?

2. D.H. has contractions 2 to 3 minutes apart and lasting 45 seconds. It is her third pregnancy (gravida 3, para 2002). Her bag of waters is intact at this time. She states that her due date is 2 days away. You determine that it is appropriate to ask for further information before a vaginal exam is done. What information do you need?

3. What assessment should you make to gain further information from D.H.?

4. Upon examination, D.H. is 80% effaced and 4 cm dilated. The fetal heart rate (FHR) is 150 beats/min and regular. She is admitted to a labor and delivery room on the unit. What nursing measures should be done at this time?

5. As part of your assessment, you review the fetal heart strip pictured below. What will you do?

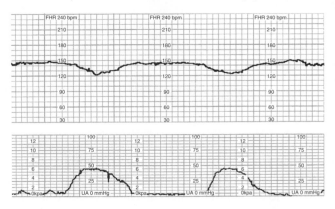

6. List the stages of labor. D.H. is in what stage of labor?

7. D.H. states that she is feeling discomfort and asks you whether there is alternative therapy available before taking medication. List at least four alternative methods to assist D.H. with controlling her discomfort.

8. As you assess both the mother and the fetus during the active stage of labor, you will look for abnormalities. Which of these are potential abnormalities during labor? (Select all that apply.)
   a. Unusual bleeding
   b. Brown or greenish amniotic fluid
   c. Contractions that last 40 to 70 seconds
   d. Sudden, severe pain
   e. Increased maternal fatigue

Although D.H. continues to use alternative therapies for discomfort, she asks for pain medication and receives a dose of meperidine (Demerol). Three hours later, D.H. is lying on her back, and during contractions you notice a few late decelerations of the FHR. You stay with D.H. to monitor her and her fetus and immediately call for someone to notify the PCP.

9. Put these actions in order of priority:

_____a. Discontinue the oxytocin infusion.

_____b. Turn D.H. onto her left side and elevate her legs.

_____c. Increase the rate of the maintenance IV fluids.

_____d. Administer oxygen at 8-10 L/min by facemask.

10. Decelerations occur in an early, variable, or late pattern. What is the significance of these patterns? State what the nurse should do for each type.

11. As you monitor D.H., you observe for prolapse of the umbilical cord. Describe what this is and what can happen to the fetus if this occurs.

12. What would be done if you noted that D.H. had a prolapsed cord?

11 Maternal/Obstetric

CASE STUDY PROGRESS

The decelerations stop, and the remainder of the labor is uneventful; D.H. has an episiotomy to allow more room for the infant to emerge and delivers a male infant.

13. What is involved in the immediate care of the newborn?

14. As you assess the newborn, you observe for CNS depressant effects that might result because the mother received an opioid during labor. Opioid antagonists such as naloxone (Narcan) can promptly reverse the CNS depressant effects in the newborn, but when is naloxone contraindicated for an infant?

15. D.H. has her episiotomy repaired and the placenta delivered. What are the signs that the placenta has released from the uterine wall?

16. What assessments are important for D.H. following delivery?

CASE STUDY OUTCOME

D.H. and her newborn baby boy are taken to the maternity unit where she begins to breastfeed him.

Case Study 116

Name _____ Class/Group _____ Date _____

Group Members _____

INSTRUCTIONS All questions apply to this case study. Your responses should be brief and to the point. When asked to provide several answers, list them in order of priority or significance. Do not assume information that is not provided. Please print or write clearly. If your response is not legible, it will be marked as? and you will need to rewrite it.

▶ Scenario

Baby H. was just born in a hospital that provides single-room maternity care (SRMC). SRMC allows the infant to remain with the parents after birth. The nurse will complete the physical assessment and observe for physiologic changes in the infant's transition from intrauterine to extrauterine life. The textbooks will tell you that the infant goes through an initial phase of reactivity 30 to 60 minutes after birth, then a sleep phase for 4 to 6 hours, then a second period of reactivity. You will see variations of the timing in actual practice.

1. What care is specific to the first period of reactivity?

2. The sleep phase and second reactive phase might occur in the SRMC or in the nursery. Identify eight assessments or tasks that the nurse needs to do during the transitional care period.

11 Maternal/Obstetric

3. You are preparing to give the injection of vitamin K (AquaMEPHYTON). The order is to give 0.5 mg subcutaneously upon arrival to the nursery. The medication comes in a solution of 1 mg/0.5 mL. Calculate how much medication you will draw up into the syringe.

4. Once the transitional care and documentation are completed, the infant might be transferred to the normal newborn nursery if the hospital does not use SRMC. What ongoing care of newborn is this nurse responsible for?

5. The laboratory also performs a Coombs' test on Baby H. What is the purpose of the Coombs' test?
   a. It is done to identify the infant's blood type.
   b. It tests for damage to the red blood cells from maternal antibodies.
   c. It checks the red blood cells for anemia.
   d. It is a test for immunity to the hepatitis virus.

6. True or False: A phenylketonuria (PKU) blood test can be done any time before an infant is discharged to home. If false, explain your rationale.

11 Maternal/Obstetric

Baby H.'s mother has decided to breastfeed her infant. She asks for assistance.

7. Identify six important points to include in your teaching plan.

8. Baby H.'s mother calls you to tell you that her baby seems too sleepy and not feeding well. What will your next action be?

CASE STUDY PROGRESS

You are meeting with Baby H.'s mother to review discharge instructions. She has many questions.

9. Baby H.'s mother asks you about cord care and circumcision care for her infant. What will you tell her?

10. Baby H.'s mother asks you how she can keep her infant from catching a cold or some other type of infection. What is the most important measure to teach her?

11 Maternal/Obstetric

11. After discharge, it is important for Baby H. to receive follow-up care. What should you teach the mother to help her understand the importance of regular visits?

12. You realize that Baby H.'s mother needs information about safety issues before being discharged. After reviewing safety issues, which statement by Baby H.'s mother indicates that she needs further instruction?
a. "I have a car seat and will use it for my baby every time we use the car."
b. "I can leave him on the infant table for just a few moments while he is a newborn."
c. "I will not drink hot coffee while holding my baby."
d. "I will check the bath water temperature before bathing him."

CASE STUDY OUTCOME

Baby H. is discharged to home with his parents.

Case Study **117**

Name _____ Class/Group _____ Date _____

Group Members _____

INSTRUCTIONS All questions apply to this case study. Your responses should be brief and to the point. When asked to provide several answers, list them in order of priority or significance. Do not assume information that is not provided. Please print or write clearly. If your response is not legible, it will be marked as? and you will need to rewrite it.

▶ Scenario

P.T. is a married 30-year-old gravida 4, para 1203 at 28 weeks' gestation. She arrives in the labor and delivery unit at a level 2 hospital complaining of low back pain and frequency of urination. She states that she feels occasional uterine cramping and believes that her membranes have not ruptured.

1. You are the charge nurse and admit P.T. Based on the information you have been given, identify the two most likely diagnoses for P.T.

2. You need additional information from P.T. to determine what you will do next. What important questions do you need to ask to differentiate what is going on with P.T.?

3. What actions would you take to help identify her underlying problem before calling the health care provider?

4. Early recognition of preterm labor is essential to successfully implement interventions. The diagnosis of preterm labor is based on what three major diagnostic criteria?

5. What is the significance of misdiagnosing preterm labor?

6. What other problems might be going on with P.T. that you should consider?

CASE STUDY PROGRESS

P.T.'s history reveals that she had one preterm delivery 4 years ago at 31 weeks' gestation. The infant girl was in the neonatal intensive care unit (NICU) for 3 weeks and discharged without sequelae. The second preterm infant, a boy, was delivered 2 years ago at 35 weeks' gestation and spent 4 days in the hospital before discharge. She has no other risk factors for preterm labor. Vital signs are normal. Her vaginal examination was essentially within normal limits: cervix long, closed, and thick; membranes intact. Abdominal examination revealed that the abdomen was nontender, with fundal height at 29 cm, fetus in a vertex presentation.

7. While you are waiting for laboratory results, what therapeutic measures do you consider?

8. When caring for a woman with symptoms of preterm labor, it is important to question the woman about whether she has symptoms when she is engaged in certain activities that might require lifestyle modifications. What activities should you assess for?

While waiting for laboratory results, you consider that if P.T. is experiencing preterm labor, she would receive antenatal glucocorticoids.

9. What is the rationale for the administration of antenatal glucocorticoids for preterm labor?
   a. To accelerate fetal lung maturity
   b. To stop uterine contractions
   c. To soften the cervix
   d. To prevent maternal infection

10. How long do these drugs take to become effective?

11. Which of these situations are considered contraindications to antenatal glucocorticoids when a woman is in preterm labor? (Select all that apply.)
   a. Cord prolapse
   b. Chorioamnionitis
   c. Presence of twin fetuses
   d. Cervical dilation of 2.5 cm
   e. Abruptio placentae

Two hours later, the laboratory results indicate a urinary tract infection. The contraction monitor indicates infrequent, mild contractions. Her physician discharges her to home on an antibiotic for the UTI.

12. What follow-up measures should be considered in providing P.T. discharge instructions?

11 Maternal/Obstetric

Case Study **118**

Name _____ Class/Group _____ Date _____

Group Members _____

INSTRUCTIONS All questions apply to this case study. Your responses should be brief and to the point. When asked to provide several answers, list them in order of priority or significance. Do not assume information that is not provided. Please print or write clearly. If your response is not legible, it will be marked as? and you will need to rewrite it.

▶ Scenario

J.F. is an 18-year-old woman, gravida 1 para 0, at 38 weeks' gestation. She felt fine until 2 days ago, when she noticed swelling in her hands, feet, and face. She complains of a frontal headache, which started yesterday and has not been relieved by acetaminophen (Tylenol) or coffee. She says she feels irritable and doesn't want the "overhead lights on." Her physician is admitting her for induction of labor. You begin to assess her.

■ Chart View

Assessment

VS: BP 152/84 mm Hg; HR 88 beats/min
Oral temperature: 98.8° F (37.1° C)
Weight: 131.4 kg (289 lb); height: 5'4"
Edema: noted in hands, feet, and face
Deep tendon reflexes (DTRs) +2, no clonus
Urine dipstick reveals proteinuria +3

1. Based on the assessment data you have obtained so far, what do you think is happening to J.F. at this time?

2. As you assess J.F. for edema in her ankles, you note that she is closest to letter B in the figure below, with edema at about 4 mm. How would you document this edema?

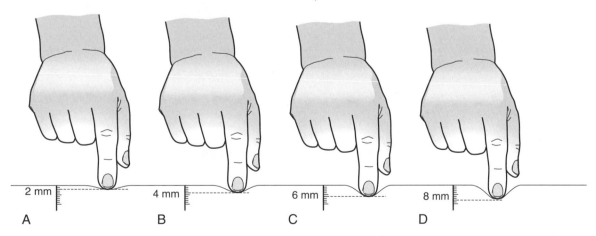

11 Maternal/Obstetric

3. What other assessment questions should you ask her at this time?

4. What information should you obtain from her obstetric record?

5. What laboratory values should be considered at this time?

6. Name at least three possible maternal and three possible fetal complications with J.F.'s diagnosis.

7. What risk factors does J.F. have that cause her to be at risk for this condition? (Select all that apply.)
   a. Obesity
   b. Nulliparity
   c. Single-fetus pregnancy
   d. Age less than 20 years
   e. Coffee drinker

8. Identify eight measures that would likely be implemented.

CASE STUDY PROGRESS

The physician orders a magnesium sulfate infusion. As you monitor J.F., you observe for signs of magnesium sulfate toxicity.

9. What are potential signs of magnesium sulfate toxicity? (Select all that apply.)
   a. Absent DTRs
   b. Increased respiratory rate
   c. Oliguria
   d. Muscle rigidity
   e. Severe hypotension

10. Four hours later, a serum magnesium level is drawn, and the results show 7.8 mEq/L. Does this result need to be reported to the physician? If so, what would you prepare to do?

11. Is there an antidote for magnesium sulfate?

11 Maternal/Obstetric

CASE STUDY PROGRESS

The magnesium sulfate infusion rate is reduced, and an oxytocin infusion has been ordered by the physician and is being given IV in increments to achieve an adequate contraction pattern. You notice on the fetal monitor strip that J.F. is experiencing seven uterine contractions in a 10-minute period over a 30-minute window, with a few FHR decelerations noted.

12. What is happening at this time?

13. What are your priority actions?

CASE STUDY PROGRESS

J.F. progresses in labor, and, at 4-cm dilation, her membranes spontaneously rupture. The small amount of amniotic fluid is green.

14. What does the green amniotic fluid indicate? What are the risks?

CASE STUDY OUTCOME

Five hours later, J.F. delivers a 6-pound, 8-ounce boy, with Apgar scores of 6 and 7.

15. What are your responsibilities at this time?

Case Study **119**

Name _____ Class/Group _____ Date _____

Group Members _____

INSTRUCTIONS All questions apply to this case study. Your responses should be brief and to the point. When asked to provide several answers, list them in order of priority or significance. Do not assume information that is not provided. Please print or write clearly. If your response is not legible, it will be marked as ? and you will need to rewrite it.

▶ Scenario

You are working as an RN in a large women's clinic. Y.L., a 28-year-old Asian woman, arrives for her regularly scheduled obstetric appointment. She is in her 26th week of pregnancy and is a primigravida. After examining the patient, the nurse-midwife tells you to schedule Y.L. for a glucose challenge test. You review Y.L.'s chart and note she is 5 feet, 3 inches and weighs 143 pounds; her prepregnancy body mass index (BMI) is 25. Her father has type 2 diabetes mellitus (DM), and both paternal grandparents had type 2 DM. You enter the room to talk to Y.L.

1. What is the purpose of a glucose challenge test?

2. When is a glucose challenge test performed?

3. What instructions would you provide Y.L. regarding the test?

■ Chart View

Laboratory Test Results		
Time of Test	Value	Normal Range
0730	109 mg/dL	under 95 mg/dL
0830	213 mg/dL	under 180 mg/dL
0930	162 mg/dL	under 153 mg/dL

4. Interpret the results of Y.L.'s test.

5. Y.L. is diagnosed with gestational diabetes mellitus (GDM). What is GDM?

11 Maternal/Obstetric

6. List five risk factors for GDM. Place a star or asterisk next to those risk factors that Y.L. has.

CASE STUDY PROGRESS

Medical nutrition therapy is the primary treatment for the management of GDM. Because treatment must begin immediately, you call the dietitian to come see Y.L. You also schedule Y.L. to meet with other members of the DM management team later in the week.

7. What is the goal of medical nutrition therapy?

8. Describe the usual diet used in treating GDM.

9. Why is medical nutrition therapy for a woman with GDM higher in fat and protein?

10. Women with GDM cannot metabolize concentrated simple sugars without a sharp rise in blood glucose. Name five examples of simple sugars you would teach Y.L. to limit.

11. Complex carbohydrates (CHO) do not cause a rapid rise in blood glucose when eaten in small amounts. Identify five foods from this group.

11 Maternal/Obstetric

During the meeting with the dietitian, Y.L. gives a diet history that is high in noodles and rice with little protein. She informs the dietitian she is lactose intolerant but can have dairy products occasionally in small portions.

12. Is it important that Y.L. take a calcium supplement along with her prenatal vitamins?

13. Y.L. is instructed to monitor her fasting blood glucose first thing in the morning and 2 hours after every meal. What are the purposes of this request?

14. Y.L. is instructed to complete ketone testing using the first-voided urine in the morning. What is the rationale for this request?

15. Y.L. asks whether having gestational diabetes will hurt her baby. How would you respond?

16. At the conclusion of the visit, you need to evaluate your teaching. Which statement made by Y.L. indicates that clarification is necessary?
    a. "I will stay on the diabetic diet described by the dietitian."
    b. "I will monitor my glucose levels at least four times each day."
    c. "I need to stop exercising because I will need more carbohydrates."
    d. "I should immediately report any ketones in my urine."

11 Maternal/Obstetric

Women's Health Disorders

12

Case Study **120**

Name _____ Class/Group _____ Date _____

Group Members _____

INSTRUCTIONS All questions apply to this case study. Your responses should be brief and to the point. When asked to provide several answers, list them in order of priority or significance. Do not assume information that is not provided. Please print or write clearly. If your response is not legible, it will be marked as ? and you will need to rewrite it.

▶ Scenario

K.W. is an 18-year-old woman who comes to Planned Parenthood for a pregnancy test because a condom broke during intercourse the night before. Her last menstrual period (LMP) was 13 days ago and was normal. She always has a monthly menstrual cycle. She is extremely nervous about pregnancy because she is beginning college on a scholarship soon. She states there have been no other acts of unprotected intercourse since her LMP. She did take oral contraceptives briefly in the past but discontinued use because of weight gain and mood swings.

1. As the nurse working in the clinic, should you run a pregnancy test?

2. K.W. asks whether she is at risk for pregnancy. How will you respond?

3. She asks what contraceptive options are available to her at this point. How will you answer?

4. K.W. says, "Are you talking about having an abortion?" Formulate a response.

CASE STUDY PROGRESS

There are three emergency contraceptive (EC) options: Plan B and ELLA, contraceptive pills containing estrogen and progesterone, and the copper intrauterine device (IUD).

5. She asks you to explain the differences among the various options. What will you tell her?

6. She asks you about side effects. What will you tell her?

7. What past medical information will you need to ask K.W. about?

8. K.W. has no contraindications to the use of hormones. Which of the previous methods of EC will you offer this patient?

9. How will you counsel K.W.?

Case Study **121**

Name _____ Class/Group _____ Date _____

Group Members _____

▶ Scenario

L.W., a 20-year-old college student, comes to the university health clinic for a pregnancy test. She has been sexually active with her boyfriend of 6 months, and her menstrual period is now 2 weeks late. The pregnancy test is positive. The patient begins to cry, saying, "I don't know what to do."

1. How will you begin to counsel L.W.?

2. What options does a woman experiencing an unplanned pregnancy have?

3. If your role is to assist her in making a choice, what information will you want L.W. to provide?

4. What are the nurse's moral and ethical obligations in this situation?

Copyright © 2013 by Mosby, an affiliate of Elsevier Inc.
Copyright © 2009, 2005, 2001, 1996, by Mosby, Inc. an affiliate of Elsevier Inc. All rights reserved.

5. L.W. asks you to tell her about abortion. What will you tell her?

6. L.W. wants you to explain the difference between vacuum aspiration and medical abortion. How would you explain this to her?

7. She tells you that she has heard that if a woman has an abortion, she might not be able to get pregnant again. How would you counsel her?

8. What types of emotional reactions do women experience after an abortion?

9. L.W. wants to know about adoption. What will you tell her?

10. L.W. asks you if there are any actions she should be doing now to take care of herself. How will you respond?

12 Women's Health

11. What factors affect carrying a pregnancy to term? L.W. asks you about the importance of prenatal care. Explain.

12. Finally, L.W. wants to know how long she has to decide.

12 Women's Health

Case Study **122**

Name _____ Class/Group _____ Date _____

Group Members _____

INSTRUCTIONS All questions apply to this case study. Your responses should be brief and to the point. When asked to provide several answers, list them in order of priority or significance. Do not assume information that is not provided. Please print or write clearly. If your response is not legible, it will be marked as ? and you will need to rewrite it.

▶ Scenario

You are working in a busy OB/GYN office, and the last patient of the day is P.B., a 36-year-old who is planning to get married soon. She wants to use birth control but is not sure what to choose. Her fiancé is in law school, and they do not have health insurance, so she is anxious not to get pregnant right away. She asks you to review the various methods and help her explore what is best for her.

1. What past medical information will you need to ask P.B. about?

2. Are there any other conditions that would influence the choice of a contraceptive method?

3. Is P.B. currently at risk for sexually transmitted infections (STIs)?

4. What lifestyle information will help you assist P.B. in choosing an appropriate method for her?

5. P.B. asks you about the effectiveness rating of available birth control methods. Categorize your response according to the following efficacy ratings: most effective (more than 99%), highly effective (97% to 99%), and moderately effective (less than 90%).

6. P.B. asks you to explain the main advantages and disadvantages of the most effective methods.

7. What are the main advantages and disadvantages of the contraceptive methods in the highly effective category?

8. What about the moderately effective birth control methods? What are the main advantages and disadvantages?

12 Women's Health

9. She wants to know about cost with each method because she will be on a tight budget, with limited insurance coverage.

10. She asks you which method you would pick. What do you tell her?

CASE STUDY PROGRESS

P.B. comes back in a week and tells you that she can get a low-cost oral contraceptive through a local store. You convey this information to the nurse practitioner, who examines P.B. and writes a prescription for a biphasic pill containing ethinyl estradiol and norethindrone. You are asked to discuss the use of the pill with P.B.

11. What key factors should you address with P.B.?

12 Women's Health

12. A few months later, K.B. calls the clinic because she realized she missed a dose of her oral contraceptive. What will you tell her? (Select all that apply.)

   a. "Take the missed pill now, along with today's pill, then resume the pack."

   b. "It is okay, you are still protected from pregnancy if you take two now."

   c. "Just throw that pill away; restart taking your pills tomorrow."

   d. "Please make an appointment so we can insert a temporary IUD."

   e. "Wait until the start of your next menses, then begin a new pack of pills."

   f. "You should use a backup form of contraception until you start your menses."

Case Study **123**

Name _____ Class/Group _____ Date _____

Group Members _____

INSTRUCTIONS All questions apply to this case study. Your responses should be brief and to the point. When asked to provide several answers, list them in order of priority or significance. Do not assume information that is not provided. Please print or write clearly. If your response is not legible, it will be marked as ? and you will need to rewrite it.

▶ Scenario

You are working as the triage nurse in the emergency department at a busy tertiary care center. A woman comes in complaining of very heavy vaginal bleeding and extreme pain. S.K. is single, 47 years of age, and has been bleeding for 24 hours, soaking a pad an hour. She works in a law firm as a paralegal and was embarrassed yesterday when she leaked around her pad and stained a chair in the conference room. She has two sexual partners currently and has been relying on condoms for birth control. She thinks her last menstrual period was 2 months ago, but they have been irregular and she is not sure. She has had some occasional spotting during the past 6 months. She states she is afraid of the amount of bleeding in the past 24 hours.

1. Identify three conditions that would require emergency care and could prove life threatening.

2. She asks you, "Could I be pregnant?" How will you respond?

3. You ask her how she would feel if she was pregnant, and she says, "It would ruin my life." She states she is a single mother with two children in junior high school. What can you tell her to help her with her obvious distress?

4. Describe the assessment you would need to perform to differentiate what might be occurring with S.K.

■ Chart View

Laboratory Test Results

Hgb	12.2 g/dL
Hct	44%
RBC	4.2 dL

Vital Signs

Blood pressure	110/68 mm Hg
Heart rate	88 beats/min
Respiratory rate	22 breaths/min

5. Interpret S.K.'s laboratory results and vital signs.

CASE STUDY PROGRESS

You determine that S.K. is stable at the present level of bleeding; she is not diaphoretic or pale. The physician orders an ultrasound (US) to determine whether she is pregnant and to evaluate some possible causes of her bleeding. During her US, her blood pressure drops to 90/42 mm Hg, and she complains of considerable cramping.

■ Chart View

Physician's Orders

Infuse 1 L of D5LR over 4 hours
Meperidine (Demerol) 25 mg IV now

6. Before administering the meperidine (Demerol), what will you ask her?

7. What precautions do you need to take while administering the meperidine (Demerol)?

8. You are preparing to infuse the D5LR. The available IV tubing supplies 15 gtt/mL. At how many gtt/min will you regulate the infusion?

CASE STUDY PROGRESS

Her US is negative for pregnancy; she does not have an ectopic or intrauterine pregnancy. The US shows a very thick endometrial lining, even after 24 hours of bleeding.

9. S.K. is obviously relieved about not being pregnant, but she expresses fear that this could be cancer. What should you tell her to reassure her?

10. S.K. asks what she can do to keep this from happening again. Please respond.

11. What risk factors will you ask her about before discussing birth control pills as a treatment option?

12 Women's Health

12. If S.K. is prescribed birth control pills for the treatment of her bleeding problem, what other risks should she be aware of if she is using the pills for birth control?

CASE STUDY PROGRESS

S.K. is more comfortable now. The physician suggests birth control pills to control her bleeding. He tells her to take one pill, four times a day for the next 5 days or until her bleeding stops. Once the bleeding has stopped, she should continue using the medication, one pill/day, for the rest of the cycle. Because she will need to continue the pills for at least 3 months, she will need to follow up with her OB/GYN.

13. What warning signs and symptoms do you want to tell her about as she starts her contraceptive pills?

14. Which statements indicate that S.K. understands the discharge instructions? (Select all that apply.)
   a. "I will call if I continue to have heavy bleeding, soaking a pad an hour."
   b. "I can take three hundred twenty-five milligrams of aspirin every six hours for the cramping pain."
   c. "If I get dizzy or feel my heart beating funny, I will come back to the ER."
   d. "I will avoid sexual intercourse until the bleeding has completely stopped."
   e. "I will try to eat more beans and spinach over the next several days."

Case Study 124

Name _____   Class/Group _____   Date _____

Group Members _____

INSTRUCTIONS All questions apply to this case study. Your responses should be brief and to the point. When asked to provide several answers, list them in order of priority or significance. Do not assume information that is not provided. Please print or write clearly. If your response is not legible, it will be marked as ? and you will need to rewrite it.

▶ Scenario

You are the nurse in a walk-in clinic. A.P. is being seen this morning for a 2-day history of diffuse but severe abdominal pain. She has complaints of nausea without vomiting; she denies vaginal bleeding or discharge. A.P. claims to have had unprotected sex with several partners recently, two of whom had penile discharge. Her last menstrual period ended 3 days ago. She has no known drug allergies and denies previous medical or psychiatric problems. Vital signs are 108/60, 110, 20, 100.6° F (38.1° C) (tympanic).

Physical examination finds that her abdomen is very tender. The slightest touch of her abdomen causes her to wince with pain. Bowel sounds are normal. Pelvic examination finds purulent material pooled in the vaginal vault, which appears to be coming from the cervix. A sample of the vaginal drainage is obtained and sent for culture. A pregnancy test is negative; a rapid diagnostic test for chlamydial infection is positive.

1. What should you teach A.P. about chlamydial infection?

2. What medical interventions can you anticipate?

3. How would you provide emotional support to A.P. at this time?

CASE STUDY PROGRESS

The physician has the option of treating A.P. by one of two different methods. First, the physician could prescribe treatment over a period of 1 week; A.P. would be given the first dose of doxycycline (Monodox) 100 mg PO, and then prescribe the same dose to be taken PO bid for 7 days. Second, the physician could prescribe a one-time dose of azithromycin (Zithromax) 1 g PO, which could be administered in the clinic.

4. Which choice is best for A.P.? Explain your reasoning.

5. You tell A.P. that chlamydial infection is a sexually transmitted infection that is mandated to be reported to the public health department. What is the purpose of reporting the infection, and what actions will be taken?

6. A.P. says she does not understand why her partners have to be told about the infection. How would you respond?

7. Based on the information A.P. has given you, you determine that she is at risk for other STIs and unplanned pregnancy. What risk assessment questions do you need to ask A.P.?

12 Women's Health

8. You ask whether someone has talked with A.P. about "safe sex." She laughs and tells you there is nothing safe about sex. Undaunted, you ask if she would be willing for you to discuss the use of condoms with her sexual partners. She tells you that she is already careful; if she does not know the guy, she uses condoms every time. How are you going to respond?

9. You ask A.P. whether she has been tested for HIV. She says no, she does not know anyone with AIDS and she does not have sex with gay men. Now what are you going to say?

10. You ask her whether she would like to be tested for HIV. It will not cost her anything, no one will know the results but her, and it is completely confidential. She agrees to the test. What counseling will you provide A.P.?

11. Describe the instructions you will give to A.P. before her leaving the clinic.

CASE STUDY PROGRESS

A.P. returns to the clinic in 1 week for her HIV test results, which are negative. Her culture results confirm the diagnosis of chlamydial infection.

12. You take this opportunity to review with A.P. regarding ways to reduce the risk of reinfection. How would you determine whether A.P. understood your teaching regarding safe sexual practices? She states that she will:
   a. inspect the genitalia of her partner before intercourse or other contact with perianal area.
   b. use a new application of spermicidal jelly instead of a condom before each encounter.
   c. douche with an over-the-counter solution within 8 hours of having intercourse.
   d. not have to worry about contacting an STI if the man states he has few partners.

12 Women's Health

12   Women's Health

Case Study 125

Name _____ Class/Group _____ Date _____

Group Members _____

INSTRUCTIONS All questions apply to this case study. Your responses should be brief and to the point. When asked to provide several answers, list them in order of priority or significance. Do not assume information that is not provided. Please print or write clearly. If your response is not legible, it will be marked as ? and you will need to rewrite it.

▶ Scenario

T.C. is a 30-year-old woman who 3 weeks ago underwent a vaginal hysterectomy and right salpingo-oophorectomy for abdominal pain and endometriosis. Postoperatively, she experienced an intra-abdominal hemorrhage, and her hematocrit (Hct) dropped from 40.5% to 21%. She was transfused with 3 units of packed RBCs. After discharge, she continued to have abdominal pain, chills, and fever and was subsequently readmitted twice: once for treatment of postoperative infection and the second time for evacuation of a pelvic hematoma. Despite treatment, T.C. continued to have abdominal pain, chills, fever, and nausea and vomiting.

T.C. has now been admitted to your unit from the post-anesthesia care unit (PACU) after an exploratory laparotomy. Vital signs (VS) are 130/70, 94, 16, 99.7° F (37.6° C) (tympanic). She is easily aroused and oriented to place and person. She dozes between verbal requests. She has a low-midline abdominal dressing that is dry and intact and a Jackson-Pratt (JP) drain that is fully compressed and contains a scant amount of bright red blood. Her Foley to down drain has clear yellow urine. She has an IV of 1000 mL D5.45NS infusing at 100 mL/hr in her left forearm, with no swelling or redness. T.C. is receiving IV morphine sulfate for pain control through a patient-controlled analgesia (PCA) pump. The settings are dose 2 mg, lock-out interval 15 minutes, 4-hour maximum dose of 30 mg. When aroused, she states that her pain is an 8 on a scale of 1 to 10. She also has 2 L oxygen by nasal cannula (O_2/NC); her Sao_2 by pulse oximeter is 93%.

1. During your assessment you note that T.C.'s respiratory rate is 16 breaths/min and shallow. Identify factors that are affecting T.C.'s respiratory status.

2. Articulate a plan for assisting T.C. in maintaining adequate ventilation.

12 Women's Health

CASE STUDY PROGRESS

The unit is busy, and you are concerned about monitoring T.C. carefully enough. Your present patient load is six; of these, two patients are newly postop and one is getting ready for discharge. You have one experienced nursing assistive personnel (NAP) to help you. You are most concerned with T.C.'s respiratory status and the possibility that she might, in her drowsy state, self-administer a dose of opioid medication that would further reduce her respiratory status (despite the lock-out time).

3. Formulate a plan of care for T.C. related to this issue.

4. Which of T.C.'s vital sign values would be most important for the NAP to report to you immediately?
   a. Temperature of 100° F (37.8° C)
   b. Blood pressure of 160/80 mm Hg
   c. Heart rate of 100 beats/min
   d. Respiratory rate of 8 breaths/min

5. Pain control using the PCA can be tricky. Throughout the first postoperative day, it has been difficult to balance T.C.'s need for pain medication and depression of her respiratory status. Discuss the concept of controlling pain with a PCA using opioids and factors that can be adjusted to better control her pain.

6. Identify three outcomes that you expect for T.C. as a result of your interventions.

7. T.C. is beginning to withdraw from conversations with you and the other staff. She sleeps most of the day and is not eating. At times, she is tearful and is irritable with her husband. You believe that she is showing signs of depression. What actions can you take to help her?

CASE STUDY PROGRESS

T.C. and her husband are talking one evening, and you overhear that they are very dissatisfied with the care provided by the physician. They believe that he has mismanaged T.C.'s care. They are discussing getting an attorney. They ask you what you think.

8. What do you do?

9. You state, "Tell me what's going on with you right now. Maybe I can help you be more comfortable." What would be the benefit of taking this approach?

12 Women's Health

10. Mr. C. says, "No one is telling us anything. My wife came in here for a simple hysterectomy. She ends up with four surgeries. She still has pain, and she is worse off than when she started. Somebody has screwed up big time. Then they have the nerve to send me a bill. This morning they demanded $185,000. I'm not paying a dime until she gets better." How are you going to respond?

Psychiatric Disorders

Case Study **126**

Name _____ Class/Group _____ Date _____

Group Members _____

INSTRUCTIONS All questions apply to this case study. Your responses should be brief and to the point. When asked to provide several answers, list them in order of priority or significance. Do not assume information that is not provided. Please print or write clearly. If your response is not legible, it will be marked as? and you will need to rewrite it.

▶ Scenario

You are the nurse working triage in the emergency department. This afternoon, a woman brings in her father, K.B., who is 72 years old. The daughter reports that, over the past year, she has noticed her father has progressively had problems with his mental capacity. These changes have developed gradually but seem to be getting worse. At times he is alert, and at other times he seems disoriented, depressed, and tearful. He is forgetting things and doing things out of the ordinary, such as placing the milk in the cupboard and sugar in the refrigerator. This morning, he thought it was nighttime and wondered what his daughter was doing at his house. He could not pour his own coffee, and he seems to be getting more agitated. K.B. reports that he has been having memory problems for the past year and, at times, has difficulty remembering the names of family members and friends. His neighbor found him down the street 2 days ago, and K.B. did not know where he was.

A review of his past medical history is significant for hypercholesterolemia and coronary artery disease. He had a myocardial infarction 5 years ago. K.B.'s vital signs today are all within normal limits.

1. What are some cognitive changes seen in a number of elderly patients?

2. You know that physiologic age-related changes in the elderly can influence cognitive functioning. Name and discuss one.

3. For each behavior listed, specify whether it is associated with delirium (DL) or dementia (DM).
   ____a. Gradual and insidious onset
   ____b. Hallucinations or delusions
   ____c. A sudden, acute onset of symptoms
   ____d. The functional impairment is progressive.
   ____e. Inability to perform ADLs
   ____f. Incoherent interactions with others
   ____g. Patients may demonstrate wandering behavior.
   ____h. Behavior disorders often worsen at night.

4. Based upon the information provided by the daughter, do you think K.B. is showing signs of delirium or dementia? Explain.

5. You know that there are four main types of dementia that result in cognitive changes. List two of these types of dementia.

6. How can the level or degree of the dementia impairment be determined?

7. A number of diagnostic tests have been ordered for K.B. From the tests listed, which would be used to diagnose dementia?
_____ Mental status examinations
_____ Toxicology screen
_____ Mini-Mental State Examination
_____ ECG
_____ EEG
_____ CMP
_____ CBC with differential
_____ Thyroid function tests
_____ Colonoscopy
_____ RPR
_____ Serum B_{12}
_____ Bleeding time
_____ HIV screening
_____ CT
_____ MRI

CASE STUDY PROGRESS

After reviewing K.B.'s history and diagnostic test results, K.B. was diagnosed with Alzheimer's dementia. The physician calls a family conference to discuss the implications with K.B. and his daughter.

13 Psychiatric

8. What neuroanatomic changes are seen in individuals with Alzheimer's disease?

9. List at least three interventions you would plan for K.B.

CASE STUDY PROGRESS

K.B. is discharged and sees his primary care physician 2 days later. K.B. receives a prescription for donepezil (Aricept) 5 mg PO/day at night. As you review the prescription with K.B.'s daughter, she tells you that she is "excited" because she did not know there were medications that could cure Alzheimer's disease.

10. How do you respond?

CASE STUDY PROGRESS

Two weeks later, K.B.'s daughter calls the physician's office and states, "I realize that the Aricept will not cure my dad, but there has been no improvement at all. Are we wasting our money?"

11. What is the best answer for her question?

Case Study **127**

Name _____ Class/Group _____ Date _____

Group Members _____

INSTRUCTIONS All questions apply to this case study. Your responses should be brief and to the point. When asked to provide several answers, list them in order of priority or significance. Do not assume information that is not provided. Please print or write clearly. If your response is not legible, it will be marked as? and you will need to rewrite it.

▶ Scenario

You are working the day shift on a medicine inpatient unit. You are discussing discharge instructions with J.B., an 86-year-old man who was admitted for mitral valve repair. His serum blood glucose had been averaging 250 mg/dL or higher for the past several months. During this admission, his dosage of insulin was adjusted, and he was given additional education in managing his diet. While you are giving these instructions, J.B. tells you his wife died 9 months ago. He becomes tearful when telling you about that loss and the loneliness he has been feeling. He tells you he just doesn't feel good lately, feels sad much of the time, and hasn't been involved in his normal activities. He has few friends left in the community because most of them have passed away. He has a daughter in town, but she is busy with her work and grandchildren. He also tells you that he has been feeling so down the past few months that he has had thoughts about suicide.

1. What other information should you ask J.B. regarding his thoughts of suicide?

2. What characteristics of J.B. put him at high risk for suicide?

3. Which psychiatric disorders can result in suicidal ideations or gestures?

4. What questions would you ask J.B. to determine whether he is clinically depressed?

13 Psychiatric

5. Ill people often have trouble sleeping, experience a change in appetite, reduce their level of activity, and have thoughts of death. How can you tell the difference between old age with illness and depression?

6. List five of the most common signs of depression.

CASE STUDY PROGRESS

You use the SAD PERSONS scale to assess J.B.'s potential for suicide and find that he is at a 4 on the 10-point scale. You are concerned about his statements.

7. What immediate interventions would you carry out for J.B.?

CASE STUDY PROGRESS

You decide to notify J.B.'s physician about your findings. The attending physician calls in a psychiatrist to evaluate J.B.

8. Identify two treatments that are available for depression.

9. Would J.B. be a candidate for electroconvulsive therapy (ECT)? Why or why not?

CASE STUDY PROGRESS

The psychiatrist on call comes in to evaluate J.B. After meeting with J.B., the psychiatrist writes an order for escitalopram (Lexapro) 10 mg daily at bedtime. J.B. is scheduled to see the psychiatrist the day after he is discharged from the hospital.

10. What special instructions will you give him regarding the Lexapro? (Select all that apply.)
   a. The full effects of the medication might not be seen for 4 to 6 weeks.
   b. The medication may cause nausea, dry mouth, sedation, and insomnia.
   c. There are no known food interactions.
   d. The herbal product, St. John's wort, will enhance the action of the Lexapro.
   e. Taking a glass of wine at bedtime will help him go to sleep.

11. Why do you think that a drug in the SSRI class was chosen over a tricyclic antidepressant or a monoamine oxidase inhibitor (MAOI)?

CASE STUDY PROGRESS

J.B.'s daughter visits him in the hospital, and they have a long talk. She is shocked when she realizes that her father is lonely to the point of considering suicide and tells you that she will do all she can to help him when he goes home.

12. What important information needs to be conveyed to J.B.'s daughter about the first few weeks of therapy with the SSRI?

13 Psychiatric

Case Study 128

Name _____ Class/Group _____ Date _____

Group Members _____

INSTRUCTIONS All questions apply to this case study. Your responses should be brief and to the point. When asked to provide several answers, list them in order of priority or significance. Do not assume information that is not provided. Please print or write clearly. If your response is not legible, it will be marked as? and you will need to rewrite it.

▶ Scenario

You are the RN case manager in an outpatient mental health clinic. S.T. is here today for her outpatient mental health appointment. She has a diagnosis of bipolar disorder and has been stable for the past 3 years. Her last episode was one of mania that required hospitalization. She is 29 years old, married, with two children ages 2 and 4. She reports that her mood is better than it has been in a long time and she has lots of energy. When asked whether she thinks this is a recurrence of mania, she says *no,* she thinks that things are just finally getting better.

1. It is common for patients with bipolar illness to deny the onset of mania because it feels good. What other information would be important to ask S.T.?

2. What other information would help determine whether S.T. is experiencing the onset of a manic or hypomanic episode?

3. Bipolar disorder is a disorder of mood, characterized by episodes of depression, mania, or hypomania. What symptoms might you see if S.T. is experiencing mania or hypomania?

4. How is hypomania different from mania?

13 Psychiatric

CASE STUDY PROGRESS

Lithium (Eskalith) is commonly used to treat bipolar disorder. S.T. has been taking lithium for several years.

5. When S.T. first started taking lithium, she would have been cautioned to report side effects. Which are common side effects of lithium? (Select all that apply.)
   a. Thirst
   b. Nausea
   c. Constipation
   d. Tremor
   e. Dizziness

6. Lithium toxicity can occur in patients taking lithium. What are the symptoms of lithium toxicity? (Select all that apply.)
   a. Vomiting
   b. Insomnia
   c. Dyspnea
   d. Diarrhea
   e. Confusion

7. S.T.'s maintenance lithium level results are reported as 1.0 mEq/L. Interpret these results.

8. What other laboratory examinations should be routinely drawn while S.T. is taking lithium?

9. What instructions should have been given to S.T. when she began lithium therapy?

10. Aside from lithium, what other medications are used to treat bipolar disorder?

11. Given her history of bipolar disorder, what should you teach S.T. to minimize mood swings?

CASE STUDY OUTCOME

S.T. is told that her lithium level is within normal limits, and states, "I feel better than I've felt in ages!" She expresses hope that this will last a long time.

13 Psychiatric

Case Study **129**

Name _____ Class/Group _____ Date _____

Group Members _____

INSTRUCTIONS All questions apply to this case study. Your responses should be brief and to the point. When asked to provide several answers, list them in order of priority or significance. Do not assume information that is not provided. Please print or write clearly. If your response is not legible, it will be marked as? and you will need to rewrite it.

▶ Scenario

You are working on an inpatient psychiatric unit and are to do an initial assessment on R.B., who has just been admitted. He has a diagnosis of schizophrenia, paranoid type. He is 22 years old and has been attending the local university and living at home with his parents. He has always been a good student and has been active socially. Last semester, his grades began declining, and he became very withdrawn. He spends most of his time alone in his room. His grooming has deteriorated; he can go days without bathing. For several weeks before admission, he insisted on keeping all of the blinds and curtains in the house closed. For the past 2 days, he has refused to eat, saying, "They have contaminated the food." As you approach R.B., you note that he appears to be carrying on a conversation with someone, but there is no one there. When you talk to him, he looks around and answers in a whisper but gives you little information. He states, "They are watching me and told me not to cooperate."

1. Explain what a "negative" symptom of schizophrenia is, and identify at least three negative symptoms of schizophrenia that R.B. might be experiencing.

2. Explain what a "positive" symptom of schizophrenia is, and identify at least two positive symptoms of schizophrenia that R.B. might be experiencing.

3. Give the definition of each of the following types of delusional thinking:
   a. Thought broadcasting
   b. Thought insertion
   c. Grandeur
   d. Ideas of reference
   e. Persecution
   f. Somatic delusions

13 Psychiatric

4. What symptoms indicate that R.B. has paranoid schizophrenia?

5. Why is it important to know R.B.'s history before he is diagnosed with schizophrenia?

6. What diagnostic screening is important in evaluating R.B.?

7. What are the most important initial interventions in treating R.B.?

CASE STUDY PROGRESS

After a full mental status assessment, the psychiatrist orders close monitoring in the inpatient setting and an antipsychotic medication.

8. Which class of antipsychotic medications is considered first-line therapy for schizophrenia?

9. K.B. will need to be monitored closely. How will this be done?

10. What types of psychosocial treatments may be used to treat R.B.'s schizophrenia?

CASE STUDY PROGRESS

R.B. is started on olanzapine (Zyprexa). You inform R.B. and his family about the common side effects of the typical antipsychotics.

11. What are the common side effects of atypical antipsychotics such as olanzapine (Zyprexa)? (Select all that apply.)
   a. Tardive dyskinesia
   b. Drowsiness
   c. Dry mouth
   d. Palpitations
   e. Nausea
   f. Weight gain

CASE STUDY PROGRESS

As you go in to give R.B. his medication, he speaks to you in fragmented sentences. "Is that a bird? The little flowers jump up and down. What says the moon?" Before you can say anything, he asks, "Do you see that bird over my bed? She is telling me not to leave this room. If I move she will swoop down and try to peck at my eyes. Be careful!"

12. Is he having an illusion or a hallucination? Explain your answer.

13. How will you respond?

CASE STUDY OUTCOME

After 2 weeks of inpatient therapy, K.B. is discharged back home to his parents and is enrolled in a day treatment program. He hopes to move to a halfway house in the community.

13 Psychiatric

Case Study **130**

Name _____ Class/Group _____ Date _____

Group Members _____

INSTRUCTIONS All questions apply to this case study. Your responses should be brief and to the point. When asked to provide several answers, list them in order of priority or significance. Do not assume information that is not provided. Please print or write clearly. If your response is not legible, it will be marked as? and you will need to rewrite it.

▶ Scenario

You are a nurse on an inpatient psychiatric unit. J.M., a 23-year-old woman, was admitted to the psychiatric unit last night after assessment and treatment at a local hospital emergency department (ED) for "blacking out at school." She has been given a preliminary diagnosis of anorexia nervosa. As you begin to assess her, you notice that she has very loose clothing, she is wrapped in a blanket, and her extremities are very thin. She tells you, "I don't know why I'm here. They're making a big deal about nothing." She appears to be extremely thin and pale, with dry and brittle hair, which is very thin and patchy, and she constantly complains about being cold. As you ask questions pertaining to weight and nutrition, she becomes defensive and vague, but she does admit to losing "some" weight after an appendectomy 2 years ago. She tells you that she used to be fat, but after her surgery she didn't feel like eating and everybody started commenting on how good she was beginning to look, so she just quit eating for a while. She informs you that she is eating lots now, even though everyone keeps "bugging me about my weight and how much I eat." She eventually admits to a weight loss of "about 40 pounds and I'm still fat."

1. How is the diagnosis of anorexia nervosa determined?

2. Identify eight clinical symptoms of anorexia nervosa. Place a star or asterisk next to those that J.M. has.

13 Psychiatric

3. What other disorders might occur along with anorexia nervosa?

4. How does bulimia nervosa differ from anorexia nervosa?

5. Name behaviors that J.M. or any other patient with anorexia may engage in other than self-starvation.

6. What common family dynamics are associated with anorexia nervosa?

You review her admission laboratory studies. An ECG has also been ordered.

■ Chart View

Admission Lab Work

Sodium	135 mEq/L
Potassium	3.4 mEq/L
Chloride	99 mEq/L
BUN	18 mg/dL
Creatinine	1.0 mg/dL
Hemoglobin	11 g/dL
Hematocrit	35%

7. Which lab results might be of concern at this time? Explain your answers.

8. What clinical symptoms of anorexia nervosa should have the highest priority? Explain your answers.

J.M.'s ECG results show normal sinus rhythm with no ST segment or other changes. You meet with J.M. to formulate a plan of care.

9. In general, the care plans for patients with anorexia are detailed and include many psychological aspects. What are they? You should be able to name at least 10.

13 Psychiatric

10. What would indicate successful treatment with J.M.?

CASE STUDY PROGRESS

After 3 weeks, you are providing discharge teaching for J.M. You ask her whether she is ready to go home. J.M. states, "I'll be so glad to get out of this place. I'm so fat and ugly. I need to lose 10 pounds. I bet I can do it in just a couple of days. Otherwise, I don't want to live anymore."

11. What will you discuss with the physician before any further discharge teaching or plans?

12. You report J.M.'s statements to the physician. What do you expect to be ordered by the physician?

13. What medications would be indicated for J.M. to assist with resolution of both her anorexia nervosa and major depression?

CASE STUDY OUTCOME

After 2 weeks, J.M. has gained 5 pounds and seems to be more willing to eat. She still expresses fears of "getting fat," but she states that she is ready to go home and back to school. The PCP arranges for J.M. to participate in an outpatient partial hospitalization program that specializes in eating disorders. J.M. expresses interest in meeting others with the same problems.

Case Study **131**

Name _____ Class/Group _____ Date _____

Group Members _____

INSTRUCTIONS All questions apply to this case study. Your responses should be brief and to the point. When asked to provide several answers, list them in order of priority or significance. Do not assume information that is not provided. Please print or write clearly. If your response is not legible, it will be marked as? and you will need to rewrite it.

▶ Scenario

You are working the afternoon shift in an inpatient psychiatric unit. The patients are in the day room watching a movie when suddenly someone starts yelling. You and other staff rush to the day room to find J.J., a 55-year-old male patient, crouched in the corner behind a chair, yelling at the other patients, "Get down. Get down quick." You and the other staff are able to calm J.J. and the other patients and take J.J. to his room. He apologizes for his outburst and explains to you that the movie brought back memories of the Gulf War. He had forgotten where he was and thought he was in combat again. He describes to you in detail the memory he had of being ambushed by the enemy and watching several of his comrades be killed. You remember hearing in report that J.J. is a Gulf War veteran.

1. You read in his medical record that J.J. has posttraumatic stress disorder (PTSD). What are common causes of PTSD, and what is the most likely cause of J.J.'s condition?

2. According to the DSM-IV-TR, name three criteria that must be present to diagnose posttraumatic stress disorder (PTSD).

3. What is the difference between PTSD and acute stress disorder, according to the DSM-IV-TR?

4. Which symptom(s) of PTSD did J.J. most likely experience?

5. What therapeutic measures can be done to help J.J. during your shift this evening?

CASE STUDY PROGRESS

While you are in J.J.'s room, he states that he would like to rest for a while, and he requests something to "calm his nerves." You check his medical record see these PRN medications listed.

■ Chart View

PRN Medications

Acetaminophen (Tylenol)
Alprazolam (Xanax)
Zolpidem (Ambien)

6. Which medication is most appropriate to administer at this time? Explain.

7. The alprazolam (Xanax) comes in different oral formulations. List each one, and state which one(s) are appropriate for J.J.'s situation.

8. What are the adverse effects of long-term use of benzodiazepine anxiolytics?

9. You decide to notify J.J.'s physician about his reaction to the movie. The physician writes an order to start paroxetine (Paxil). How does this medication differ from the alprazolam?

CASE STUDY PROGRESS

J.J. asks you whether there are other things he can do, in addition to medications, to help his anxiety.

10. List some relaxation techniques that could be implemented or taught to J.J. to help relieve his anxiety.

11. To what other treatment modalities could J.J. be referred after his hospitalization to help treat his PTSD and related problems?

Over the next 2 weeks, J.J. participates in individual and group therapy sessions and tells you that he is beginning to be able to face what happened to him years ago. He tells you that he feels "encouraged" and wants to help others with the same problems.

13 Psychiatric

Case Study **132**

Name _____   Class/Group _____   Date _____

Group Members _____

INSTRUCTIONS All questions apply to this case study. Your responses should be brief and to the point. When asked to provide several answers, list them in order of priority or significance. Do not assume information that is not provided. Please print or write clearly. If your response is not legible, it will be marked as? and you will need to rewrite it.

▶ Scenario

J.G., a 49-year-old man, was seen in the emergency department (ED) 2 days ago, diagnosed with alcohol intoxication, and released after 8 hours to his brother's care. He was brought back to the ED 12 hours ago with an active gastrointestinal (GI) bleed and is being admitted to the intensive care unit (ICU); his diagnosis is upper GI bleed and alcohol intoxication.

You are assigned to admit and care for J.G. for the remainder of your shift. According to the ED notes, his admission vital signs were BP 84/56 mm Hg, P 110 bpm, R 26, and he was vomiting bright red blood. He was given IV fluids and transfused 6 units of packed red blood cells (PRBCs) in the ED. On initial assessment, you note that J.G.'s VS are blood pressure BP 154/90 mm Hg, P 110 bpm; he has a slight tremor in his hands, and he appears anxious. He complains of a headache and appears flushed. You note that he has not had any emesis and has not had any frank red blood in his stool or melena (black tarry stools) over the past 5 hours. In response to your questions, J.G. denies that he has an alcohol problem but later admits to drinking approximately a fifth of vodka daily for the past 2 months. He reports that he was drinking vodka just before his admission to the ED. He admits to having had seizures while withdrawing from alcohol in the past.

■ Chart View

Admission Lab Work	
Hgb	10.9 g/dL
Hct	23%
ALT (SGPT)	69 units/L
AST (SGOT)	111 units/L
GGT	75 units/L
Serum alcohol (ETOH)	291 mg/dL

1. Which data from your assessment of J.G. are of concern to you?

2. What do the admission laboratory results indicate?

3. Which of the previous lab results specifically reflects chronic alcohol ingestion?

13 Psychiatric

4. What are two most likely causes of J.G.'s symptoms?

5. What is the most likely time frame for someone to have withdrawal symptoms after abrupt cessation of alcohol?

CASE STUDY PROGRESS

You note that J.G.'s physician has not diagnosed J.G. as having alcohol dependence, and his orders do not include treatment for alcohol withdrawal.

6. As an RN, what action is necessary before you continue to care for J.G.?

7. According to the DSM-IV-TR, what is the difference between alcohol dependence and alcohol abuse?

8. What would be helpful for J.G.'s physician to know regarding J.G.'s substance abuse history?

CASE STUDY PROGRESS

J.G.'s physician comes to the ICU to assess J.G. and tells you to "watch out" because J.G. is about to go into alcohol withdrawal delirium. The physician writes several medication orders.

9. What medications are commonly prescribed for patients withdrawing from alcohol? (Select all that apply.)
   a. Benzodiazepines, such as chlordiazepoxide (Librium)
   b. Naltrexone (Revia), an opioid-reversal agent
   c. Acamprosate (Campral), an alcohol deterrent agent
   d. Clonidine (Catapres), an alpha-adrenergic blocker
   e. Antiepileptic drugs, such as carbamazepine (Tegretol)
   f. Disulfiram (Antabuse), an alcohol deterrent agent
   g. Atenolol (Tenormin), a beta-adrenergic blocker

13 Psychiatric

10. Explain the rationale for each of the drugs used during acute alcohol withdrawal.

11. What chronic health problems are associated with alcoholism?

12. What lab tests might the physician order to assess for nutritional deficiencies or other medical problems J.G. is experiencing?

13 Psychiatric

CASE STUDY PROGRESS

J.G. experiences alcohol withdrawal delirium that lasts for 36 hours before subsiding. He did not experience any seizures this time. As his medical condition stabilizes, he is transferred out of the ICU to the hospital's psychiatric unit. He tells you that he is "ready to go home" and does not want to "touch another drink" but admits that he needs help.

13. What medications might be prescribed to J.G. to assist him with sobriety? What is the usual treatment regimen, and what side effects and precautions should you educate the patient about concerning each?

14. What types of education and referral will be done before J.G.'s discharge from the hospital?

15. J.G. is referred to the local Alcoholics Anonymous (AA) program. What strategy can be implemented to increase his likelihood of attendance to these meetings?

CASE STUDY OUTCOME

J.G.'s AA sponsor meets with him while J.G. was still in the hospital, and the meeting went well. The day after his discharge from the hospital, J.G. attends his first AA meeting with his sponsor.

13 Psychiatric

Case Study **133**

Name _____ Class/Group _____ Date _____

Group Members _____

INSTRUCTIONS All questions apply to this case study. Your responses should be brief and to the point. When asked to provide several answers, list them in order of priority or significance. Do not assume information that is not provided. Please print or write clearly. If your response is not legible, it will be marked as? and you will need to rewrite it.

▶ Scenario

It is 1000 hours in the emergency department (ED) when the ambulance brings in G.G., a 35-year-old man who is having difficulty breathing. He complains of chest pain and tightness, dizziness, palpitations, nausea, paresthesia, and feelings of impending doom and unreality; he is having trouble thinking clearly. He tells you, "I don't think I'm going to make it. I must be having a heart attack." He is diaphoretic and trembling. His vital signs are 184/92, 104, 28, 98.4° F (36.9° C). This episode began at work during a meeting at approximately 0920 and became progressively worse. A co-worker called 911 and stayed with the patient until medical help arrived. The patient has no history of cardiac problems.

1. What initial steps would the nurse take, and what orders would the nurse expect to receive?

CASE STUDY PROGRESS

After a full medical workup, it is determined that G.G. is stable. His shortness of breath and anxiety are resolved after he is given lorazepam (Ativan) 1 mg IV push (IVP). There is no evidence of any physical disorder, and the diagnosis of panic attack has been made. G.G. admits to having had three similar episodes in the past 2 weeks; however, they were not nearly as severe or long lasting.

2. How do you think this diagnosis was determined?

3. G.G. asks whether there is something wrong with his memory because he has been having trouble remembering things. What effect does panic disorder have on memory?

CASE STUDY PROGRESS

G.G. shares with the ED staff that he has been under severe stress at work and home. He tells them he is going through a divorce, he lost a child last summer in a motor vehicle accident, and his company is downsizing. He will probably be out of a job soon. He hasn't been sleeping well for the past couple of months and has lost about 20 pounds.

4. Identify five additional triggers that could cause anxiety to build to the point of panic.

5. G.G. wants to know what causes panic attacks or panic disorder. Using etiologic theories regarding anxiety, what will you tell him?

6. G.G. has questions regarding the differences between panic attacks and panic disorder. According to the DSM-IV-TR, what are the differences?

CASE STUDY PROGRESS

G.G.'s condition is stable, and the ED physician discusses what has happened with G.G. The physician gives G.G. a prescription for a "week's worth" of medication and instructs G.G. to see his primary care physician for further treatment and evaluation.

7. The physician gave G.G. a prescription for alprazolam (Xanax) to last one week and instructs G.G. to see his primary care physician for further treatment and evaluation. Why do you think the physician gave G.G. a prescription for only 1 week of Xanax?

8. What medications are used to treat panic attacks? What will your patient teaching include?

CASE STUDY PROGRESS

G.G. tells you all about his worries with his job and all that has happened to him in the past year. He tells you that he appreciates you listening to him. He expresses fear of panic attacks returning.

9. What techniques to help him cope will you discuss with him?

10. What actions or interventions are most indicated in the treatment of panic disorder?

CASE STUDY OUTCOME

G.G. makes an appointment with his company's Employee Assistance Program to take advantage of the resources offered for counseling to help him work with his coping strategies. In addition, his primary care physician started him on a low dose of an SSRI. After a few months, G.G.'s panic attacks have become very rare and he works on preparing a résumé to seek new employment before his company has another round of job cuts.

Alternative Therapies

Case Study **134**

Name _____ Class/Group _____ Date _____

Group Members _____

INSTRUCTIONS All questions apply to this case study. Your responses should be brief and to the point. When asked to provide several answers, list them in order of priority or significance. Do not assume information that is not provided. Please print or write clearly. If your response is not legible, it will be marked as ? and you will need to rewrite it.

▶ **Scenario**

J.B., a 45-year-old woman, is an office manager for a busy law firm and single mother of two children. While cleaning a shower stall, she experienced a sharp pain in her lower back. Over the next few hours, her lower back became increasingly more painful. By the time she picked up the children from their sporting event and drove to the nearest walk-in medical clinic, she had a sharp shooting pain into her right buttocks. Her spinal x-rays were not significant, and she was diagnosed with acute musculoskeletal strain, instructed to take a nonsteroidal anti-inflammatory medication, such as ibuprofen (Advil or Motrin) and given a prescription for hydrocodone 5 mg/acetaminophen 500 mg (Lortab) PO q6h prn for severe pain. She was instructed to rest her back for the next 24 hours. Monday morning she called in sick to work because she couldn't think clearly because of the pain medication. She developed stomach pain, and her back pain was only slightly improved. She called a friend who had experienced a similar episode and related a favorable outcome after being treated with acupuncture. J.B. comes to your alternative medicine clinic for her acupuncture appointment.

1. As you complete her intake interview, she asks, "What is acupuncture?" What will you tell her?

2. J.B. wants to know how acupuncture works. How will you explain acupuncture to her?

3. J.B. asks how acupuncture can help her back pain. Explain how acupuncture differs from traditional Western medicine in the treatment of back pain.

4. J.B. asks, "What does it feel like? Does it hurt?" How will you respond?

5. J.B. asks, "Does insurance cover the cost?" Provide a response.

6. List possible risks and complications of acupuncture.

7. What conditions can be treated with acupuncture?

8. J.B. asks where she could find an acupuncture practitioner.

Case Study 135

Name _____ Class/Group _____ Date _____

Group Members _____

INSTRUCTIONS All questions apply to this case study. Your responses should be brief and to the point. When asked to provide several answers, list them in order of priority or significance. Do not assume information that is not provided. Please print or write clearly. If your response is not legible, it will be marked as ? and you will need to rewrite it.

▶ Scenario

One month ago, J.P., a 50-year-old man, came to the outpatient clinic with complaints of mild shortness of breath and some mild intermittent chest pain. He described himself as a high-stress, type A personality who owns his own business and works long hours. He has smoked one pack of cigarettes per day for the past 30 years. He has tried to quit several times and was successful for as long as 6 months at a time, but when business became stressful, he started smoking again. J.P. said he has been trying to lose the extra 30 pounds he is carrying but stated it is difficult to exercise because of the long hours of work. The cardiac workup is negative for coronary artery disease, and he has returned for a follow-up visit. During the discussion about lifestyle changes, J.P. expresses interest in medical hypnosis for stress management, smoking cessation, and weight loss. He would like more information. You are the case manager for the clinic and meet with J.P. to discuss medical hypnosis.

1. J.P. asks, "What is hypnosis?" What will you tell him?

2. J.P. asks what you mean by *trance state*. Explain the term.

3. J.P. wants to know what you mean by subconscious mind. Explain.

4. J.P. asks, "How does hypnosis work to help someone change a subconscious belief?" How will you respond?

14 Alternative Therapies

5. J.P. states he has seen TV shows where people did silly things on stage. He wants to know how medical hypnosis is different from TV hypnosis. Explain.

6. J.P. asks how you can tell that hypnosis will work for a patient. Please respond.

7. J.P. wants to know how hypnosis is done and what happens during a session. You inform him that medical hypnosis has several components: patient preparation and education, establishing a rapport and trusting relationship, induction and deepening, hypnotic suggestions, and reawakening from the trance state. Briefly explain each step.

8. J.P. asks what types of medical conditions can be helped by hypnosis. How will you respond?

14 Alternative Therapies

9. J.P. asks whether hypnosis is contraindicated for anyone. What will you tell him?

10. J.P. apologizes for being full of questions but wants to know whether hypnosis can be done in a group or one on one only. How will you respond?

11. J.P. asks you how he would go about finding a hypnotist. What will you tell him?

12. J.P. states he would like to read more about hypnosis on the Internet. List three credible websites you could give him.

14 Alternative Therapies

Patients with Multiple Disorders 15

Case Study **136**

Name _____ Class/Group _____ Date _____

Group Members _____

INSTRUCTIONS All questions apply to this case study. Your responses should be brief and to the point. When asked to provide several answers, list them in order of priority or significance. Do not assume information that is not provided. Please print or write clearly. If your response is not legible, it will be marked as? and you will need to rewrite it.

▶ Scenario

You are working in the emergency department (ED) of a community hospital when the ambulance arrives with A.N., an 18-year-old woman who was caught in a house fire. She was sleeping when the fire started and managed to make her way out of the house through thick smoke. The emergency medical system crew initiated humidified oxygen at 15 L/min per nonrebreather mask and started a 16-gauge IV with lactated Ringer's solution. On arrival to the ED, her vital signs are 100/66, 125, 34, Sao_2 93%. An additional 16-gauge IV is inserted. She appears anxious and in pain.

1. As you perform your initial assessment, you note superficial partial-thickness burns on A.N.'s right anterior leg, left anterior and posterior leg, and anterior torso. Shade the affected areas, then using the "rule of nines," calculate the extent of A.N.'s burn injury.

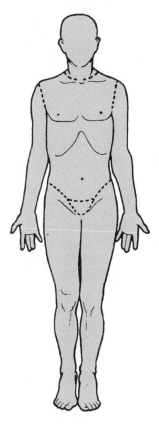

15 Multiple Disorders

2. Because you are concerned about possible smoke inhalation, what signs will you monitor A.N. for?

■ Chart View

Laboratory Test Values

Hgb	20 g/dL
Hct	51%
K	4.9 mEq/dL
Na	133 mEq/dL
Cl	100 mEq/dL
Glu	159 mg/dL
BUN	28 mg/dL
Cre	1.0 mg/dL

3. Interpret A.N.'s laboratory results.

4. A.N. is undergoing burn fluid resuscitation using the standard Baxter (Parkland) formula. She was admitted at 0400. She weighs 110 pounds. Calculate her fluid requirements, specify the fluids used in the Baxter (Parkland) formula, specify how much will be given, and indicate what time intervals will be used.

15 Multiple Disorders

5. A.N. is in severe pain. What is the drug of choice for pain relief following burn injury, and how should it be given?

CASE STUDY PROGRESS

A.N. does not exhibit any signs of smoke inhalation injury and is admitted to the medical unit for further treatment. As her nurse, you are concerned about meeting her needs for infection prevention, skin integrity, nutrition, fluids, and psychological support.

6. Because of her significant burn injury, A.N. is at high risk for infection. What measures will you institute to prevent this?

7. A.N.'s burns are to be treated by the open method with topical application of silver sulfadiazine (Silvadene). When caring for A.N., which interventions will you perform? (Select all that apply.)
   a. Maintain the room temperature at 85° F (29.4° C).
   b. Use clean technique when changing A.N.'s dressings.
   c. Monitor CBC frequently, particularly the white blood cells.
   d. Do not allow her to bathe for the initial 72 hours following injury.
   e. Apply a $\frac{1}{16}$-inch film of medication, covering entire burn.
   f. Shave all hair within the wound beds.

15 Multiple Disorders

8. A.N. has one area of circumferential burns on her right lower leg. What complication is she in danger of developing, and how will you monitor for it?

9. What interventions will facilitate maintaining A.N.'s peripheral tissue perfusion?

10. A special burn diet is ordered for A.N. She has always gained weight easily and is concerned about the size of the portions. What diet-related teaching will you provide?

11. Describe interventions that you could use to assist in meeting A.N.'s nutrition goals.

■ Chart View

Vital Signs

Blood pressure	90/50 mm Hg
Heart rate	110 beats/min
Respiratory rate	24 breaths/min

CASE STUDY PROGRESS

Eighteen hours after the injury, the NAP reports these vital signs for A.N. and states that the urine output for the past hour was 20 mL.

12. What do you suspect is occurring, and why does this concern you?

13. What treatment do you anticipate?

■ **Chart View**

Laboratory Test Values

Hgb	24 g/dL
Hct	59%
K	5.3 mEq/dL
Na	128 mEq/dL
Cl	92 mEq/dL
Glu	122 mg/dL
BUN	38 mg/dL
Cre	1.9 mg/dL

14. The physician orders a new set of lab work. Compare A.N.'s current lab results with those from admission.

15. Tissues under and around A.N.'s burns are severely swollen. She looks at you with tears in her eyes and asks, "Will they stay this way?" What is your answer?

16. A.N. is concerned about visible scars. What will you tell her to allay her fears?

15 Multiple Disorders

Case Study 137

Name _____ Class/Group _____ Date _____

Group Members _____

INSTRUCTIONS All questions apply to this case study. Your responses should be brief and to the point. When asked to provide several answers, list them in order of priority or significance. Do not assume information that is not provided. Please print or write clearly. If your response is not legible, it will be marked as? and you will need to rewrite it.

▶ Scenario

You are admitting a 30-year-old woman, J.L., to your telemetry unit with the diagnosis of status post-cardiac transplantation and fever of unknown origin. She was healthy until the birth of her only child at 27 years of age. She developed idiopathic cardiomyopathy after childbirth and underwent cardiac transplantation 10 months ago. All of her endomyocardial biopsies have been negative for signs of rejection; her last one was 3 weeks ago. She is currently maintained on a regimen of baby aspirin, multivitamins, tacrolimus (Prograf), nifedipine (Procardia), and metolazone (Zaroxolyn).

1. Admitting has assigned J.L. to a semiprivate room. Her roommate is on day 4 of IV antibiotic treatment for pneumonia and now has a near normal WBC count. Is this assignment appropriate?

2. Fever is a sign of two major complications of organ transplantation. What are they?

3. What is the purpose of tacrolimus (Prograf), and what role does that play in your assessment?

4. Compare and contrast the signs and symptoms of organ rejection and sepsis that you need to assess for in J.L.

CASE STUDY PROGRESS

While you are assessing J.L., she tells you that she always urinates frequently because of her diuretics. However, she has experienced burning with urination for the past 2 days. You decide to collect a urine specimen for laboratory analysis.

15 Multiple Disorders

5. What are the possible causes of the burning, and what type of urine specimen should you obtain?

■ Chart View

Urinalysis

pH	7.8
WBC	12
RBC	≤2
Bacteria	↑ than 100,000 colonies

Urine C&S

S. aureus	↑ than 100,000 colonies
Amoxicillin	R
Ceftriaxone	R
Ciprofloxacin	R
Doxycycline	S
Trimethoprim-sulfa	R
Nitrofurantoin	R
Vancomycin	S

6. Interpret J.L.'s UA and culture and sensitivity results.

CASE STUDY PROGRESS

J.L.'s BUN and creatinine are within normal limits, and the physician determines that an infection, and not renal dysfunction, is the reason for J.L.'s symptoms. The physician orders IV vancomycin (Vancocin) 500 mg every 8 hours, and he sends J.L. to interventional radiology for placement of a peripherally inserted central catheter (PICC). Her first dose of vancomycin arrives from the pharmacy just as J.L. returns to the floor.

7. What other information do you need to know before you begin the vancomycin (Vancocin)?

8. What interventions do you need to implement to safely administer vancomycin? (Select all that apply.)
   a. Obtain a trough level 6 hours after each infusion
   b. Administer each infusion over a minimum of 1 hour
   c. Hold the infusion if J.L. complains of tinnitus
   d. Assess for the onset of hypertension during the infusion
   e. Monitor urine output, BUN, and creatinine levels
   f. Anticipate replacing the PICC line every 48 hours

9. Describe the transmission-based precautions you need to institute for J.L.

10. Considering J.L.'s urinary infection and her immunosuppressed status, what other interventions should you implement when caring for J.L.?

15 Multiple Disorders

CASE STUDY PROGRESS

After 7 days, J.L. shows a positive response to antibiotic therapy, and she is preparing for discharge. She will continue her pre-hospital drug regimen, with the addition of an oral antibiotic.

11. J.L. tells you that her husband's parents have given her son a pet cat. She jokingly says, "They gave him the play and me the work! My husband is going to have to help. I'm not up to looking after a cat, too." What job does her husband need to do, and why?

12. You would like to teach J.L. some practical things she can do to protect herself from infection. List five.

13. What information would you want to review with J.L. regarding the signs and symptoms of infection and when to seek treatment?

Case Study **138**

Name _____ Class/Group _____ Date _____

Group Members _____

INSTRUCTIONS All questions apply to this case study. Your responses should be brief and to the point. When asked to provide several answers, list them in order of priority or significance. Do not assume information that is not provided. Please print or write clearly. If your response is not legible, it will be marked as? and you will need to rewrite it.

▶ Scenario

You are working evenings on an orthopedic floor. One of your patients, J.O., is a 25-year-old man who was a new admission on day shift. He was involved in a motor vehicle accident (MVA) during a high-speed police chase on the previous night. His admitting diagnosis is status post (S/P) open reduction internal fixation (ORIF) of the right femur, multiple rib fractures, sternal bruises, and multiple abrasions. He speaks some English but is more comfortable with his native language. He is under arrest for narcotics trafficking, so one wrist is shackled to the bed and a guard is stationed outside his room continuously. Another drug dealer told him he is "coming to get him." Hospital security is aware of the situation.

Your initial assessment reveals stable vital signs (VS) of 116/78, 84, 16, 98.6° F. His only complaint is pain, for which he has a patient-controlled analgesia (PCA) pump. Lungs are clear to auscultation. His abdomen is soft and nontender. He has a nasogastric tube connected to intermittent low wall suction. His IV of D5LR is infusing in the proximal port of a left subclavian triple-lumen catheter at 75 mL/hr; the remaining two ports are heparin-locked. His right femur is connected to skeletal traction. The dressing is dry and intact over the incision site. J.O.'s right leg is connected to 10 pounds of skeletal traction.

1. J.O. has not had a cigarette since the accident. He is irate because the day nurse would not let him smoke. What is your major concern about J.O.'s smoking?

2. Do you think J.O. would be a good candidate for a nicotine patch? Why or why not? State your rationale.

3. J.O. has an antiembolism stocking ordered for his left leg. What is the rationale for putting stockings on this leg only?

4. J.O. has a Foley catheter inserted to drain his urine. What would you assess for in relation to the Foley catheter?

15 Multiple Disorders

5. In view of the threat made on J.O.'s life and his vulnerable situation, what precautions should the nursing unit take to protect him?

The nurse in the emergency department phones to tell you that J.O.'s immunization status could not be determined when he arrived, so no tetanus immunization was given. When you ask J.O. the date of his last tetanus shot, you find out that he was born and raised in Colombia and immigrated to the United States 5 years ago. He does not know whether he has ever had a tetanus shot. You inform the physician, and he orders diphtheria/tetanus toxoid 0.5 mL IM and tetanus immune globulin (HyperTET) 250 units deep IM.

6. Why is J.O. getting two injections?

7. When you give J.O. the tetanus injections, you find J.O. in the position illustrated below. Are any of these findings of concern to you? If so, how would you fix it?

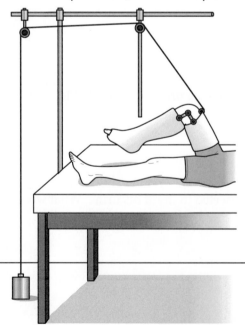

8. While assessing distal to the fractured femur, you note that his toes are slightly cool to the touch. What other assessment findings should be gathered?

At 2100, J.O.'s guard summons you to his room. J.O. is pale, slightly confused, and complaining of chest pain and dyspnea. VS are 90/60, 120, 28, 100.0° F (37.8° C), and Sao₂ of 84%. His pulse is weak and thready, and there are petechiae on his chest. You immediately suspect a fat embolism.

9. Explain the pathophysiology of a fat embolism.

10. List the priority actions you should take next and the rationale for each.

■ **Chart View**

Arterial Blood Gases on 2 L Nasal Cannula

pH	7.32
$Paco_2$	53 mm Hg
HCO_3	22 mmol/L
Pao_2	84 mm Hg

15 Multiple Disorders

11. Interpret J.O.'s ABG results.

The physician comes and examines J.O. He writes the following orders, then leaves, stating he will be back in 1 hour to check on J.O.

■ **Chart View**

Physician's Orders

Bed rest
Oxygen (O_2) to maintain Sao_2 of 90%
Change D5LR IV rate to 125 mL/hr
ECG monitoring
Repeat arterial blood gases (ABGs) in 1 hour
CBC with differential and serum lipase now
STAT CXR
Methylprednisolone (Solu-Medrol) 12 mg IVP now
Furosemide (Lasix) 60 mg IV push now
Digoxin 0.25 mg IV push now

12. Describe a plan for implementing these orders in order of priority.

13. What is the expected outcome associated with each of the medications ordered for J.O.?

■ **Chart View**

Arterial Blood Gases on 10 L Face Mask

pH	7.29
$Paco_2$	56 mm Hg
HCO_3	22 mmol/L
Pao_2	74 mm Hg

15 Multiple Disorders

14. J.O. is placed on oxygen at 10 L via face mask. ABGS are redrawn after 1 hour. Interpret the results.

15. What intervention do you anticipate, based on your interpretation of these values?

CASE STUDY PROGRESS

The physician returns to reexamine J.O. Because J.O.'s status is deteriorating, despite the application of oxygen and the administration of the IV medications, the physician writes to transfer J.O. to the ICU for ventilator support.

16. You accompany J.O. on the transfer to the ICU. Why would you do this, and what information would you provide to the ICU nurse?

CASE STUDY OUTCOME

J.O. recovered for several weeks in the hospital before being sent to jail to await trial. Shortly before his trial date, he was found stabbed to death in his cell. Although there was an investigation, the murder weapon was never found, and no one was ever charged in his death.

15 Multiple Disorders

Case Study **139**

Name _____ Class/Group _____ Date _____

Group Members _____

INSTRUCTIONS All questions apply to this case study. Your responses should be brief and to the point. When asked to provide several answers, list them in order of priority or significance. Do not assume information that is not provided. Please print or write clearly. If your response is not legible, it will be marked as? and you will need to rewrite it.

▶ Scenario

You are working on a telemetry unit and have just received a transfer from the ICU. The 50-year-old male patient, T.A., is postoperative day 2 from a repair of an abdominal aortic aneurysm (AAA) measuring 8 cm in diameter. He is an attorney with an active practice. Before surgery, he routinely took medication for gastritis and has a 10-year history of type 2 diabetes mellitus (DM) requiring insulin the past 6 months to control glucose levels. Despite this, T.A. considered himself to be healthy before diagnosis of the aneurysm. The ICU tells you during report that since surgery, T.A. has experienced some weakness of his lower extremities and decreasing urinary output.

1. T.A. has questions about his surgery. He asks you, "I was fine before surgery. I'd still be fine now if I hadn't been operated on, wouldn't I?" Based on your knowledge of AAA, what will your response be?

2. Why are you concerned about the weakness in T.A.'s legs?

3. You are performing your initial assessment of T.A.'s legs. What findings should you record?

4. Four hours after admission to your floor, you note that T.A. has had a urinary output of 75 mL of dark amber urine. Why are you concerned?

5. You examine the catheter and tubing for obstructions, and there are none. What other assessments do you need to gather?

15 Multiple Disorders

CASE STUDY PROGRESS

You notify the physician of the decrease in urine output. The physician orders a STAT electrolyte panel and asks you to call him with the results.

■ Chart View

Laboratory Test Results

Potassium	5.3 mEq/L
Sodium	132 mEq/L
BUN	48 mg/dL
Creatinine	2.4 mg/dL

6. Interpret T.A.'s laboratory results.

CASE STUDY PROGRESS

The physician determines that T.A. is in the beginning phases of acute renal failure. T.A. is sent to radiology for placement of a dialysis catheter. Upon T.A.'s return, the physician updates T.A.'s medical orders.

7. Indicate the expected outcome for T.A. that is associated with each of the following medications he is receiving.

■ Chart View

Medication Administration Record

Lantus (insulin glargine) 30 units subcut daily
NovoLog (insulin aspart) subcut per sliding scale ac/hs
Imipenem–cilastatin sodium (Primaxin) 1 g IVPB q8h
Dopamine IV infusion at 2 mcg/kg/hr
Furosemide (Lasix) 20 mg IV push q8h
Sevelamer hydrochloride (RenaGel) 800 mg PO with meals
Sodium polystyrene sulfonate (Kayexalate) 1 g PO bid

8. The dialysis catheter is inserted into T.A.'s left subclavian vein. You are preparing to administer the IV antibiotic and find that his only other IV access, a peripheral line, is the site of the dopamine infusion. What will you do?

9. T.A. is placed on a fluid restriction and a renal diet. T.A. asks what he is going to be able to eat and drink on this diet. What is your reply?

10. As you plan your care of T.A. for the remainder of the shift, identify which aspects of his care you can delegate to the nursing assistive personnel (NAP). (Select all that apply.)
a. Evaluate T.A.'s intake and output trends for the past 48 hours.
b. Obtain and record an accurate daily weight.
c. Monitor T.A.'s lung sounds every 4 hours.
d. Measure vital signs every 2 hours.
e. Assist him with oral hygiene as needed.
f. Assess T.A.'s glucose level before dinner.

11. You note that T.A.'s blood glucose levels have ranged from 62 to 387 mg/dL over the past 3 days. He comments, "That's funny, you're giving me almost twice the amount of insulin that I give myself at home. I don't understand why it's not working." How should you respond?

12. Explain the relationship between his blood glucose readings and wound healing.

15 Multiple Disorders

CASE STUDY PROGRESS

On return from his first dialysis, T.A. complains of headache and severe nausea. He is restless and slightly confused, and he has an elevated blood pressure.

13. What is the significance of these findings?

14. You notify the physician. What will you do in the interim before the physician returns your call?

15. T.A. has an episode of severe vomiting. His abdominal wound dehisces, and a loop of his intestines eviscerates. Another staff member has summoned the physician. What care will you render before the physician's arrival?

CASE STUDY OUTCOME

Following the repair of the evisceration, T.A. returns to the ICU. During the remainder of his hospitalization, he experiences delayed wound healing and difficulties with maintaining fluid and electrolyte balance between his dialysis treatments. His kidneys eventually regain function, and he spends 2 more weeks on the rehab unit before being discharged with home health assistance for wound care.

Case Study **140**

Name _____ Class/Group _____ Date _____

Group Members _____

▶ Scenario

You are a nurse working in the medical ICU and take the following report from the emergency depart-ment (ED) nurse: "We have a patient for you; R.L. is an 89-year-old frail woman who has been in a nurs-ing home. Her admitting diagnosis is sepsis, pneumonia, and dehydration, and she has a known stage III right hip pressure ulcer. Past medical history includes remote cerebrovascular accident with residual right-sided weakness and paresthesia, remote myocardial infarction, and peripheral vascular disease. Her vital signs are 98/62, 88 and regular, 38 and labored, 100.4° F (38° C). Lab work is pending; she has oxygen at 10 L via face mask, an IV of D5.45NS at 100 mL/hr, and an indwelling Foley. The infectious disease doc-tor has been notified, and respiratory therapy is with the patient—they are just leaving the ED and should arrive shortly."

1. Knowing that R.L. is frail, has right-sided weakness, and a pressure ulcer, what consults would you initiate?

2. You conduct a skin assessment. What areas of R.L.'s body will you pay particular attention to?

CASE STUDY PROGRESS

During your admission skin assessment, you note that she has very dry, thin, almost transparent skin. She has limited mobility from her stroke and is currently bedridden. There are several areas of ecchymosis on her upper extremities. She is alert and oriented to person only.

3. What major factors increase risk for the development of pressure-induced ulcers?

4. What are the advantages of using a validated risk assessment tool to document a patient's skin condition on admission?

5. Evaluate R.L. on the Norton Risk Assessment Scale.

Norton scale

		Physical condition	Mental condition	Activity	Mobility	Incontinent	
		Good 4 Fair 3 Poor 2 Very bad 1	Alert 4 Apathetic 3 Confused 2 Stupor 1	Ambulant 4 Walk/help 3 Chairbound 2 Bed rest 1	Full 4 Slightly limited 3 Very limited 2 Immobile 1	Not 4 Occasional 3 Usually/urine 2 Doubly 1	Total score
Name	Date						

6. Given R.L.'s Norton score, describe specific measures you would implement in her care to prevent further skin breakdown.

As you are completing R.L.'s assessment, an enterostomal therapy (ET) and wound nurse specialist comes in. She knows R.L. from a prior admission; as soon as she received the wound care consult, she ordered a specialty mattress. She states an air overlay should be delivered to your unit before your shift ends.

7. Why is a specialty bed or mattress used for immobile or compromised patients?

8. Why do patients placed on specialty mattresses or beds remain at risk for breakdown?

9. What are the essential points all nurses should know about a specialty bed?

10. Why do the heels have the greatest incidence of breakdown, even when the patient is on the most advanced specialty bed?

11. What intervention can you initiate to protect R.L.'s heels?

12. Compare and contrast friction and shear.

15 Multiple Disorders

13. What interventions are needed to reduce the possibility of shear?

14. What risk factor does using a draw sheet prevent or minimize?

15. While caring for R.L., it is important for you to instruct the NAP to: (Select all that apply.)
    a. keep R.L.'s head of bed below a 30-degree angle.
    b. assist with hygiene measures when incontinent.
    c. develop an every 2-hour turn schedule.
    d. assess R.L.'s skin status every shift.
    e. use the appropriate sheets on the airflow bed.
    f. empty and measure output in the urine collection device.

CASE STUDY PROGRESS

The wound nurse gently removes the old dressing, using the push-pull method and adhesive remover wipes. After she takes off the outside dressing, often called a *secondary dressing*, she pulls out the primary dressing and states that she has a tunneled wound that was "packed" too hard.

16. What problems can packing a wound too full create?

17. The nurse systematically assesses the ulcer and confirms the presence of a stage III wound. What does it mean to "stage a pressure ulcer"?

18. What is a tunneling wound? What are risk factors associated with tunneling?

19. For each of the four stages of pressure ulcers, describe the tissues involved and what you would expect the skin to look like.

CASE STUDY PROGRESS

After the wound nurse performs a set of cultures, you watch as she dresses the wound. The wound nurse charts the findings and makes formal recommendations for management of the wound to the primary care provider.

20. Describe the technique for packing a tunneled wound.

21. What factors influence the selection of wound dressing?

22. Describe five different types of wound dressings, including specific uses of each.

15 Multiple Disorders

Emergency Situations

16

Case Study 141

Name _____ Class/Group _____ Date _____

Group Members _____

INSTRUCTIONS All questions apply to this case study. Your responses should be brief and to the point. When asked to provide several answers, list them in order of priority or significance. Do not assume information that is not provided. Please print or write clearly. If your response is not legible, it will be marked as? and you will need to rewrite it.

▶ Scenario

You are on duty in the emergency department (ED) when a "code blue" is called overhead. As the code nurse, you grab the crash cart and run to the code, which is in the employee lounge of the operating room. On the couch, you find a nurse, Z.H., unconscious, cyanotic, and barely breathing. Her respirations are 8 breaths per minute and shallow. She is intubated and an IV line is started with 0.9% normal saline. You attach ECG leads to her chest and find the following:

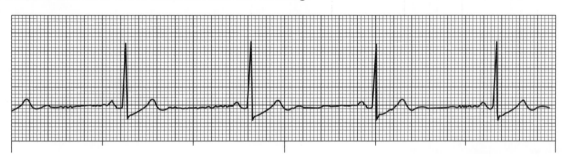

1. What is your interpretation of Z.H.'s rhythm?

CASE STUDY PROGRESS

Z.H. is given an ampule of 50 mL D50W, 0.4 mg naloxone (Narcan), and 0.5 mg atropine IV push. Her respirations improve slightly, and pulse increases to 56 beats/min. She is transported to the ED.

2. Describe the purpose of administering the combination of D50W, atropine, and naloxone (Narcan).

16 Emergency

3. What treatment will Z.H. require in the ED?

4. Within 30 minutes of receiving the naloxone (Narcan), Z.H. is starting to respond. You need to continue to observe her closely because: (Select all that apply.)
   a. multiple doses of naloxone (Narcan) increase Z.H.'s risk of developing pulmonary edema.
   b. adverse effects of naloxone (Narcan) are atrial fibrillation and ventricular dysrhythmias.
   c. the opioid effect associated with the drug overdose might return after the naloxone (Narcan) is metabolized.
   d. reversing the effects of the drug overdose too quickly causes a rebound decline in the level of consciousness.

CASE STUDY PROGRESS

After an additional dose of 0.4 mg naloxone (Narcan), Z.H.'s level of consciousness improves and she is able to be extubated.

5. What information do you want to obtain for Z.H.?

6. In response to your questions, Z.H. tells you that she took fentanyl (Duragesic). She then asks you to call a friend to come stay with her. What information would you give her friend over the phone?

7. The friend asks you what is wrong. How do you respond?

16 Emergency

Once stabilized, Z.H. is admitted to the ICU for 24-hour observation and then transferred to the chemical dependency unit.

8. What is a chemically impaired nurse?

9. What is the profile of an impaired nurse? List five characteristics.

10. One of Z.H.'s colleagues calls on the phone to ask how she is. She tells you that she thought something was wrong with Z.H. because her behavior was so erratic, but "I had no idea it was drugs. I didn't think Z.H. would ever do anything like that!" What are the visible signs of a chemically impaired nurse?

11. State four problems associated with impaired nurses who are practicing.

16 Emergency

12. Z.H. asks what is going to happen to her career. What are the regulatory issues related to impaired nurses that will guide your response?

CASE STUDY PROGRESS

Z.H. successfully completes treatment and continues to practice as a nurse. She is now serving as a sponsor for another nurse undergoing treatment for chemical dependency.

16 Emergency

Case Study 142

Name _____ Class/Group _____ Date _____

Group Members _____

INSTRUCTIONS All questions apply to this case study. Your responses should be brief and to the point. When asked to provide several answers, list them in order of priority or significance. Do not assume information that is not provided. Please print or write clearly. If your response is not legible, it will be marked as? and you will need to rewrite it.

▶ Scenario

You are the nurse on a medical unit taking care of a 40-year-old man, A.A., who has been admitted with peptic ulcer disease secondary to chronic alcoholism. He also has a history of "street" drug abuse. You enter A.A.'s room and find him having a generalized convulsive (tonic-clonic) seizure.

1. List five things you would do in order of priority.

2. Describe status epilepticus.

3. Given A.A.'s history, state at least two possible causes for his tonic-clonic seizure.

CASE STUDY PROGRESS

The rapid response team is called, and the attending physician orders the following:

■ Chart View

Medication Administration Record

Thiamine (vitamin B₁) 100 mg IM now

50% glucose, 1 50-mL IV bolus now

Lorazepam (Ativan) 4 mg IV now over 2-5 minutes

16 Emergency

4. Indicate the expected outcome for A.A. associated with each medication.

5. List one thing you would be particularly alert for when giving lorazepam (Ativan) intravenously.

6. The lorazepam (Ativan) is supplied in a single-use vial. How many milliliters will A.A. receive? Shade in the dose on the syringe.

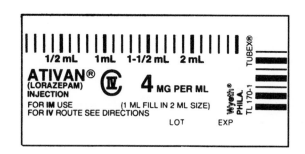

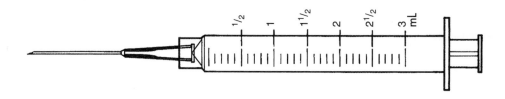

CASE STUDY PROGRESS

A.A.'s seizure activity has not subsided. The physician orders an additional 4 mg of IV lorazepam (Ativan), without effect. Fifteen minutes have now elapsed since you initially found A.A. having seizure activity.

7. What is the significance of this time lapse?

8. The physician decides to administer propofol (Diprivan) and intubate A.A. to support his airway. What is propofol (Diprivan), and why is it being administered to A.A.?

16 Emergency

9. The physician orders phenytoin (Dilantin) 15 mg/kg IV loading dose to be given at a rate of 50 mg/min. What is the rationale behind administering phenytoin (Dilantin)?

10. A.A. weighs 143 pounds. How much phenytoin (Dilantin) will you administer?

11. As you prepare to administer the phenytoin (Dilantin), you see that A.A. has D5W infusing at 75 mL per hour. Why does this concern you and what are your options?

12. A.A. is transported to the ICU, and his seizure activity ceases. What are the main complications of status epilepticus that the nurse will monitor for?

13. Identify nursing interventions that are appropriate for A.A. at this time.

16 Emergency

CASE STUDY PROGRESS

A.A.'s seizure is successfully treated with lorazepam (Ativan) and phenytoin (Dilantin), and he has no further seizure activity. A.A. decides to enter a detoxification program; however, insurance approval has not been received and A.A. is being discharged. As you are writing up his discharge papers, you overhear A.A. telling his girlfriend to have his car brought to the hospital so he can drive home.

14. How will you respond to this situation?

CASE STUDY OUTCOME

A.A. receives insurance approval for a detoxification program and enters 3 days later. He successfully completes the program and remains free of drug and alcohol use.

Case Study **143**

Name _____ Class/Group _____ Date _____

Group Members _____

INSTRUCTIONS All questions apply to this case study. Your responses should be brief and to the point. When asked to provide several answers, list them in order of priority or significance. Do not assume information that is not provided. Please print or write clearly. If your response is not legible, it will be marked as? and you will need to rewrite it.

▶ Scenario

You are the charge nurse on the intermediate cardiac care unit in a large hospital. One of the patients on the unit is R.J., who was admitted at 1300 following an auto accident in which he sustained a chest contusion and fractures of the fourth and fifth ribs on his left side. At about 2000 hours, his wife runs up to you at the nurses' station and says, "I think my husband just had a heart attack. Come quick!" She follows you into his room, where you find him face down on the floor. He is breathing and is cyanotic from the neck up. His pulse is rapid but very weak.

1. What will your first action be?

2. What immediate care will you provide to R.J.?

3. Given R.J.'s admitting diagnosis, what differential diagnoses do you consider?

4. Suddenly, you remember R.J.'s wife, who is anxiously hovering over you in the room. What are you going to do?

CASE STUDY PROGRESS

The code team arrives. R.J.'s trauma surgeon is making rounds on your unit when the code is called, and he runs to the room. R.J. is intubated, and the normal saline lock is changed to an IV of lactated Ringer's at "wide open." The trauma surgeon recognizes Beck's triad and calls for a cardiac needle and syringe. He inserts the needle below the xiphoid process and aspirates 75 mL of unclotted blood.

5. What is Beck's triad, and what causes it?

6. Explain the rationale for the surgeon performing a pericardiocentesis.

7. What is the significance of the surgeon aspirating unclotted blood?

8. The physician orders dopamine IV to "begin at 4 mcg/kg/min and titrate to maintain a systolic BP over 100 mm Hg." What is the rationale for this order?

9. Describe how you will titrate the dopamine infusion.

10. Identify four assessment findings that would indicate that R.J. is responding to your immediate actions.

CASE STUDY PROGRESS

R.J. is transferred to the thoracic intensive care unit (TICU) for observation.

11. As the team prepares R.J.'s transfer, you go to find R.J.'s wife to thank her for alerting you to the emergency so promptly and to tell her what has happened. Briefly, and in lay terms, how would you explain what happened to her husband?

12. As you both get up to leave, Mrs. J. suddenly turns pale and says she feels very dizzy. What are you going to do?

16 Emergency

Case Study **144**

Name _____ Class/Group _____ Date _____

Group Members _____

INSTRUCTIONS All questions apply to this case study. Your responses should be brief and to the point. When asked to provide several answers, list them in order of priority or significance. Do not assume information that is not provided. Please print or write clearly. If your response is not legible, it will be marked as? and you will need to rewrite it.

▶ Scenario

You are the nurse on duty on the intermediate care unit, and you are scheduled to take the next admission. The emergency department (ED) nurse calls to give you the following report: "This is Barb in the ED, and we have a 42-year-old man, K.L., with lower GI (gastrointestinal) bleeding. He is a sandblaster with a 12-year history of silicosis. He is taking 40 mg of prednisone per day. During the night, he developed severe diarrhea. He was unable to get out of bed fast enough and had a large maroon-colored stool in the bed. His wife 'freaked' and called the paramedics. He is coming to you. His vital signs (VS) are stable—110/64, 110, 28—and he's a little agitated. His temperature is 98.2° F (36.8° C). He has not had any stools since admission, but his rectal exam was guaiac positive and he is pale but not diaphoretic. We have him on 5 L O_2/NC. We started a 16-gauge IV with lactated Ringer's at 125 mL/hr. He has an 18-gauge Salem Sump to continuous low suction; that drainage is also guaiac positive. We have done a CBC with differential, chem 14, coagulation times, a T&C (type and crossmatch) for 4 units RBCs, arterial blood gases, and a urinalysis (UA). He's all ready for you."

1. How do you prepare for this patient's arrival?

CASE STUDY PROGRESS

K.L. arrives on your unit. As you help him transfer from the ED stretcher to the bed, K.L. becomes very dyspneic and expels 800 mL of maroon stool.

2. What are the first three actions you should take?

CASE STUDY PROGRESS

K.L. reports that he is getting nauseated but not thirsty. VS are 92/58, 116, 32.

3. What additional interventions do you need to institute?

16 Emergency

4. What assessment indicators would you monitor in K.L.?

5. While caring for K.L., which of these care activities can be safely delegated to the nursing assistive personnel (NAP)? (Select all that apply.)
a. Initiating a pulse oximetry monitoring
b. Measuring K.L.'s vital signs every 15 minutes
c. Obtaining consent from K.L. for a possible blood transfusion
d. Assessing K.L.'s peripheral circulation
e. Emptying each Foley catheter collection bag each hour
f. Monitoring K.L.'s hemoglobin and hematocrit levels

■ Chart View

Arterial Blood Gases

pH	7.47
$Paco_2$	33 mm Hg
Pao_2	65 mm Hg
HCO_3	23 mmol/L
Sao_2	91%

Complete Blood Count

Hgb	7.8 g/dL
Hct	23%

6. Interpret the preceding arterial blood gases (ABGs). What do they tell you?

7. Discuss K.L.'s hemoglobin and hematocrit results.

CASE STUDY PROGRESS

The gastroenterologist is notified by K.L.'s physician and schedules an immediate colonoscopy and endoscopy. You accompany K.L. to the endoscopy suite and give him midazolam (Versed) and morphine sulfate
IV during the procedures.

8. Given the above history, what do you think significantly contributed to the GI bleed?

9. What are midazolam (Versed) and morphine sulfate, and why are they being given to K.L.?

CASE STUDY PROGRESS

During the colonoscopy, K.L. begins passing large amounts of bright red blood. He becomes more pale
and diaphoretic and begins to have an altered level of consciousness.

10. Identify five immediate interventions you should initiate.

11. You are preparing to administer the first of 2 units of packed RBCs. Evaluate each of the
    following statements about the safe administration of blood. Enter "T" for true or "F" for
    false. Discuss why the false statements are incorrect.
    ____1. Prime the correct tubing and filter with normal saline.
    ____2. Verify K.L.'s identification with secretary in the endoscopy suite.
    ____3. Obtain baseline vital signs before starting the transfusion.
    ____4. Begin the transfusion at a rate of 125 mL per hour.
    ____5. Take K.L.'s vital signs 30 minutes after starting the transfusion.
    ____6. Complete the transfusion within 6 hours of receiving the unit.

16 Emergency

CASE STUDY PROGRESS

The physician is able to find the site of the bleeding and cauterize the affected vessels. There is no further evidence of active bleeding. K.L. is transferred back to the unit. His condition is stabilized with fluids, blood, and fresh frozen plasma (FFP). He received esomeprazole (Nexium) 40 mg IV push (IVP) and is placed on 40 mg PO bid.

12. Later, when he seems to be feeling better, K.L. tells you he is really embarrassed about the mess he made for you. How are you going to respond to him?

CASE STUDY OUTCOME

The physician concludes that the GI hemorrhage was prednisone-induced. Because the prednisone was being used to suppress the progression of silicosis, the physician will attempt to decrease his maintenance dose of prednisone while monitoring his respiratory status.

Case Study **145**

Name _____ Class/Group _____ Date _____

Group Members _____

INSTRUCTIONS All questions apply to this case study. Your responses should be brief and to the point. When asked to provide several answers, list them in order of priority or significance. Do not assume information that is not provided. Please print or write clearly. If your response is not legible, it will be marked as? and you will need to rewrite it.

▶ Scenario

J.R. is a 28-year-old man who was doing home repairs. He fell from the top of a 6-foot stepladder, striking his head on a large rock. He experienced a momentary loss of consciousness. By the time his neighbor got to him, he was conscious but bleeding profusely from a laceration over the right temporal area. The neighbor drove him to the emergency department of your hospital. As the nurse, you immediately apply a cervical collar, lay him on a stretcher, and take J.R. to a treatment room.

1. Differentiate between a primary and secondary head injury.

2. What steps will you take to assess J.R.?

3. List at least five components of a neurologic examination.

4. What is the most sensitive indicator of neurologic change?

CASE STUDY PROGRESS

You complete your neurologic examination and find the following: Glasgow Coma Scale (GCS): 15; pupils: equal, round, reactive to light; and full sensation intact. J.R. complains of a headache and is becoming increasingly drowsy. As the radiology technician performs a portable cross-table lateral cervical spine x-ray, J.R. begins to speak incoherently and appears to drift off to sleep.

16 Emergency

5. What are the next actions you will take?

You find that J.R. has become unresponsive to verbal stimuli and responds to painful stimuli by abnormally flexing his extremities (decorticate movement). He has no verbal response. The right pupil is larger than the left and does not respond to light.

6. What is J.R.'s GCS score at this time? Indicate what this means.

7. You summon the physician. Based on the GCS score, what are the next steps you will take?

8. What is a normal intracranial pressure (ICP), and why is increased ICP so clinically important?

9. Identify at least five signs and symptoms of increased ICP.

10. The physician orders a 25% mannitol solution IV. What is mannitol, and why is it being administered to J.R.?

J.R. is transported to radiology for a CT, where he is found to have a large epidural hematoma on the right with a hemispheric shift to the left. He will be taken straight to the operating room (OR) for evacuation of the hematoma. While en route from the CT scan to the OR, the physician instructs the respiratory therapist to initiate hyperventilation of the patient to "blow off more CO_2."

11. What is the rationale for this action?

12. While he is in surgery, J.R.'s family arrives at the ED with their faith healer. They ask that their faith healer anoint J.R. and pray over him. What should the nurse say?

CASE STUDY PROGRESS

After J.R.'s surgery he is admitted to the neurological intensive care unit (NICU).

13. What assessment indicators will be closely monitored in J.R.?

14. J.R. has ICP monitoring in place with an intraventricular catheter. Nursing interventions related to J.R.'s care while the catheter is in place include: (Select all that apply.)
   a. continuously monitoring the ICP waveforms.
   b. using aseptic technique when setting up the device.
   c. maintaining a cerebral perfusion pressure of 60 mm Hg.
   d. leveling the transducer even with the foramen of Monroe.
   e. administering prophylactic antibiotic therapy.
   f. notifying the physician if the ICP is greater than 30 mm Hg.

16 Emergency

15. List four medication classifications that NICU nurses could use to decrease or control increased ICP and the rationale for using each.

16. Explain at least eight independent nursing interventions and the rationale for each that would be used to prevent increased ICP in the first 48 postoperative hours.

16 Emergency

Case Study **146**

Name _____ Class/Group _____ Date _____

Group Members _____

INSTRUCTIONS All questions apply to this case study. Your responses should be brief and to the point. When asked to provide several answers, list them in order of priority or significance. Do not assume information that is not provided. Please print or write clearly. If your response is not legible, it will be marked as? and you will need to rewrite it.

▶ Scenario

You are working in an outpatient clinic when a mother brings in her 20-year-old daughter, C.J., who has type 1 diabetes mellitus (DM) and has just returned from a trip to Mexico. She has had a 3-day fever and diarrhea with nausea and vomiting (N/V). She has been unable to eat and has tolerated only sips of fluid. Because she was unable to eat, she did not take her insulin.

Because C.J. is unsteady, you bring her to the examining room in a wheelchair. While assisting her onto the examining table, you note her skin is warm and flushed. Her respirations are deep and rapid, and her breath is fruity and sweet-smelling. C.J. is drowsy and unable to answer your questions. Her mother states, "She keeps telling me she's so thirsty, but she can't keep anything down."

1. List four pieces of additional information you need to elicit from C.J.'s mother.

CASE STUDY PROGRESS

The mother tells you the following:

  "Blood glucose monitor has been reading 'high.'"

  "C.J. has had sips of ginger ale but that's all."

  "She has been vomiting about every other time she drinks."

  "When she first got home, she went [voided] a lot, but yesterday she hardly went at all, and I don't think she has gone today."

  "She went to bed early last night, and I could hardly wake her up this morning. That's why I brought her in."

2. Describe the pathophysiology of diabetic ketoacidosis (DKA).

16 Emergency

▪ Chart View

Vital Signs

Blood pressure	90/50 mm Hg
Heart rate	124 beats/min
Respiratory rate	36 and deep
Temperature	101.3° F (38.5° C) (tympanic)

Laboratory Test Values

Glucose	777 mg/dL
Potassium	5.8 mEq/L

3. Are these VS appropriate for a woman of C.J.'s age? Why or why not? Discuss your rationale.

4. Explain the rationale for C.J.'s other presenting signs and symptoms.

5. A decision has been made to transport C.J. by ambulance to the local emergency department (ED). After evaluating C.J., the ED physician writes the following orders. Carefully review each order. Mark with an "A" if the order is appropriate; mark with an "I" if inappropriate. For each order you mark as "I," explain why it is inappropriate, and correct the order.

_____1. 1000 mL lactated Ringer's (LR) IV STAT

_____2. 36 units NPH (Humulin N) and 20 units regular (Humulin R) insulins subcut now

_____3. CBC with differential; complete metabolic panel (CMP); blood cultures × 2 sites; clean-catch urine for urinalysis (UA) and culture and sensitivity (C&S); stool for ova and parasites, *Clostridium difficile* toxin, and C&S; serum lactate, ketone, and osmolality; arterial blood gases (ABGs) on room air

_____4. 1800-calorie, carbohydrate-controlled diet

_____5. Ambulate in hall three times daily

_____6. Acetaminophen (Tylenol) 650 mg orally q 4 hours as needed

_____7. Furosemide (Lasix) 60 mg IV push now

_____8. Urinary output every hour

_____9. VS every shift

16 Emergency

6. List five additional interventions and the rationale for the use of each that need to be performed for C.J.

7. Which of these ABG results would you expect to see in C.J.?
   a. pH 7.40, Pao_2 88, $Paco_2$ 34, HCO_3 23
   b. pH 7.48, Pao_2 90, $Paco_2$ 30, HCO_3 28
   c. pH 7.27, Pao_2 90, $Paco_2$ 50, HCO_3 20
   d. pH 7.26, Pao_2 94, $Paco_2$ 23, HCO_3 18

CASE STUDY PROGRESS

All orders have been corrected and initiated. C.J. has received fluid resuscitation and is on a sliding-scale insulin drip via infusion pump. After several hours, her latest labs are:

16 Emergency

■ **Chart View**

Laboratory Test Results

Na	149 mmol/L
K	3.0 mmol/L
Cl	119 mmol/L
Total CO_2	21 mmol/L
BUN	12 mg/dL
Creatinine	1.2 mg/dL
Glucose	307 mg/dL

8. The physician orders a change in the insulin drip infusion, decreasing it from 6 units to 4 units per hour. The label on the bag infusing reads, "100 units regular (Humulin R) insulin in 250 mL of normal saline." At how many milliliters per hour will you set the infusion pump?

9. What is the rationale behind using an infusion pump for the insulin drip?

10. Based on C.J.'s lab results, what changes in her IV fluids do you anticipate, and why?

11. C.J. is ready for transport to the medical ICU. C.J.'s mother is beginning to realize that C.J. is more acutely ill than she thought. She leaves the room and begins to cry. How would you handle this situation?

12. C.J.'s mother asks where she can get more information on how C.J. can manage her diabetes. What are some resources she might find useful?

CASE STUDY OUTCOME

C.J. is transported to the MICU in slightly improved condition. She continues to improve and is discharged from the hospital 3 days later.

Case Study **147**

Name _____ Class/Group _____ Date _____

Group Members _____

INSTRUCTIONS All questions apply to this case study. Your responses should be brief and to the point. When asked to provide several answers, list them in order of priority or significance. Do not assume information that is not provided. Please print or write clearly. If your response is not legible, it will be marked as? and you will need to rewrite it.

▶ Scenario

T.R. is a 22-year-old college senior who lives in the dormitory. His friend finds him wandering aimlessly about the campus appearing pale and sweaty. He engages T.R. in conversation and walks him to the campus medical clinic, where you are on duty. The friend explains to you how he found T.R. and states that T.R. has diabetes mellitus (DM) and takes insulin. T.R. is not wearing a medical warning tag. It is 1015.

1. What do you think is going on with T.R.?

2. What is the first action you would take?

3. If no glucose meter were available, would you treat T.R. on the assumption that he is hyperglycemic or hypoglycemic? Explain your rationale.

4. T.R.'s glucose reading is 50 mg/dL. What would your next action be?

5. When you enter the room to administer the juice, T.R. is unresponsive. What should you do?

6. T.R. is breathing at 16 breaths/min, has a pulse of 85 beats/min and regular, but remains unresponsive. Because outpatient resources vary, describe what your next action would be if (1) your clinic is well equipped for emergencies or (2) your clinic has no emergency supplies.

16 Emergency

647

CASE STUDY PROGRESS

A few minutes after dextrose is administered, T.R. begins to awaken. He becomes alert and asks where he is and what happened to him. You orient him, and then explain what has transpired.

7. What questions would you ask to find out what precipitated these events?

8. What further action do you need to take?

CASE STUDY PROGRESS

T.R. tells you he took 35 units glargine (Lantus) insulin and 12 units of regular (Humulin R) insulin at 0745. He says he was late to class, so he just grabbed an apple on the way. He adds that he has had two similar low-blood sugar episodes in the past. He treated them by eating a candy bar and then ate a meal. He says he is on a 2000-calorie, carbohydrate (CHO)–controlled diet but has been checking his blood glucose levels every "couple of days" only.

9. Based on your knowledge of the types of insulin T.R. is receiving, when would you expect T.R. to experience a hypoglycemic reaction?

10. What common mistake in previously treated episodes of hypoglycemia did T.R. make?

11. List at least four important points that you would stress in discussing your teaching plan with T.R.

12. You will recognize that T.R. understands your teaching regarding hypoglycemia if he states:
   a. "If I am too sick to eat, I will not take either insulin until I feel better."
   b. "I will exercise just before eating and taking insulin so I do not get cramps."
   c. "I need to eat within thirty minutes of taking regular (Humulin R) insulin."
   d. "Only certain types of alcoholic drinks will affect my blood glucose levels."

16 Emergency

Case Study **148**

Name _____ Class/Group _____ Date _____

Group Members _____

INSTRUCTIONS All questions apply to this case study. Your responses should be brief and to the point. When asked to provide several answers, list them in order of priority or significance. Do not assume information that is not provided. Please print or write clearly. If your response is not legible, it will be marked as? and you will need to rewrite it.

▶ Scenario

S.K., a 51-year-old roofer, was admitted to the hospital 3 days ago after falling 15 feet from a roof. He sustained bilateral fractured wrists and an open fracture of the left tibia and fibula. He was taken to surgery for open reduction internal fixation (ORIF) of all of his fractures. He is recovering in your orthopedic unit. You have instructions to begin getting him out of bed and into the chair today. When you enter the room to get S.K. into the chair, you notice that he is agitated and dyspneic. He says to you, "My chest hurts really badly. I can't breathe."

1. Identify five possible reasons for S.K.'s symptoms.

CASE STUDY PROGRESS

You auscultate S.K.'s breath sounds. You find that they are diminished in the left lower lobe (LLL). S.K. is diaphoretic and tachypneic and has circumoral cyanosis. His apical pulse is irregular and 110 beats/min.

2. List in order of priority three actions you should take next.

3. Using SBAR, what information will you provide to the physician when you call?

CASE STUDY PROGRESS

The physician orders the following: arterial blood gases (ABGs), chest x-ray (CXR), ECG, and a helical (spiral) CT of the lungs.

16 Emergency

■ Chart View

ABGs

pH	7.49
$Paco_2$	30.6 mm Hg
Pao_2	52 mm Hg
HCO_3	24.2 mmol/L
Sao_2	83%
A-a oxygen gradient	32 mm Hg

4. Interpret S.K.'s ABG results with the rationale for your interpretations.

5. Based on the ABGs and your assessment findings, what do you think is wrong with S.K.?

6. The physician writes the following orders for S.K. Review each order. Mark with an "A" if the order is appropriate; mark with an "I" if the order is inappropriate. Correct all inappropriate orders, and provide rationales for your decisions.

_____1. Transfer to MICU

_____2. Heparin 20,000 units IV push now, then 20,000 units in 1000 mL/D5W to run at 1000 units/hr

_____3. PT/INR and PTT q4h; call house officer with results

_____4. 3 L oxygen by nasal cannula

_____5. Patient-controlled analgesia (PCA) pump with morphine sulfate: loading dose 10 mg; dose 2 mg; lock-out time 15 minutes; maximum 4-hour dose 30 mg

_____6. Streptokinase 250,000 IU IV over 30 minutes, then 100,000 IU/hr for 24 hours

_____7. Prednisolone (Solu-Cortef) 1 g IV push now

_____8. Albuterol (Proventil) metered-dose inhaler (MDI), two puffs q6h

All orders have been corrected. S.K.'s helical CT scan confirms the diagnosis of pulmonary embolism (PE) in the LLL, and heparin therapy is initiated. Repeat ABGs show the following values:

■ Chart View

ABGs

pH	7.45
Pa_{CO_2}	35 mm Hg
Pa_{O_2}	82 mm Hg
HCO_3	24.1 mmol/L
Sa_{O_2}	90%
A-a oxygen gradient	28 mm Hg

7. What do these gases generally indicate?

8. The physician orders furosemide (Lasix) 20 mg IV push now. What is the expected outcome associated with administering furosemide (Lasix) to S.K.?

■ Chart View

Laboratory Test Values

PTT	70 seconds
INR	1.4

9. Coagulation times are redrawn after S.K. has been on heparin therapy for 4 hours. What changes, if any, do you anticipate, based on your interpretation of these values?

10. List six independent nursing interventions that would be implemented for S.K. and the rationale for each.

16 Emergency

11. What instructions would you give to the NAP who is assisting with S.K.'s care? (Select all that apply.)
    a. Use care when repositioning S.K.; make sure you have adequate help.
    b. Use a rectal thermometer when taking S.K.'s vital signs.
    c. Immediately report any signs of bleeding.
    d. Use a sponge-toothed applicator when helping S.K. with oral care.
    e. Use an electric razor when shaving S.K.
    f. Position S.K. with the head of the bed elevated, on his left side.

CASE STUDY PROGRESS

S.K. is watched closely for the next several days for the onset of pulmonary edema. Heparin therapy, oxygen, pulse oximetry, daily CXRs and ABG analysis, and pain management are continued. When he is stable, S.K. is transferred back to your orthopedic unit.

12. The next day, S.K. suddenly explodes and throws the physical therapist out of his room. He yells, "I'm sick and tired of having everyone tell me what to do." How are you going to deal with this situation?

Case Study **149**

Name _____ Class/Group _____ Date _____

Group Members _____

▶ Scenario

D.V. is a 38-year-old woman who had a ruptured appendix 10 days ago with subsequent peritonitis. She was discharged to home care yesterday, on postoperative day 9, with a left peripherally inserted central catheter (PICC) for IV antibiotic therapy. You work for the home care department of the hospital. You have been assigned to D.V.'s case, and this is your first home visit. You are to do a full assessment on D.V. During the assessment, you notice a large ecchymotic area over the right upper arm. You ask her whether she fell and hit her arm. She tells you, "The nurses took my blood pressure so many times it bruised."

1. Do you accept D.V.'s explanation? Why or why not?

2. In examining D.V. further, you find a fine, non-raised, dark red rash over her trunk (petechiae). What questions would you ask D.V. to elicit additional information?

CASE STUDY PROGRESS

D.V. had not noticed the petechiae before you pointed it out. She states that the rash does not itch or cause pain and that she has never had one like it before.

3. What other information would you want to gather?

CASE STUDY PROGRESS

Her vital signs are within normal limits except for a temperature of 99.8° F (37.7° C). The abdominal wound is not discolored or draining; however, her abdomen is tender to light palpation. The rash is confined to the trunk. There is oozing of serosanguineous fluid around the PICC insertion site. She has no other signs of bleeding. You make a decision to call the physician regarding your findings.

16 Emergency

4. What information will you relay to the physician?

CASE STUDY PROGRESS

The physician orders blood to be drawn for coagulation studies and a CBC with differential. He says he would like to evaluate D.V. for disseminated intravascular coagulation (DIC).

5. What laboratory tests would you expect to see performed in coagulation studies?

6. You give D.V. a dose of her antibiotic and draw her blood. You tell her that you will return in 6 hours to give her another dose of antibiotics. She asks you, "What is going on?" How would you respond?

CASE STUDY PROGRESS

You drop the blood off at the hospital and proceed to your next visit. When you return to the car, you see that D.V. sent you a text wanting you to "come back now." When you return to D.V.'s home, she greets you at the door. She is upset and ushers you to the bathroom, where you find blood in the toilet. She tells you that she went to the bathroom and urinated blood. She also shows you a tissue in which she has bloody-appearing sputum and some bloody drainage from the blood draw 2 hours earlier. You call 911 immediately to have D.V. taken to the emergency department (ED) and notify the physician of your actions. You call the ED and give report to the triage nurse on duty.

7. What are you going to tell the triage nurse?

8. Are D.V.'s presenting signs and symptoms consistent with DIC? Explain.

■ Chart View

Laboratory Test Values

PT	19 seconds
aPTT	96 seconds
D-dimer	4.8 mcg/mL
Fibrinogen	56 mg/dL
WBC	12,500/mm³
Platelet count	46,000/mm³

9. Interpret D.V.'s laboratory values.

10. D.V. is diagnosed with DIC. List at least three priority needs for D.V.

D.V. is stabilized with oxygen, fluids, and blood products, and medication therapy is initiated. She is transferred to the ICU in guarded condition.

16 Emergency

Case Study **150**

Name _____ Class/Group _____ Date _____

Group Members _____

INSTRUCTIONS All questions apply to this case study. Your responses should be brief and to the point. When asked to provide several answers, list them in order of priority or significance. Do not assume information that is not provided. Please print or write clearly. If your response is not legible, it will be marked as? and you will need to rewrite it.

▶ Scenario

You are the trauma nurse working in the emergency department (ED) of a busy tertiary care facility. You receive a call from the paramedics that they are en route to your facility with the victim of gunshot wounds to the chest and abdomen. The paramedics have started two large-bore IV lines with lactated Ringer's and oxygen by mask at 15 L/min. The patient has a sucking chest wound on the left and a wound in the right upper quadrant (RUQ) of the abdomen. Vital signs in the field are 80/36, 140, and 42. The patient is diaphoretic, very pale, and confused. The estimated time of arrival is 4 minutes.

1. List at least six things you will do to prepare for this patient's arrival.

CASE STUDY PROGRESS

On arrival, your patient, B.W., is cyanotic and in severe respiratory distress. When he is transferred to the trauma stretcher, you notice that there is an occlusive dressing over the sucking chest wound. It is taped down on all sides.

2. Is taping the occlusive dressing on all sides appropriate? Explain.

3. Who usually responds to a trauma code, and what are the functions of the people from the various departments?

16 Emergency

4. Prioritize the actions of the physicians and nurses in the trauma situation.

5. Based on B.W.'s vital signs and condition, what are the priority interventions at this time?

CASE STUDY PROGRESS

Treatments aimed toward stabilizing B.W.'s respiratory and volume status are started. You begin the secondary survey.

6. Describe the actions that you will perform as part of the secondary survey.

7. During your assessment, you note the following ecchymotic area on B.W.'s abdomen. What might this signify?

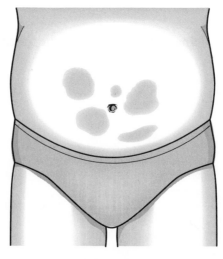

16 Emergency

8. B.W.'s abdomen has become distended and rigid. What are the possible reasons for the abdominal distention and rigidity?

9. You report your findings to the physician, who orders a focused abdominal sonography for trauma (FAST). Why would this procedure be appropriate for B.W.?

CASE STUDY PROGRESS

The FAST is positive, and B.W. is sent for a CT of the abdomen, which shows a large liver laceration. The surgeon needs to take B.W. to the operating room (OR) for an exploratory laparotomy with repair of liver laceration.

10. Because B.W. is not currently able to give consent for surgery, how will consent be obtained?

11. When you return from transporting the patient to the OR, B.W.'s wife is in the ED, upset and frightened. The social worker has been called to another emergency. What information do you need to obtain from B.W.'s wife?

12. How would you support her?

16 Emergency

Appendix: Abbreviations and Acronyms

AA	Alcoholics Anonymous	bid	twice daily
AAA	abdominal aortic aneurysm	BiPAP	CPAP with mask over both mouth and nose
ABCs	airway, breathing, circulation(s)		
ABGs	arterial blood gases	BM	bowel movement
ABI	ankle-brachial index	BMI	body mass index
A/C	assist-controlled	BMP	basic metabolic panel
ac	before meals	BNP	brain natriuretic peptide
ACE	angiotensin-converting enzyme	BOW	bag of waters
		BP	blood pressure
AD	autonomic dysreflexia	bpm	beats per minute
ADL	activities of daily living	BR	bed rest
ad lib	as directed	BRP	bathroom privileges
A-fib	atrial fibrillation	BS	bowel sounds; breath sounds
AIDS	acquired immunodeficiency syndrome	BSC	bedside commode
		BSE	breast self-examination
AKA	above-the-knee amputation	BSF	basilar skull fracture
ALS	amyotrophic lateral sclerosis	BUN	blood urea nitrogen
ALT (SGPT)	alanine transaminase (*formerly* serum glutamic pyruvic transaminase)	CABG	coronary artery bypass graft
		CAD	coronary artery disease
		C&DB	cough and deep breathe
ALP	alkaline phosphatase	Ca	Calcium
AM	morning	CAP	community-acquired pneumonia
AMA	against medical advice		
ANA	antinuclear antibody	CBC	complete blood count
ANC (AGC)	absolute neutrophil count	CBC with diff	complete blood count with differential
Anti-Sm	anti-smooth muscle antibody		
aPTT	activated partial thromboplastin time	C/C	chief complaint
		CCU	coronary care unit
ARB	angiotensin II receptor blocker	CDC	Centers for Disease Control and Prevention
ARDS	adult respiratory distress syndrome		
		CDE	certified diabetes educator
ARF	acute respiratory failure	CEA	carcinoembryonic antigen
ART	antiretroviral therapy	CF	cystic fibrosis
ASA	aspirin	CHO	carbohydrate(s)
AST (SGOT)	aspartate transaminase (*formerly* serum glutamic oxaloacetic transaminase)	Chol	cholesterol
		CI	cardiac index
		CK (CPK)	creatinine phosphokinase
ATB	antibiotic	CK-MM, CK-MB	CK isoenzymes
AV	atrioventricular; arteriovenous		

Cl	Chloride		DVT	deep vein thrombosis
CMP	complete metabolic panel (profile)		Dx	diagnosis
			EBL	estimated blood loss
CMV	cytomegalovirus		EC	emergency contraception
CNS	central nervous system		ECF	extended care facility
CO	cardiac output; carbon monoxide		ECG	electrocardiogram
			echo	echocardiogram; cardiac ultrasound (sonogram)
C/O	complaint(s) of, complaining of			
CO_2	carbon dioxide		*E. coli*	*Escherichia coli*
COPD	chronic obstructive pulmonary disease		ECT	electroconvulsive therapy
			ED	emergency department; erectile dysfunction
CP	cerebral palsy			
CPAP	continuous positive airway pressure		EDC	estimated date of confinement
			EEG	electroencephalogram
CPP	cerebral perfusion pressure		EF	ejection fraction
CPR	cardiopulmonary resuscitation		EMG	electromyogram
CRF	chronic renal failure		EMS	emergency medical system
CRP	C-reactive protein		EMT	emergency medical technician
C&S	culture and sensitivity		ENT	ear, nose, and throat
CSF	cerebrospinal fluid		EOMs	extraocular movements
CT	chest tube		ER	estrogen receptor
CT scan	computed tomography scan		ERCP	endoscopic retrograde cholangiopancreatogram
CV	cardiovascular			
CVA	cerebrovascular accident; costovertebral angle		ESR	erythrocyte sedimentation rate
			ET	enterostomal therapist; eustachian tube
CVC	central venous catheter			
CVP	central venous pressure		ETOH	alcohol
CWOCN	certified wound, ostomy, continence nurse		ETT	endotracheal tube
			EVD	extraventricular drain
CXR	chest x-ray		FBG	fasting blood glucose
DC; D/C	discontinue		FDA	U.S. Food and Drug Administration
DD	down drain			
DEXA scan	duel-energy x-ray absorptiometry		FFP	fresh frozen plasma
			FHR	fetal heart rate
DIC	disseminated intravascular coagulation		Fio_2	fraction of inspired oxygen
			FOC	frontal occipital circumference
DKA	diabetic ketoacidosis		Fr	French
DM	diabetes mellitus		FSH	follicle-stimulating hormone
DME	durable medical equipment		ft	feet
DNA	deoxyribonucleic acid		F/U	follow-up
DOB	date of birth		FUO	fever of unknown origin
DOE	dyspnea on exertion		GBS	Guillain-Barré syndrome
DPT	diphtheria, pertussis, tetanus		GCS	Glasgow Coma Scale
			GDM	gestational diabetes mellitus
DRE	digital rectal examination		GERD	gastroesophageal reflux disease
DSA	digital subtraction angiography		GFR	glomerular filtration rate
DSM-IV-TR	*Diagnostic and Statistical Manual of Mental Disorders*		GGT	gamma-glutamyl transferase (transpeptidase)
DTs	delirium tremens		GI	gastrointestinal
DTRs	deep tendon reflexes		gtt	drop

GU	genitourinary	JVD	jugular venous distention
HbA1C	hemoglobin A1C; glycosylated hemoglobin test	K	potassium
		KCl	potassium chloride
hCG	human chorionic gonadotropin	KUB	kidney, ureters, and bladder x-ray
HCl	hydrochloric acid		
HCO_3	bicarbonate ion	KVO	keep vein open
Hct	hematocrit	L	left; liter
HCTZ	hydrochlorothiazide	lab(s)	laboratory; laboratory tests
HCV	hepatitis C virus	LAD	left anterior descending coronary artery
HD	hemodialysis		
HDL	high-density lipoprotein	lb	pound(s)
HEENT	head, eyes, ears, nose, throat	LBBB	left bundle branch block
HF	heart failure	LDH	lactic (lactate) dehydrogenase
Hgb	hemoglobin	LDL	low-density lipoprotein
H/H	hemoglobin/hematocrit	LFTs	liver function tests
HHN	hand-held nebulizer	LLL	left lower lobe (of lungs)
HIPAA	Health Insurance Portability and Accountability Act	LLQ	left lower quadrant (of abdomen)
HIV	human immunodeficiency virus	LMP	last menstrual period
		LOC	level of consciousness
HLA	human leukocyte antigen	LPN	licensed practical nurse
HMO	health maintenance organization	LR	lactated Ringer's *or* Ringer's lactate
HOB	head of bed	LTBI	latent tuberculosis infection
HPV	human papillomavirus	LUQ	left upper quadrant (of abdomen)
hsCRP	highly sensitive C-reactive protein		
		LV	left ventricle
HTN	hypertension	LWS	low wall suction
IADL	instrumental activities of daily living	MAOI	monoamine oxidase inhibitor
		MD	doctor of medicine
IBD	inflammatory bowel disease	MDI	multiple-dose injection; metered-dose inhaler
IBS	irritable bowel syndrome		
ICD; AICD	implantable cardioverter defibrillator; automatic ICD	meds	medications
		mg	milligram
ICP	intracranial pressure	MG	myasthenia gravis
ICU	intensive care unit	MI	myocardial infarction
IICP	increased intracranial pressure	MICU	medical intensive care unit
IM	intramuscular	mL	milliliter
in	inch(es)	MNT	medical nutrition therapy
INR	International Normalized Ratio	MRI	magnetic resonance imaging
I&O	intake and output	MS	multiple sclerosis
IS	incentive spirometer	MUGA	multiple gated acquisition
IT	intrathecal	MVP	mitral valve prolapse
IUD	intrauterine device	Na	sodium
IV	intravenous	NAP	unlicensed nursing assistive personnel
IVF	intravenous fluid		
IVP	intravenous push; intravenous pyelogram	NC	nasal cannula
		NG	nasogastric
IVPB	intravenous piggyback	NGT	nasogastric tube
JP	Jackson-Pratt	NH_3	ammonia

NICU	neonatal intensive care unit; neurological intensive care unit	PEFR	peak expiratory flow rate
NKA	no known allergies	PEG	percutaneous endoscopic gastrostomy tube
NKDA	no known drug allergies	PEJ	percutaneous endoscopic jejunostomy tube
NPH	neutral protamine Hagedorn (a modified insulin)	peri	perineal (related to perineum)
NPO	nothing by mouth	PERRL(A)	pupils equal, round, and reactive to light (accommodation)
NS	normal saline		
NSAIDs	nonsteroidal anti-inflammatory drugs	PET	positron emission tomography
		PFM	peak flow meter
NTG	nitroglycerin	PFT	pulmonary function test
N/V	nausea and vomiting	pH	negative logarithm of the hydrogen ion concentration— acidity/basicity of the blood
O_2	oxygen		
OB	obstetric		
OB/GYN	obstetrician/gynecologist	PICC	peripherally inserted central catheter
OM	otitis media		
OR	operating room	PICU	pediatric intensive care unit
ORIF	open reduction internal fixation	PIH	pregnancy-induced hypertension
OSA	obstructive sleep apnea		
OT; OTR	occupational therapist (therapy); registered occupational therapist	PKU	phenylketonuria
		PM	afternoon or evening
		PMH	past medical history
OTC	over the counter	PMI	point of maximal impulse
P	pulse	PO	by mouth
PA	physician's assistant	POD	postoperative day
PACs	premature atrial contractions	postop	postoperatively
$Paco_2$	partial pressure of carbon dioxide in arterial blood	PPD	purified protein derivative (test for TB); packs per day (cigarettes)
PACU	post-anesthesia care unit		
Pao_2	partial pressure of oxygen in arterial blood	PRBCs	packed red blood cells
		preop	preoperatively
PAF	paroxysmal atrial fibrillation	prn	as needed
Pap	Papanicolaou smear	PSA	prostate-specific antigen
PAP	pulmonary artery pressure	PT; RPT	physical therapist (therapy); registered physical therapist
PCA	patient-controlled analgesia		
PCI	percutaneous coronary intervention	PT or PT/INR	prothrombin time, prothrombin time/ International Normalized Ratio
PCP	primary care provider; *Pneumocystis jiroveci* (formerly *carinii*) pneumonia	PTCA	percutaneous transluminal coronary angioplasty
		PTSD	posttraumatic stress disorder
PCTA	percutaneous coronary angioplasty	PTT; aPTT	partial thromboplastin time; activated partial thromboplastin time
PCWP	pulmonary capillary wedge pressure		
PD	Parkinson's disease	PUD	peptic ulcer disease
PE	pulmonary embolus (embolism)	PVCs	premature ventricular contractions
		PVD	peripheral vascular disease
PEEP	positive end-expiratory pressure	PVR	postvoiding residual
PEF	peak expiratory flow	q	every (e.g., q2h)

R	right; respirations	SVR	systemic vascular resistance
RA	room air; rheumatoid arthritis	T&A	tonsillectomy and adenoidectomy
RAI	radioactive iodine	TAH	total abdominal hysterectomy
RBCs	red blood cells	TB	tuberculosis
RCA	right coronary artery	T&C	type and crossmatch
RD	registered dietitian	T	temperature
RDS	respiratory distress syndrome	Td	tetanus/diphtheria (vaccine)
RLL	right lower lobe (of lung)	TED	thromboembolic deterrent
RLQ	right lower quadrant (of abdomen)	TF	tube feeding
RML	right middle lobe (of lung)	TIA	transient ischemic attack
RN	registered nurse	TIBC	total iron binding capacity
R/O	rule out	tid	3 times per day
ROM	range of motion	TJC	The Joint Commission
RPR	rapid plasma reagin (test for syphilis)	TLS	tumor lysis syndrome
RSV	respiratory syncytial virus	TNM	tumor, node, metastasis
RT	respiratory therapist (therapy)	TPA	tissue plasminogen activator
R/T	related to	TPN	total parenteral nutrition
RUQ	right upper quadrant (of abdomen)	Trig	triglycerides
SAH	subarachnoid hemorrhage	TRH	thyrotropin-releasing hormone
SaO_2	arterial oxygen saturation	TSH	thyroid-stimulating hormone
SBAR	situation, background, assessment, recommendation	TURP	transurethral resection of the prostate
SBO	small bowel obstruction	UA	urinalysis
SCD	sickle cell disease; sequential compression device	UDS	urinary drainage system
SCI	spinal cord injury	UGI	upper gastrointestinal
sed rate	erythrocyte sedimentation rate	UI	urinary incontinence
SIADH	syndrome of inappropriate antidiuretic hormone	UOP	urinary output
SICU	surgical intensive care unit	URI	upper respiratory tract infection
SL	sublingual	US	ultrasound
SLE	systemic lupus erythematosus	UTI	urinary tract infection
SLP	speech-language pathologist	V-fib	ventricular fibrillation
SOB	short (shortness) of breath	VLDL	very-low-density lipoprotein
S/P	status post	VP	ventriculoperitoneal
SRMC	single-room maternity care	$\dot{V}/\dot{Q}$ scan	ventilation-perfusion scan (of lungs)
S/S	signs and symptoms	VS	vital signs
SSRI	selective serotonin reuptake inhibitor	V_T	tidal volume
S/T	secondary to	V-tach	ventricular tachycardia
STAT	immediately	WBCs	white blood cells
STI	sexually transmitted infection	WNL	within normal limits
Subcut	subcutaneous	WNR	within normal range
		W/O	without
		yo	year-old

Illustration Credits

Case Study 7
(p. 32) From Ignatavicius DD, Workman ML: *Medical-surgical nursing*, ed 6, St. Louis, 2010, Saunders.

Case Study 8
(p. 38) Modified from Lilley LL, Rainforth Collins S, Harrington S, et al: *Pharmacology and the Nursing Process*, ed 6, St. Louis, 2011, Mosby.

Case Study 10
(p. 43) Modified from Huszar R: *Basic dysrhythmias: interpretation and management—revised reprint*, ed 3, St. Louis, 2007, Mosby.

Case Study 11
(p. 49) From Gray Morris D: *Calculate with confidence*, ed 5, St. Louis, 2010, Mosby.

Case Study 13
(p. 58) Modified from Fuller JK: *Surgical technology: principles and practice*, ed 5, St. Louis, 2010, Saunders.

Case Study 25
(p. 114) Modified from Linton AL: *Introduction to medical-surgical nursing*, ed 4, St. Louis, 2007, Saunders.

Case Study 29
(p. 135, both figures) From Brown M, Mulholland JM: *Drug calculations: process and problems for clinical practice*, ed 8, St. Louis, 2008, Mosby.

Case Study 31
(p. 146) From Aehlert B: *ECGs made easy*, ed 4, St. Louis, 2011, Mosby/JEMS.

Case Study 48
(p. 218) From Gray Morris D: *Calculate with confidence*, ed 5, St. Louis, 2010, Mosby.

Case Study 72
(p. 323) From Urden LD, Stacy KM, Lough ME: *Critical care nursing: diagnosis and management*, ed 6, St. Louis, 2010, Mosby.

Case Study 75
(p. 338) From Lewis SL, Dirksen SR, Heitkemper MM, et al: *Medical-surgical nursing: assessment and management of clinical problems*, ed 8, St. Louis, 2011, Mosby.

Case Study 96
(p. 431) From Gray Morris D: *Calculate with confidence*, ed 5, St. Louis, 2010, Mosby.

Case Study 102
(p. 456) From Gray Morris D: *Calculate with confidence*, ed 5, St. Louis, 2010, Mosby.

Case Study 108
(p. 485) From Gray Morris D: *Calculate with confidence*, ed 5, St. Louis, 2010, Mosby.

Case Study 111
(p. 500) Modified from Harkreader H, Hogan MA: *Fundamentals of nursing: caring and clinical judgment*, ed 2, St. Louis, 2004, Saunders.

Case Study 115
(p. 514) Modified from Perry SE, Hockenberry MJ, Lowdermilk DL, et al: *Maternal child nursing care*, ed 4, St. Louis, 2010, Mosby.

Case Study 118
(p. 525) From Perry SE, Hockenberry MJ, Lowdermilk DL, et al: *Maternal child nursing care*, ed 4, St. Louis, 2010, Mosby.

Case Study 136
(p. 599) Modified from Ignatavicius DD, Workman ML: *Medical-surgical nursing*, ed 6, St. Louis, 2010, Saunders.

Case Study 140
(p. 620) From Norton D, McLaren R, Exton-Smith AN: *An investigation of geriatric nursing problems in hospital*, Edinburgh, 1975, Churchill Livingstone.

Case Study 141
(p. 625) From Aehlert B: *ECGs made easy*, ed 4, St. Louis, 2011, Mosby/JEMS.

Case Study 142
(p. 630, both figures) From Gray Morris D: *Calculate with confidence*, ed 5, St. Louis, 2010, Mosby.